Gastrointestinal Radiology THE REQUISITES

SERIES EDITOR **James H. Thrall,** MD
Radiologist-in-Chief
Department of Radiology
Massachusetts General Hospital
Boston, Massachusetts

OTHER VOLUMES IN THE REQUISITES SERIES

Pediatric Radiology

Neuroradiology

Thoracic Radiology

Cardiac Radiology

Genitourinary Radiology

Nuclear Medicine

Mammography

Musculoskeletal Radiology

Ultrasound

Gastrointestinal Radiology

THE REQUISITES

ROBERT D. HALPERT, MD
Professor of Radiology
H. Lee Moffitt Cancer Center and Research Institute
The University of South Florida
Tampa, Florida

PHILIP GOODMAN, MD
Associate Professor of Radiology
University of Texas Medical Branch
Galveston, Texas

*with **386** illustrations*

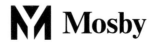
Mosby

St. Louis Baltimore Boston Chicago London Philadelphia Sydney Toronto

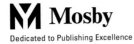

Mosby

Dedicated to Publishing Excellence

Publisher: George S. Stamathis
Editor: Anne S. Patterson
Developmental Editor: Maura K. Leib
Project Manager: Carol Sullivan Wiseman
Production Editor: Catherine Schwent
Designer: Susan Lane

Printed in the United States of America

Mosby—Year Book, Inc.
11830 Westline Industrial Drive
St. Louis, Missouri 63146

Library of Congress Cataloging in Publication Data

Halpert, Robert D.
    Gastrointestinal radiology : the requisites / Robert D. Halpert,
Philip Goodman.
        p.   cm. — (Requisites in radiology series)
    Includes index.
    ISBN 0-8016-6382-2 : $65.00
    1. Gastrointestinal system—Radiography.   I. Goodman, Philip.
    II. Title.   III. Series.
    [DNLM: 1. Gastrointestinal System—radiography.   W1 100 H195g]
RC804.R6H27 1993
616.3'307572—dc20
DNLM/DLC   92-49533
for Library of Congress   CIP

        96   97   CL / MY   9   8   7   6   5   4   3   2

To my wife
Sylvia
whose love, patience, and support make all things possible,
and to my children
Heather Anne, Stephenie, Janie, Emily, Maggie, and Robbie
who were willing, for a limited period of time,
to share their Dad with this venture.

R.D.H.

To my parents
Dr. Morris *and* **Lillian Goodman**
for their love and support,
and to my friend
Dr. Benjamin Eisenberg
of Geneva, New York, for his encouragement.

P.G.

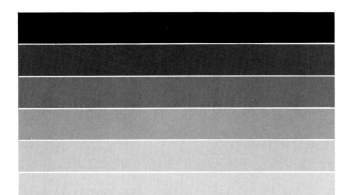

Foreword

Gastrointestinal Radiology: The Requisites is the first book in a new series primarily designed to present core material in major subspecialty areas of radiology for the resident in radiology and for the practicing radiologist seeking a concise review.

Radiology residents are faced at two times in their careers with the need for a concise book providing the core material, the "requisites", of each important subspecialty area. The first time occurs early in the residency program. Most radiology residencies are now designed in a format of subspecialty-based rotations. The resident must go from little or no radiological knowledge of the area to a useful working knowledge in the short period embraced by the subspecialty rotation. Later in the residency when reviewing for inservice and other examinations the resident is again faced with the need for a concise text so that multiple sub-specialty areas can be reasonably reviewed in the always limited time available.

These observations were the basis for creating *The Requisites in Radiology* series. One book specifically written for each of the major subspecialty areas is planned. The length of each book will be dictated by the material requiring coverage, but the goal is to provide the resident with a text that might be reasonably read within several days at the beginning of each subspecialty rotation and perhaps reread several times during both initial and subsequent rotations. The books are not intended to be exhaustive but should provide the basic conceptual, factual, and interpretive material required for clinical practice. Each book will be written by a nationally recognized authority in the respective subspecialty area and, as a completely new series, each author has the opportunity to present material in the context of today's contemporary practice of radiology rather than grafting information about

new imaging modalities and approaches onto text material originally developed for conventional radiography.

Drs. Halpert and Goodman have succeeded outstandingly in capturing the philosophy of the "requisites" concept in this initial offering in the series. The structure of their book at the chapter level is by anatomic region. Each chapter begins with a brief overview of examination techniques. These discussions include information on the reasons for using specialized maneuvers and different imaging modalities as well as an overview of how to actually perform the respective examinations. Thereafter, each chapter is organized in a logical and straightforward manner on the basis of radiographical findings and their differential diagnosis. This approach defines a particular strength of their book: the reader encounters the gastrointestinal tract and its diseases the way they are encountered by the radiologist in clinical practice. Appropriately performed examinations reveal patterns of abnormality that must first be recognized and then evaluated for etiology. Knowledge of the radiological differential diagnosis, coupled with clinical context, brings the observer to the most likely possibilities.

Although examination of the gastrointestinal tract remains heavily oriented toward studies using barium contrast media, all contemporary imaging modalities have become important. Drs. Halpert and Goodman do an excellent job of discussing the roles of cross-sectional imaging techniques that have assumed prominence in evaluating the extraluminal and solid organ components of the gastrointestinal tract.

I believe the resident in radiology wil find *Gastrointestinal Radiology: The Requisites* to be a concise and useful introduction to the subject. Residents, fellows, and practicing radiologists should also find this a very manageable text for a review of the subject. I further hope that surgeons and internists and their resident and fellowship trainees interested in the gastrointestinal tract will find this to be a user-friendly text with which to begin their understanding of the radiology of gastrointestinal disease.

James H. Thrall, MD

Radiologist-in-Chief
Massachusetts General Hospital
Professor of Radiology
Harvard Medical School

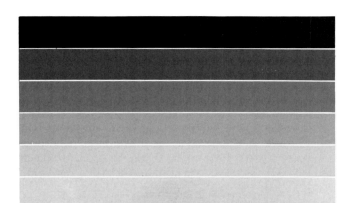

Preface

In August of 1879, while attending the Annual Meeting of the American Association for the Advancement of Science in Saratoga, New York, the renowned physician, Sir William Osler chanced to meet the inventor, Thomas Edison. Edison, having a passing interest in the medical applications of his inventions, suggested to Osler that it might be possible to "illumine the interior of the body by passing a small electric burner into the stomach." Sir William's response is not recorded, but his account of the encounter suggests some degree of amusement at the prospect of passing a tube with a light on the end into the stomach.

Nevertheless, Edison's words were prophetic and 114 years later, endoscopic direct visualization of the mucosal surface has established itself as the standard of gastrointestinal (GI) diagnosis following several decades of virtual domination of this field by radiologists. However, the expected demise of radiological imaging of the gastrointestinal tract has not occurred. Instead, a collaborative, complimentary relationship between endoscopy and radiological imaging of the gut has evolved, spurred on and encouraged by the profound effect of cost constraint and the increasing diagnostic sensitivity and relatively low cost of the radiological procedures.

Barium studies have decreased but not disappeared since the advent of widely available endoscopy. Moreover, the technical refinement of low-cost barium examinations may, in all likelihood, carve out a well-defined niche as a screening examination for many patients.

In addition, the development of other imaging methods has tremendously enhanced the role of imaging in GI diagnosis. Without doubt, the use of computer-assisted tomography, real-time ultrasound, and to some extent, magnetic resonance imaging has greatly impacted gastrointestinal imaging. Indeed, modern cross-sectional multiplanar imaging has opened the abdomen for radiological inspection in a way that had been hitherto unattainable. Enhanced liver diagnosis and evaluation of the spleen, pancreas, lymphatics, and the structures surrounding the gut are now possible and signal the beginning of yet a new era in abdominal imaging and diagnosis.

In recent decades, our clinical colleagues have developed what they refer to as the *problem-oriented approach* to patient care and patient records. This refers to an orderly approach to patient diagnosis and management wherein the problems of greatest concern are appropriately weighted, while diagnoses of lesser importance are not lost sight of or neglected in the process. The goal is to establish a global perspective of patient care. Moreover, it should also facilitate a more readable and organized medical record.

In a similar fashion, we have tried to view the "radiological terrain" through the eyes of a first year resident, a resident preparing for boards, or possibly a radiologist desiring to acquire a concise and abbreviated review of the specialty of gastrointestinal imaging. It would seem appropriate, from our view, to develop a problem-oriented approach to radiology to best address all of these demands and to attempt to present radiological problem solving (diagnosis) in an organized prioritized fashion.

This is generally referred to in radiology as the pattern approach. However, in keeping with a patient-orientated perspective on the practice of radiology, I would prefer to call these radiological patterns of disease, "problems". The irregular thickened gastric fold, from the referring physician's point of view (and especially the patient's perspective) is not a pattern, but a problem! For the attending radiologist, the issue is one of problem solving. Although some may see this as nothing more than hair splitting and semantics (and they may be correct), it is, nevertheless, an accurate reflection of a philosophical perspective on the practice of radiology, no doubt left over from my days as a general practitioner.

The advantage of this approach, as opposed to the disease-oriented method, is to allow a closer paralleling of the real day-to-day world of radiology, and as a result, be of more practical value. The disadvantage is in the complexities of presenting material. In terms of writing a textbook, it is easier to describe a disease and all its radiological presentations, than to start with the radiological problem and work backward toward a reasonable differential diagnosis. The former is the organizational basis of almost all reference texts, while the latter is the daily experience of most radiologists. However, in the problem-oriented clinical management of a patient, problems often overlap, or the same disease may result in several very different problems. In the same way, a disease may have several radiological presentations. Gastric carcinoma, for example, may present as a problem of gastric folds, gastric mass, or ulceration. Hence, the inherent weakness in such a presentation of material.

Accordingly, we have tried to avoid undue redundancy while at the same time overlapping wherever necessary. Usually, the more in depth discussion will be reserved for the most common radiological problem posed by the disease entity.

Robert D. Halpert, MD
Philip Goodman, MD

I greatly acknowledge those people whose efforts and contributions were insrumental in the completion of this project: Sally Hammer who devoted many hours to the preparation of the manuscript; Drs. Robert A. Clark and Steven S. Morse, my colleagues at the H. Lee Moffitt Cancer Center and Research Institute who so willingly shared their material.

R.D.H.

I owe deep thanks to many people.

My secretary, Vicki McDowell, spent many hours patiently transforming my scribbles into manuscript pages. Victor Luciano and John Ellis provided photographic services, and Heather Anne Halpert assisted with line drawings. Dr. Melvyn Schreiber and Dr. Rajendra Kumar of the University of Texas Medical Branch in Galveston and Dr. Howard Gorell of Lakeland, Florida graciously contributed unique films from their personal collections.

I am grateful to my teachers at Rochester General Hospital and the Hospital of the University of Pennsylvania and to my colleagues at the University of Texas Medical Schools in Houston and Galveston. I am also indebted to Drs. Robert Halpert and James Thrall for inviting me to participate in this exciting project and to Anne Patterson and her colleagues at Mosby–Year Book for their help in the final preparation of the book.

P.G.

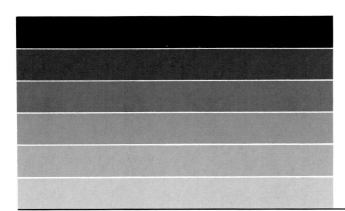

Contents

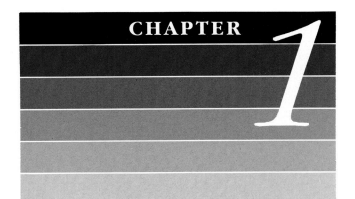

CHAPTER 1

Esophagus and Gastroesophageal Junction

EXAMINATION TECHNIQUES

Radiographic examination of the esophagus encompasses both conventional fluoroscopic studies and various cross-sectional imaging methods. Esophagram or barium swallow is most often performed as a biphasic examination in which both double- and single-contrast techniques are employed. In the upright position, the patient ingests an effervescent agent followed by a cup of high-density barium. Films obtained during this time demonstrate the esophageal lumen distended with gas and the mucosal surface coated with barium (Fig. 1-1). This double-contrast phase of the examination is especially useful for showing fine mucosal detail, such as superficial nodules or ulcerations. When pooling of barium prevents visualization of the distal esophagus, a tube esophagram can be performed by injecting air directly into the esophageal lumen through a tube. If the esophagram is performed as part of an upper gastrointestinal (UGI) series, double-contrast films of the stomach and duodenum are obtained immediately following double-contrast films of the esophagus.

Single-contrast examination of the esophagus is usually performed with the patient in the right anterior oblique (RAO) prone position. Esophageal peristalsis is observed fluoroscopically after the patient has taken a single swallow of low-density barium. Films are then obtained as the patient continues to drink the cup of low-density barium (Fig. 1-2). This single-contrast phase of the examination is especially useful for evaluating esophageal motility and distensibility and for detecting certain abnormalities of the distal esophagus, including sliding hiatal hernia and mucosal ring (B-ring).

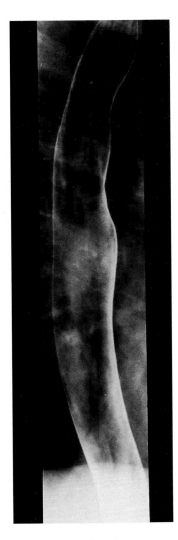

Fig. 1-1   Double-contrast film of the thoracic esophagus.

1

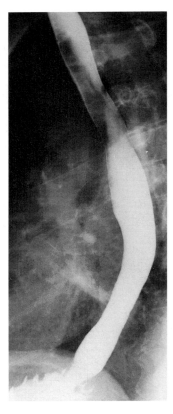

Fig. 1-2 Single-contrast film of the thoracic esophagus.

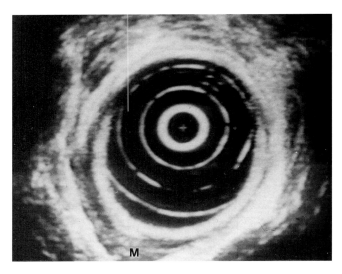

Fig. 1-3 Endoscopic ultrasound shows a hypoechoic mural mass *(M),* representing esophageal carcinoma.

Spontaneous gastroesophageal reflux may also be observed fluoroscopically during the single-contrast phase of the examination. Provocative maneuvers to increase intraabdominal pressure and thereby elicit reflux are sometimes performed, but the significance of reflux induced by these maneuvers remains controversial. Mucosal-relief views of the collapsed esophagus show the longitudinal fold pattern and may be useful for demonstrating esophageal varices. Although esophagram is usually performed as part of a complete UGI series, it is sometimes requested as an isolated examination in patients with dysphagia or other complaints localized to the esophagus. However, all esophagrams should include evaluation of the proximal stomach because stomach lesions may cause dysphagia, chest pain, or other symptoms suggesting esophageal disease.

Detailed examination of the pharynx and cervical esophagus may be incorporated into the routine esophagram in patients with cervical dysphagia or other symptoms localized to the neck. This is performed during the double-contrast phase with the patient in an upright position. Rapid-sequence films (three exposures per second) or a video recording are obtained in frontal and lateral projections while the patient drinks high-density barium. This allows dynamic evaluation of swallowing function and detection of physiological abnormalities, such as incomplete cricopharyngeal relaxation. Frontal and lateral spot films are then obtained while the patient phonates to distend the hypopharynx. The distention and mucosal coating seen on these spot films provides detailed anatomical information that might be obscured by barium on rapid-sequence or video filming.

In cases of suspected esophageal perforation, water-soluble contrast material is recommended because leakage of barium into the mediastinum may induce mediastinitis. If water-soluble contrast material does not demonstrate an esophageal perforation, the study should be repeated using barium because a small leak of water-soluble contrast material may be difficult to visualize. Water-soluble contrast material is hyperosmolar, therefore it can induce pulmonary edema when introduced into the respiratory tract, either by aspiration from the hypopharynx or extension through an esophagorespiratory fistula. However, low-osmolality, water-soluble contrast material does not cause pulmonary edema and can be used safely in patients with suspected esophageal perforation who are at risk of aspirating or who are known to have an esophagorespiratory fistula.

Computed tomography (CT) is the most commonly used cross-sectional technique for evaluating the esophagus. CT is most helpful for demonstrating the extraluminal component of esophageal disease. This includes staging of esophageal carcinoma (wall thickening, invasion of adjacent structures, and distant metastases) and evaluation of esophageal trauma (extension to mediastinum or pleural cavity). Magnetic resonance imaging (MRI) offers cross-sectional evaluation with the advantages of multiplanar capabilities and lack of ionizing radiation. Although MRI has been of limited usefulness because of motion artifact, image quality is improving with the use of cardiorespiratory gating techniques. Endoscopic ultrasound, in which a transducer is endoscopically placed into the esophageal lumen, can differentiate the individual layers of the esophageal wall and has been especially useful in evaluating the depth of esophageal tumors (Fig. 1-3).

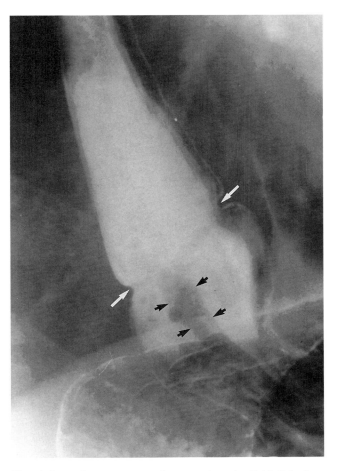

Fig. 1-4   Inflammatory esophagogastric polyp/fold *(black arrows)* in a small hiatal hernia. A nonobstructing B-ring *(white arrows)* is also present.

SOLITARY MUCOSAL MASSES

Nonneoplastic
   Inflammatory esophagogastric polyp/fold
Neoplastic
   Carcinomas
   Adenomas
   Papillomas

Nonneoplastic

Inflammatory esophagogastric polyp/fold is a prominent fold extending from the gastric cardia into the distal esophagus. This fold often has a protuberant tip that may simulate an esophageal polyp (Fig. 1-4). This polyp/fold complex (sometimes referred to as a sentinel polyp) is usually associated with gastroesophageal reflux. If the polypoid tip is larger than 2.5 cm in diameter or appears irregular, a biopsy is indicated to exclude adenocarcinoma of the gastroesophageal junction.

Neoplastic

Primary squamous cell carcinoma of the hypopharynx or esophagus can present as a solitary mucosal mass, either small and plaquelike or large and polypoid (Figs. 1-5 and 1-6). Ulceration of the mass can occur in both small and large lesions.

Squamous cell carcinoma represents up to 95% of esophageal carcinomas. The most common risk factors for development of squamous cell carcinoma of the esophagus are cigarette smoking and alcohol ingestion. Other risk factors include the following:
- Chronic food stasis (achalasia)
- Chronic inflammation and scarring (lye stricture or radiation)
- Tylosis (a rare genetic disease of the skin characterized by palmar and plantar hyperkeratosis)
- Plummer-Vinson syndrome (association of cervical esophageal webs, iron-deficiency anemia, and dysphagia)
- Sprue

Squamous cell carcinomas of the head and neck are also associated with an increased incidence of subsequent squamous cell carcinoma of the esophagus, resulting from either common risk factors (e.g., cigarettes and alcohol) or radiation used to treat the original tumor.

Adenocarcinoma of the esophagus accounts for less than 5% of esophageal carcinomas. Most cases represent either superior extension of gastric adenocarcinoma or malignant transformation of gastric-type epithelium in Barrett's esophagus. Adenocarcinoma develops in approximately 10% of patients with Barrett's

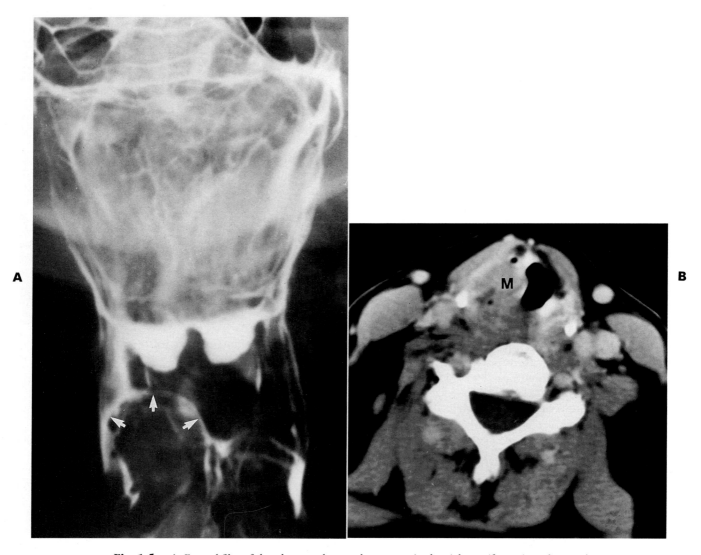

Fig. 1-5   **A,** Frontal film of the pharynx shows a large mass in the right pyriform sinus *(arrows)* representing squamous cell carcinoma. **B,** CT shows the soft tissue mass *(M)* obliterating the right pyriform sinus.

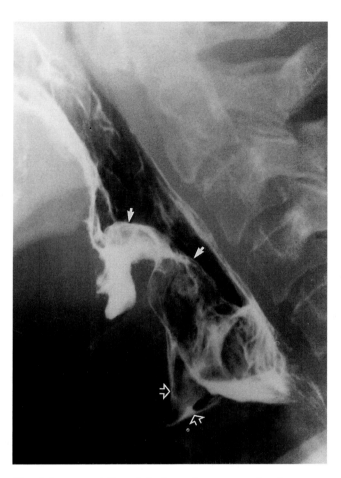

Fig. 1-6 Lateral film of the hypopharynx reveals a large mass involving the epiglottis and aryepiglottic fold *(arrows)*, representing squamous cell carcinoma. Barium is also seen in the larynx and supraglottic portion of the airway *(open arrows)*.

esophagus, suggesting the need for regular surveillance of this condition.

Spindle-cell carcinoma represents an uncommon variant of squamous cell carcinoma that has undergone focal mesenchymal metaplasia. This typically appears as a bulky, polypoid intraluminal mass. Carcinosarcoma, oat cell carcinoma, and primary malignant melanoma of the esophagus are rare epithelial malignancies that appear morphologically similar to spindle-cell carcinoma.

Adenomas and papillomas are uncommon, benign tumors of the esophagus that arise from columnar and squamous epithelium, respectively.

MULTIPLE MUCOSAL MASSES

Nonneoplastic
  Candida esophagitis
  Reflux esophagitis
  Glycogenic acanthosis
  Crohn's disease
  Pemphigoid and epidermolysis bullosa
  "Hairy" esophagus
Neoplastic
  Papillomatosis
  Superficial spreading carcinoma
  Cowden's syndrome
  Leukoplakia

Nonneoplastic

Fungal esophagitis caused by *Candida albicans* is most commonly seen in patients with acquired immune deficiency syndrome (AIDS) or patients with other immunocompromising diseases. This fungus causes whitish, slightly raised plaques that may also involve the pharynx or tongue (oral thrush). In the esophagus, these plaques resemble small mucosal nodules that often occur in longitudinal columns (Figs. 1-7 and 1-8). Patients with esophageal stasis, such as those with achalasia or scleroderma, are also at risk for developing *Candida* esophagitis.

Reflux esophagitis may occur in patients with gastroesophageal reflux as a result of sensitivity of the esophageal mucosa to the acidic gastric fluid. Because reflux usually does not extend beyond the distal esophagus, esophagitis is most commonly confined to this area. Abnormal esophageal motility and mucosal edema are early signs of reflux esophagitis, with erosions, ulcerations, and stricture formation occurring with prolonged or severe reflux.

Glycogenic acanthosis is a benign degenerative condition of the esophagus seen in middle-aged and elderly people. Focal deposits of glycogen form discrete plaques that appear as mucosal nodules on contrast studies (Fig. 1-9). This does not cause dysphagia and is usually an incidental finding.

Filiform polyps are a rare manifestation of Crohn's disease of the esophagus. These thin, tubular or branching mucosal polyps resemble those seen in the colon or ileum in the healing stage of inflammatory bowel disease.

Subepidermal bullae or blebs in the esophagus may be associated with cutaneous lesions in both benign mucous membrane pemphigoid and epidermolysis bul-

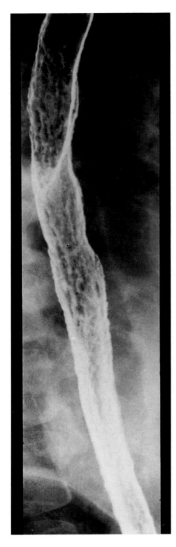

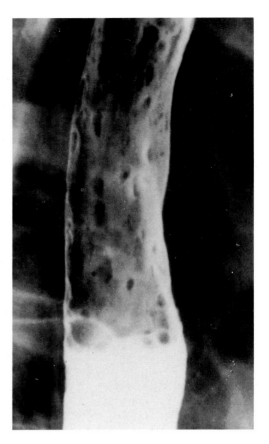

Fig. 1-8 Diffuse mucosal nodularity represents esophageal candidiasis in a patient with AIDS.

Fig. 1-7 Diffuse mucosal plaques in a patient with AIDS and esophageal candidiasis.

losa. These appear initially as small mucosal nodules but subsequently undergo inflammation, ulceration, and fibrosis with stricture formation.

Following pharyngoesophageal reconstructive surgery, hair follicles from the skin graft may appear as multiple small mucosal masses ("hairy" or hirsute esophagus).

Neoplastic

Papillomatosis is a rare condition characterized by multiple esophageal papillomas. These benign epithelial growths are usually solitary, but they can be multi-

ple in squamous papillomatosis, an unusual genetic disease, or in acanthosis nigricans, a disease in which esophageal papillomas occur in association with focal thickening and hyperpigmentation of the skin.

Superficial spreading carcinoma is an unusual form of squamous cell carcinoma characterized by small mucosal nodules. These tumors are limited to the mucosal and submucosal layers of the esophagus, but metastasis to adjacent lymph nodes may be present.

Cowden's syndrome is a rare genetic disease in which tiny hamartomas may cause diffuse mucosal nodularity of the GI tract, including the esophagus. This disorder is often associated with various tumors of the skin, breast, and thyroid gland.

Leukoplakia represents small, whitish plaques resulting from hyperplasia of squamous epithelium. This rare cause of esophageal nodularity has an uncertain malignant potential, although it appears histologically identical to the more common premalignant leukoplakia of the oropharynx.

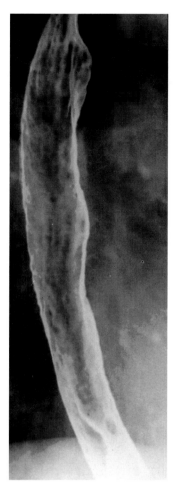

Fig. 1-9   Diffuse mucosal nodularity represents glycogenic acanthosis.

SUBMUCOSAL MASSES

Nonneoplastic
    Varices
    Cysts
Neoplastic
    Mesenchymal tumors
    Kaposi's sarcoma
    Fibrovascular polyp
    Lymphoma
    Metastases

Nonneoplastic

Esophageal varices represent dilated veins in the submucosal layer of the esophageal wall. The more common uphill varices involve the distal esophagus and result from elevated portal venous pressure, usually secondary to cirrhosis of the liver. This causes in-

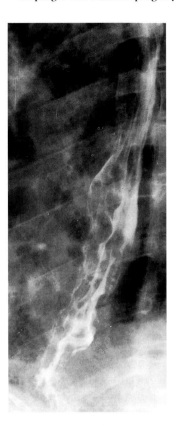

Fig. 1-10   Collapsed view of the distal esophagus demonstrates typical serpentine appearance of varices.

creased blood flow through the coronary (left gastric) vein into the distal esophageal venous plexus that then empties through the azygous system into the superior vena cava. Gastric fundal varices are sometimes associated with distal esophageal varices.

The less common downhill varices involve the proximal thoracic esophagus and result from obstruction of the superior vena cava. Collateral blood flow bypasses the obstruction and enters the superior vena cava through the azygous system, thereby sparing the distal esophageal veins. However, an obstruction involving either the azygous system or the superior vena cava inferior to its junction with the azygous vein leads to collateral blood flow through the coronary and portal veins into the inferior vena cava. This results in varices involving the entire length of the thoracic esophagus.

On contrast studies, esophageal varices are best demonstrated with the patient in the horizontal position because in the upright position gravity decreases distention of esophageal veins and can render varices invisible. The optimal technique for detecting varices is to have the patient take a single swallow of high-density barium. Continuous drinking may overcompress the varices; a single swallow will usually demonstrate the smooth, serpentine submucosal masses typical of varices (Fig. 1-10). Mucosal relief views of the collapsed esophagus are also useful for demonstrating this appearance.

On CT, varices can appear as thickening of the esophageal wall or as adjacent lobulated soft tissue masses. Bolused IV contrast material may be necessary to differentiate enhancing varices from nonenhancing neoplastic or inflammatory disease. Angiography is also useful for demonstrating esophageal varices and may be combined with interventional techniques for treating acute variceal bleeding.

Esophageal cysts may be congenital (foregut duplication cysts) or acquired (retention cysts). Duplication cysts are usually asymptomatic and, though usually discovered in childhood, are first noted in adults in 30% of cases. They appear as a round, soft tissue density mediastinal mass on chest films and as a submucosal mass on esophagrams. Retention cysts, rare lesions that arise from dilated mucous glands in the distal esophagus, have a similar radiographic appearance.

Neoplastic

Leiomyoma is the most common benign neoplasm of the esophagus. This smooth muscle tumor produces a focal rounded impression (Fig. 1-11). Although usually solitary, multiple leiomyomas of the esophagus occur in up to 3% of cases. Leiomyomas occasionally contain mottled calcifications.

Other benign submucosal tumors of the esophagus are uncommon. Like leiomyomas, they arise from mesenchymal tissues and appear radiographically as smooth, rounded masses. These tumors include hemangiomas, lipomas, neurofibromas, and granular cell tumors.

Kaposi's sarcoma is a vascular tumor that was originally described as a rare cutaneous lesion affecting elderly men of Mediterranean descent. However, it is now recognized as a common lesion involving the skin, GI tract, and respiratory tract of patients with AIDS.

Fibrovascular polyp, an unusual benign tumor, originates in the wall of the proximal esophagus and elongates to form a smooth intraluminal mass. This mass may extend inferiorly to occupy the entire esophageal lumen or may be regurgitated into the pharynx and cause asphyxiation.

Primary malignant neoplasms (sarcomas) and secondary malignancies (lymphoma, leukemia, and hematogenous metastases) are rare causes of discrete submucosal masses in the esophagus.

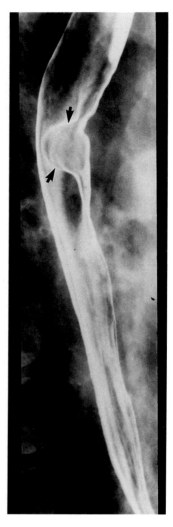

Fig. 1-11   Smooth submucosal mass *(arrows)* in the upper thoracic esophagus represents a leiomyoma.

EXTRINSIC PROCESSES

Cervical Esophagus
    Postcricoid defect
    Cricopharyngeus muscle
    Cervical spine
    Thyroid
    Other soft tissue masses
Thoracic Esophagus
    Normal impressions
    Abnormal vessels
    Mediastinal adenopathy
    Spinous osteophytes
    Cardiac impressions
    Lung tumor

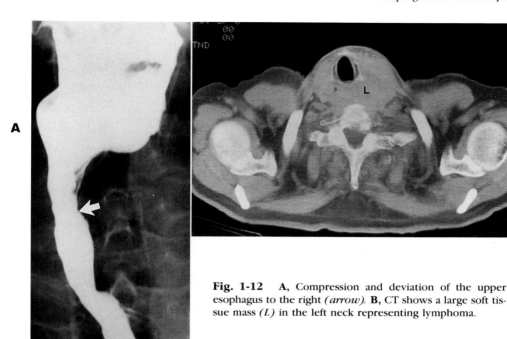

Fig. 1-12   **A,** Compression and deviation of the upper esophagus to the right *(arrow)*. **B,** CT shows a large soft tissue mass *(L)* in the left neck representing lymphoma.

Cervical Esophagus

Postcricoid defect is a normal indentation on the anterior aspect of the hypopharynx at approximately the level of the C4 vertebra. This was originally felt to represent a venous plexus but is now considered to result from redundant mucosa. This incidental finding may simulate a superficial neoplasm.

Incomplete relaxation of the cricopharyngeus muscle can cause transient extrinsic impression on the posterior aspect of the cervical esophagus at the level of the C5 or C6 vertebra. This localized esophageal dysmotility can cause significant dysphagia.

Anterior osteophytes of the cervical spine and rarely anterior herniation of an intervertebral disc may cause focal impressions on the posterior wall of the cervical esophagus. Focal or diffuse enlargement of the thyroid gland can deviate and compress the esophagus. Retropharyngeal tumor, hematoma, or abscess may displace the hypopharynx and cervical esophagus anteriorly. Cervical adenopathy and parathyroid enlargement may also lead to extrinsic compression of the cervical esophagus (Fig. 1-12).

Thoracic Esophagus

The most commonly noted normal extrinsic impressions on the thoracic esophagus are the aortic arch and left main bronchus (Fig. 1-13). Abnormal vessels, such as a right aortic arch, aneurysm or ectasia of the tho-

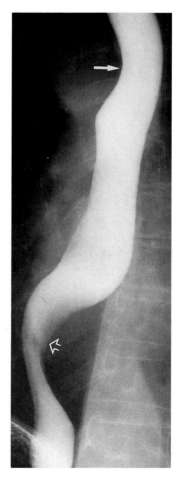

Fig. 1-13   Esophageal compression by the aortic arch *(arrow)* and tortuous descending thoracic aorta *(open arrow)*.

racic aorta, and aberrant subclavian artery, may also compress or displace the esophagus (Fig. 1-14).

Mediastinal adenopathy causes impressions along the anterior aspect of the midesophagus, and spinous osteophytes result in one or more focal impressions on the posterior esophageal wall. Cardiac impressions on

the esophagus can be focal (left atrial enlargement) or more diffuse (generalized cardiomegaly and pericardial effusion) (Fig. 1-15). An adjacent lung tumor may compress and deviate the esophagus; pulmonary volume loss as a result of fibrosis typically causes ipsilateral retraction of the esophagus.

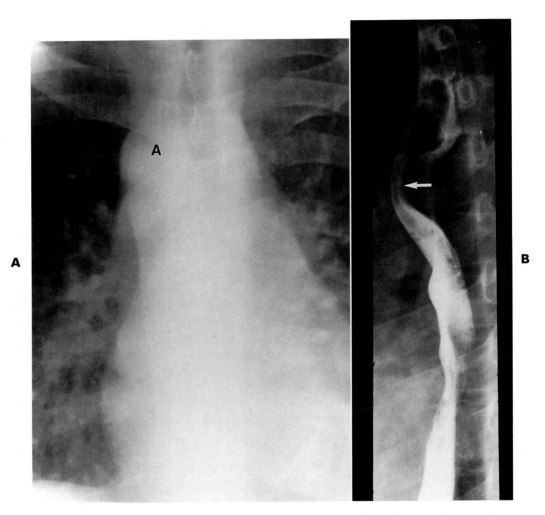

Fig. 1-14   **A,** Chest film shows a right aortic arch *(A).* **B,** Lateral view from esophagram shows smooth posterior compression of the upper thoracic esophagus *(arrow)* by aberrant left subclavian artery.

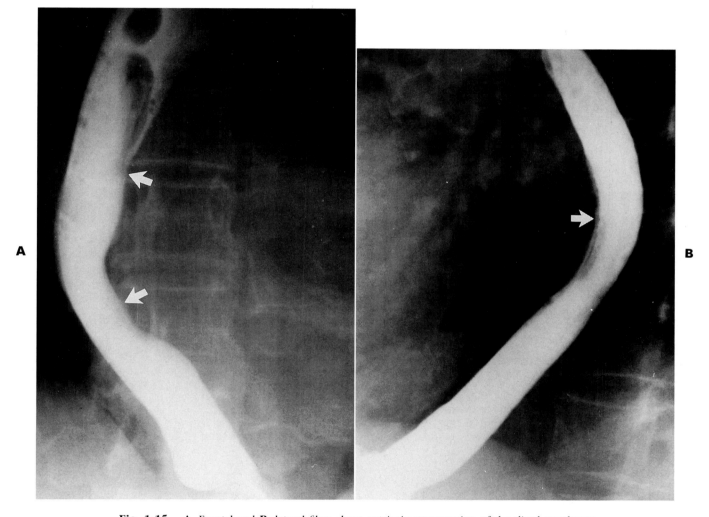

Fig. 1-15   **A,** Frontal and **B,** lateral films show extrinsic compression of the distal esophagus *(arrows)* by an enlarged left atrium.

ULCERATIONS AND FISTULAS

Nonneoplastic
   Infections
   Inflammation (noninfectious)
   Aortoesophageal fistula
   Trauma
Neoplastic
   Carcinoma
   Metastases
   Lymphoma

Nonneoplastic

Infectious causes of esophageal ulceration include viruses, fungi, and bacteria. Viral esophagitis most often

affects immunocompromised patients, particularly those with AIDS. Herpes simplex virus and cytomegalovirus (CMV) both cause solitary or multiple discrete shallow ulcers on a normal esophageal mucosal background (Fig. 1-16). The ulcers of CMV may be quite large. Human immunodeficiency virus (HIV) itself has been reported to produce giant esophageal ulcers identical to those caused by CMV.

Tuberculous esophagitis usually occurs in patients with pulmonary or mediastinal tuberculosis and may result from contiguous extension of disease or from swallowing infected sputum. Esophageal ulcerations, sinus tracts, and nodularity are typically noted (Fig. 1-17). This is being reported with increasing frequency in patients with AIDS and may result in esophagorespiratory fistulas. Esophageal ulceration caused by atypical mycobacteria has also been described in AIDS.

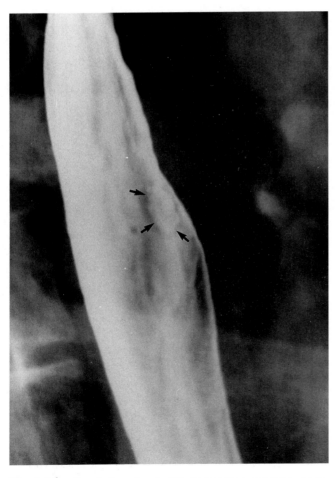

Fig. 1-16   Focal ulceration in the midesophagus *(arrows)* represents CMV esophagitis in a patient with AIDS.

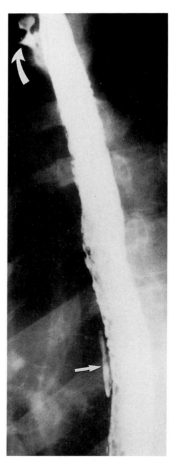

Fig. 1-17   Sinus tract *(curved arrow)* and longitudinal ulceration *(arrow)* in a patient with AIDS and mycobacterial esophagitis. (From Goodman P, Pinero SS, Rance RM, et al: Mycobacterial esophagitis in AIDS, *Gastrointest Radiol* 14:103-105, 1989.)

In *Candida* esophagitis, confluence of fungal plaques may allow barium to penetrate between the plaques, resulting in pseudoulceration. True ulceration may also occur in severe esophageal candidiasis and can be focal or diffuse.

Reflux esophagitis can cause erosions or ulcerations in the distal esophagus as a result of irritation of the esophageal mucosa by gastric acid. Conditions predisposing to development of severe reflux esophagitis include bile reflux esophagitis, Zollinger-Ellison syndrome, and prolonged nasogastric intubation. Bile reflux esophagitis is a particularly severe form of reflux esophagitis seen most often in patients with previous partial or complete gastric resection in whom alkaline bile from the proximal small bowel refluxes into the esophagus. This may lead to esophageal ulceration and stricturing. This complication can be avoided by surgically diverting the flow of bile away from the gastric remnant or esophagus (revision of gastroduodenostomy or creation of Roux-en-Y enteroenterostomy). Zollinger-Ellison syndrome, when complicated by gastroesophageal reflux, may also lead to severe reflux esophagitis because of the acidic gastric fluid in this condition.

Prolonged nasogastric intubation, by not allowing complete closure of the lower esophageal sphincter around the indwelling tube, permits continuous reflux to occur. The tube also alters esophageal peristalsis, preventing rapid clearance of the refluxed material from the esophagus. This may eventually result in diffuse esophageal narrowing.

Barrett's esophagus is a condition in which esophageal squamous epithelium undergoes metaplasia to a gastric-type columnar epithelium. This occurs in about 10% of patients with reflux esophagitis and is felt to be directly related to reflux disease. Although Barrett's esophagus is usually seen in the distal esophagus (where reflux most often occurs), it may also involve the mid or upper thirds of the esophagus with areas of intervening normal esophageal mucosa. Radiographic manifestations of Barrett's esophagus include mucosal nodularity, a reticular mucosal pattern (on double-contrast films), focal ulceration, and focal narrowing or stricture formation.

Certain oral medications may cause focal irritation and ulceration of the esophagus by prolonged contact with the esophageal mucosa (Fig. 1-18). This is most often seen with tetracycline and its derivatives and has also been reported with quinidine, potassium chloride, and several other medications. The tablet, especially when taken at bedtime with a small amount of water, may lodge in the esophagus at the level of the aortic arch or distal esophagus. The focal esophagitis will usu-

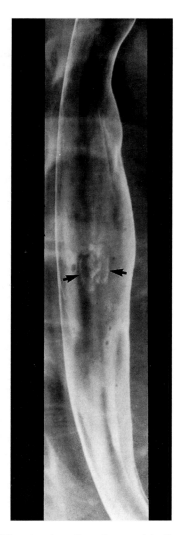

Fig. 1-18   Discrete ulcerations *(arrows)* in the midesophagus caused by the ingestion of antibiotic capsules.

ally heal following discontinuation of the offending medication.

Corrosive esophagitis resulting from the ingestion of lye or other caustic substances often leads to severe edema and ulceration of the esophagus in the acute stage, followed by stricture formation after healing occurs. Contrast studies are not usually performed in the acute stage of a severe corrosive esophagitis.

In acute alcoholic esophagitis, superficial ulcerations are seen in the midesophagus and distal esophagus shortly after alcoholic binges.

Although the esophagus is relatively radioresistant, radiation therapy to the mediastinum may cause esophagitis and esophageal ulcerations. This occurs in the acute stage and may lead to stricture formation following healing. The location of inflammatory changes conforms to the radiation port used.

Changes of radiation esophagitis are typically seen after doses of 4500 to 6000 rads over a 6- to 8-week period and are even more common following combination radiation therapy and chemotherapy. Following radiation therapy, esophagorespiratory fistulas may develop in patients with mediastinal adenopathy compressing the esophagus, presumably as a result of tumor necrosis induced by radiation. Similarly, patients who undergo external beam or intracavitary radiation therapy for primary esophageal carcinoma, may develop necrosis of the tumor with subsequent ulceration or formation of an esophagorespiratory fistula.

Esophageal involvement occurs in approximately 3% of patients with Crohn's disease of the ileum or colon and may be seen as aphthous or longitudinal ulcers. Crohn's disease of the esophagus rarely occurs in the absence of ileal or colonic disease.

Behçet's disease is an unusual condition of unknown etiology that is characterized by oral and genital ulcerations, ocular inflammation, and vascular thrombosis. Focal ulcerations have been reported in the esophagus, colon, and ileum.

Benign mucous membrane pemphigoid and epidermolysis bullosa are rare skin diseases that may be associated with ulcerations, webs, and strictures in the pharynx and esophagus. As noted, the initial finding in these conditions is multiple mucosal nodules.

Eosinophilic esophagitis is a rare cause of esophageal ulcerations. This disease, like eosinophilic gastroenteritis, is associated with eosinophilic infiltration, peripheral eosinophilia, and a history of allergies. In addition to ulcerations, esophageal nodularity and stricture formation may occur in this disease.

Aortoesophageal fistula is an unusual complication of thoracic aortic aneurysms or aortic grafts. Erosion into the esophagus causes hematemesis, usually followed within hours to days by massive bleeding.

Trauma may lead to ulceration, laceration, or perforation of the esophagus. This includes iatrogenic causes, such as instrumentation, endoscopic perforation of an esophageal diverticulum, and sclerotherapy of esophageal varices with resultant ulceration. Taco chips or corn chips may lacerate the esophagus, and impacted foreign bodies may cause focal irritation and ulceration. Vomiting can lead to mucosal disruption (Mallory-Weiss tear) or transmural perforation (Boerhaave's syndrome) of the distal esophagus.

Neoplastic

Focal necrosis and ulceration are not unusual in primary squamous cell carcinoma of the esophagus. However, extensive ulceration (in which the tumor is almost completely ulcerated) is uncommonly seen radiographically. Primary esophageal adenocarcinoma arising in Barrett's epithelium may also undergo focal ulceration. Other malignant lesions that may appear ulcerated include metastases and lymphoma.

DYSMOTILITY

Cervical Esophagus
   Neuromuscular abnormalities
   Incomplete cricopharyngeal relaxation
Thoracic Esophagus
   Neuromuscular abnormalities
   Esophagitis
   Systemic diseases
   Drug-induced

Normal esophageal motility or peristalsis refers to the coordinated propulsion of a bolus from the pharynx to the stomach. This process is regulated by complex neuromuscular interactions and appears radiographically as a continuous, smooth, wavelike contraction. Whereas a primary wave is initiated by the act of swallowing, a secondary wave is produced in response to the bolus itself.

Cervical Esophagus

Diseases of striated muscle, such as dermatomyositis and muscular dystrophy, can affect motility of the cervical esophagus because this portion of the esophagus is composed of striated muscle rather than smooth muscle. Various neuromuscular abnormalities including brainstem infarction, multiple sclerosis, and pseudobulbar palsy can cause dysmotility of the cervical esophagus because swallowing function is controlled by the central nervous system, cranial nerves, and peripheral autonomic nerves. Myasthenia gravis, a disorder involving the neuromuscular junction, can also affect cervical esophageal motility.

The cricopharyngeus muscle, as the lower portion of the inferior constrictor muscle, forms the posterior wall of the pharyngoesophageal junction. During swallowing, the cricopharyngeus muscle normally relaxes to allow the food bolus to pass from the pharynx into the esophagus. If this muscle remains contracted during swallowing, it causes a smooth, rounded impression at the level of the C5-C6 disc space that may persist for a variable length of time (Fig. 1-19). This is an important cause of dysphagia and may lead to the formation of a Zenker's diverticulum by creating increased intraluminal pressure in the hypopharynx. In-

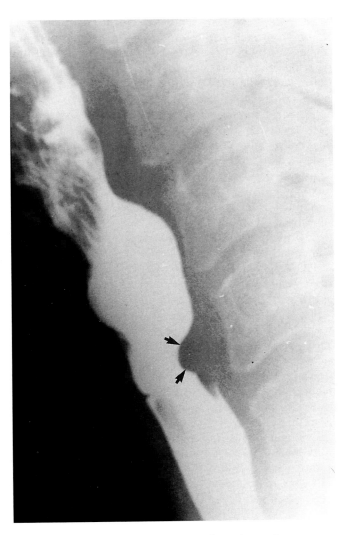

Fig. 1-19   Lateral view of the cervical esophagus shows prominence of the cricopharyngeus muscle *(arrows).*

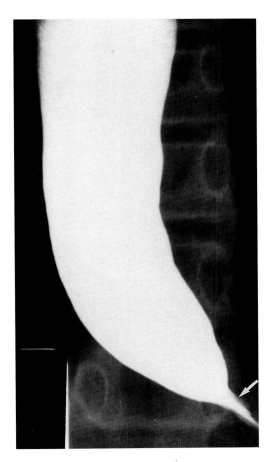

Fig. 1-20   Esophageal dilatation with smooth distal tapering *(arrow)* represents achalasia.

complete cricopharyngeal relaxation may develop as a protective mechanism in patients with gastroesophageal reflux to prevent aspiration of gastric contents. Prominence of the cricopharyngeus muscle can also be seen following laryngectomy.

Thoracic Esophagus

Scleroderma is a systemic disorder of connective tissue in which smooth muscle is replaced by fibrous tissue. In the esophagus, the proximal third that is composed of striated muscle is unaffected while the distal two thirds, composed of smooth muscle, displays abnormal motility. Typically the esophagus appears dilated and the gastroesophageal junction is widely patent. Gastroesophageal reflux is common and may be

marked. Because of the long-standing reflux and the delayed clearance of refluxed material by the flaccid esophagus, reflux esophagitis usually develops. This may be severe with resultant stricture formation or development of Barrett's esophagus. Mixed connective tissue diseases that often include scleroderma may also demonstrate these findings.

Achalasia is a disease of the myenteric plexus of the esophagus in which peristalsis is diffusely decreased or absent and the lower esophageal sphincter fails to relax. The esophagus is often dilated and may appear on frontal chest films as an air- or fluid-filled tubular structure in the medial right hemithorax (with an air-fluid level present on upright films). Contrast studies show dilution of barium by retained fluid in the esophagus. Peristaltic contractions appear disordered in the early stage of the disease and diminished or absent in later stages. The distal esophagus demonstrates smooth, tapered narrowing caused by the contracted lower esophageal sphincter (Fig. 1-20). In the upright posi-

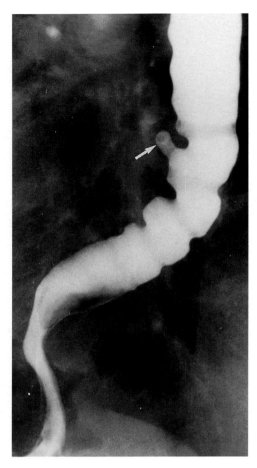

Fig. 1-21   Tertiary contractions and a pulsion diverticulum *(arrow)* in the distal esophagus.

Secondary achalasia simulates primary achalasia but results from malignancy and usually has an abrupt onset later in life. The decreased peristalsis and smooth tapering of the distal esophagus in secondary achalasia typically result from tumor infiltrating the myenteric plexus of the distal esophagus. This can occur in invasive gastric carcinoma, lymphoma, and metastatic disease involving the gastroesophageal junction. Other suggested pathogenetic mechanisms in secondary achalasia include paraneoplastic syndrome and central nervous system lesions affecting the vagal nerve nuclei.

Chagas' disease, an infectious disease seen in Brazil and other tropical areas, also mimics idiopathic achalasia. Chagas' disease is caused by *Trypanosoma cruzi,* a protozoan transmitted to humans by the reduviid bug, and affects the esophagus, duodenum, colon, and heart.

Diffuse esophageal spasm and related disorders (i.e., presbyesophagus and corkscrew esophagus) cause a spectrum of esophageal dysmotility. Disordered peristalsis is often reflected by the presence of tertiary waves (Fig. 1-21). These nonpropulsive, sometimes bizarre-appearing contractions may be associated with significant dysphagia.

Abnormal esophageal motility is one of the earliest findings in reflux esophagitis and in other inflammatory causes of esophagitis, such as radiation and caustic ingestion.

Systemic diseases that may cause esophageal dysmotility include myxedema, thyrotoxicosis, amyloidosis, and diabetes mellitus.

Drugs, particularly atropine and other anticholinergics, also can cause esophageal dysmotility.

tion, gravity may partially overcome the decreased peristalsis and the tightened sphincter to allow intermittent passage of small amounts of contrast material into the stomach. However, in the horizontal position, little, if any, contrast material passes into the stomach.

Primary or idiopathic achalasia usually has its onset in early adulthood and results in dysphagia, regurgitation, and other complications of esophageal stasis including bad breath, aspiration pneumonia, and esophageal candidiasis. In cases of long-standing achalasia, there is an increased incidence of squamous cell carcinoma of the esophagus, probably secondary to chronic mucosal irritation by retained food. Diagnosis of superimposed carcinoma in achalasia is rarely made before the tumor has become large and invasive. Early radiological detection is limited by the patient's underlying chronic dysphagia, the markedly dilated esophageal lumen, and the presence of food and debris within the esophagus.

NARROWED ESOPHAGUS

Neoplasms
Infections
Inflammation (noninfectious)
Neuromuscular, motility abnormalities
Hematoma
Extrinsic compression

Narrowing of the esophagus may result from intrinsic or extrinsic causes. Narrowing can be further characterized as focal or diffuse, mild or severe, and smooth or irregular.

Esophageal neoplasms, especially squamous cell carcinoma, are common causes of focal esophageal narrowing. The most typical appearance of esophageal squamous cell carcinoma on contrast studies is an abrupt irregular narrowing by an annular mass (Fig. 1-22). CT is used to evaluate the primary lesion and to determine depth of invasion and presence of regional adenopathy and distant metastases. Contiguous extension of tumor may involve the tracheobronchial tree, aorta, pleura, or pericardium and is demonstrated by infiltration of paraesophageal fat planes. However, this may be overestimated in the absence of fat planes secondary to cachexia or fibrosis. Lymphatic extension of tumors, though usually present when adjacent lymph nodes appear enlarged, may be underestimated (if malignant nodes do not appear enlarged) or, less commonly, overestimated (if nodes are enlarged because of benign disease).

MRI has been limited in evaluation of esophageal carcinoma because of motion artifact but may play a more important role with the development of cardiorespiratory gating techniques.

Esophageal adenocarcinoma arising in Barrett's epithelium can cause irregular luminal narrowing similar to that seen in squamous cell carcinoma.

Metastatic disease to the esophagus occurs through contiguous or hematogenous spread of tumor. Direct invasion can involve the cervical esophagus (laryngeal carcinoma and thyroid carcinoma), midesophagus (lung carcinoma and mediastinal adenopathy), or distal esophagus (superior extension of gastric carcinoma) (Fig. 1-23). Radiographic findings include esophageal obstruction, displacement, narrowing, ulceration, and fistula formation. Hematogenous metastasis to the esophagus (breast carcinoma and malignant melanoma) is less common than contiguous spread but may also produce a variety of radiographic findings including focal narrowing and submucosal masses.

Lymphoma affects the esophagus in less than 1% of cases and is more often a result of extrinsic compression by mediastinal adenopathy than of intrinsic esophageal involvement. Esophageal lymphoma has many different radiographic appearances and may simulate achalasia, varices, contiguous extension of gastric carcinoma, and hematogenous metastases. It may also cause luminal narrowing or a polypoid mass, either of which may be associated with ulceration.

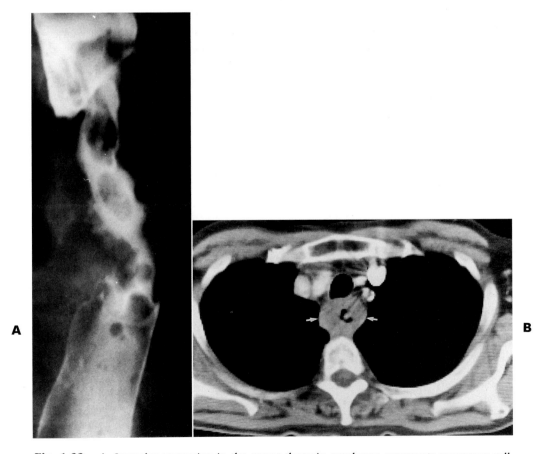

A

B

Fig. 1-22 **A,** Irregular narrowing in the upper thoracic esophagus represents squamous cell carcinoma. **B,** CT demonstrates marked circumferential wall thickening *(arrows)* as a result of tumor infiltration.

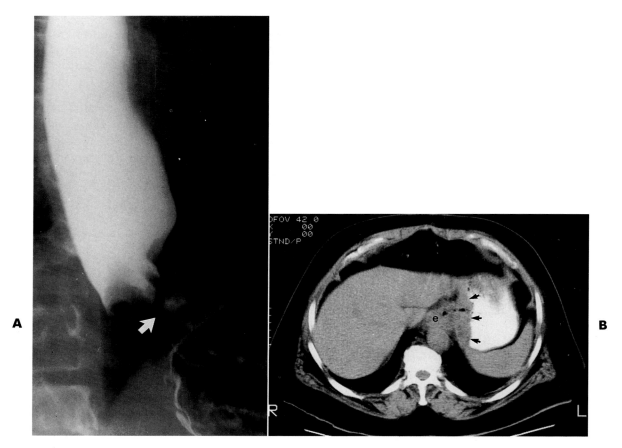

Fig. 1-23   **A,** Narrowing of the distal esophagus *(arrow)* with an overhanging proximal margin represents adenocarcinoma. **B,** CT shows soft tissue mass involving the distal esophagus *(e)* and gastric cardia *(arrows).*

Leiomyomas or other benign esophageal neoplasms, when of sufficient size, can cause smooth compression and narrowing of the esophageal lumen.

Another intrinsic cause of esophageal narrowing is inflammatory stricture formation. Infectious causes of stricturing include tuberculosis, candidiasis, and rarely syphilis. Noninfectious, inflammatory strictures may result from gastroesophageal reflux (and disorders associated with reflux), Barrett's esophagus, corrosive ingestion, and radiation (Figs. 1-24 to 1-28). Less common causes include Crohn's disease, benign mucous mem-brane pemphigoid, epidermolysis bullosa, eosinophilic esophagitis, graft-versus-host disease, and prior sclero-therapy for varices (Fig. 1-29).

Motility abnormalities may focally narrow the esophagus by causing tertiary contractions (diffuse esophageal spasm) or incomplete relaxation of the dis-tal esophageal sphincter (achalasia). Traumatic intra-mural hematoma of the distal esophagus can also cause focal narrowing.

Extrinsic compression by adjacent benign or malig-nant processes typically causes smooth, eccentric nar-rowing.

verticulum most likely results from increased intraluminal pressure in the hypopharynx and may be associated with incomplete relaxation of the cricopharyngeus muscle. When small, Zenker's diverticulum extends directly posteriorly and is best visualized in the lateral projection on contrast examination (Fig. 1-31). With continued increased pressure, the diverticulum may enlarge and extend laterally. Complications associated with Zenker's diverticulum include dysphagia, bad breath, and aspiration pneumonia, and iatrogenic perforation of the diverticulum at endoscopy is a recognized danger. Less commonly, diverticula can arise from the lateral aspects of the pharyngoesophageal junction.

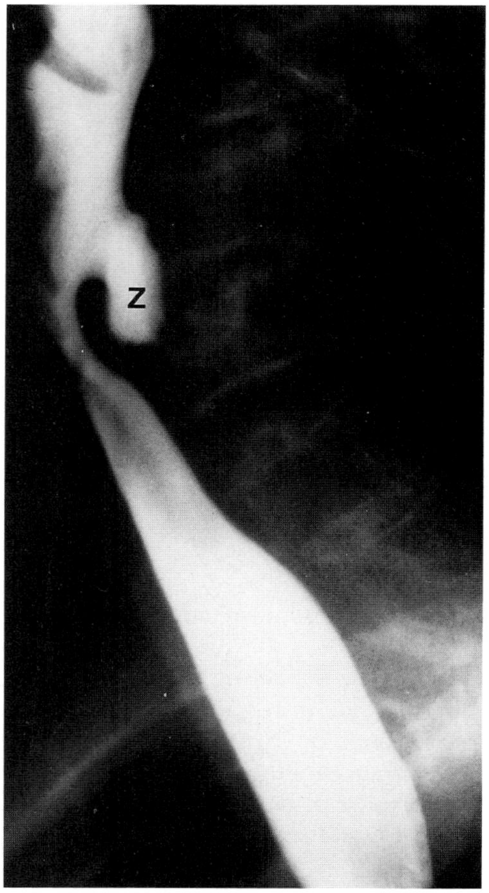

Midesophageal diverticula often occur at the anterior aspect of the esophagus at the level of the carina (Fig. 1-32). These may represent traction diverticula resulting from retraction of the esophageal wall by healed granulomatous disease of the mediastinum. However, recent studies suggest that most midesophageal diverticula are caused by increased intraluminal

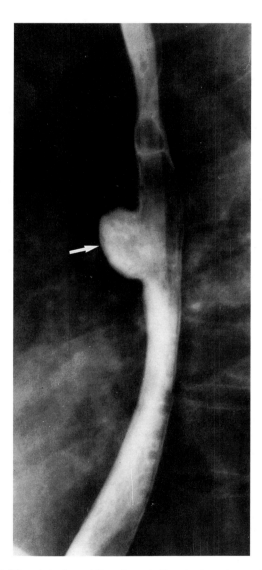

Fig. 1-31   Lateral view of the cervical esophagus shows a Zenker's diverticulum (Z).

Fig. 1-32   Anterior midesophageal diverticulum (arrow).

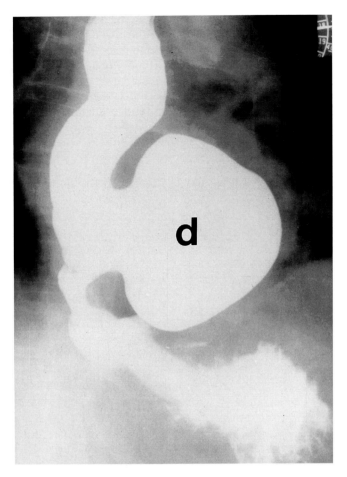

Fig. 1-33   Large epiphrenic diverticulum *(d)*.

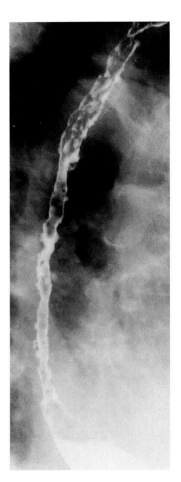

Fig. 1-34   Long stricture of the thoracic esophagus with numerous intramural pseudodiverticula.

pressure and therefore represent pulsion diverticula. On contrast examination, traction diverticula, which contain a muscular wall, typically have an angular contour and can contract, whereas pulsion diverticula, which lack a muscular wall, have a rounded configuration and do not contract.

Epiphrenic diverticula are located in the distal esophagus near the gastroesophageal junction (Fig. 1-33). These pulsion diverticula result from abnormal intraluminal pressure and may be associated with tertiary contractions of the esophagus. Accidental entry of the endoscope into an epiphrenic diverticulum may lead to perforation.

Esophageal intramural pseudodiverticulosis is an unusual condition in which dilated mucous glands in the esophageal wall may simulate true diverticula on contrast studies (Fig. 1-34). The pseudodiverticula are usually flask shaped and of uniform depth. They may be solitary or multiple, and distribution may be segmental or diffuse. This condition is most often associated with esophageal strictures, although the diverticula may be located proximal or distal to the stricture site. Intramural pseudodiverticulosis usually occurs as a rare sequela of esophagitis.

Intraluminal esophageal diverticulum represents a transient artifact that results from barium mixing with retained fluid or debris in the esophagus. This appears similar to an intraluminal duodenal diverticulum ("windsock") on contrast examination but is not associated with an intraluminal membrane.

FOLDS

Normal
   Longitudinal
   Transverse
Thickened
   Esophagitis
   Varices
   Varicoid carcinoma
   Lymphoma

Normal

Longitudinal folds extend along the entire length of the esophagus and are best demonstrated on collapsed views. Transverse folds also occur normally, though seen less often than longitudinal folds. These thin, transient folds represent contraction of the muscularis mucosa of the esophageal wall (Fig. 1-35). This is sometimes referred to as a feline esophagus because the transverse folds resemble those seen normally in the esophagus of a cat.

Thickened

Thickening of longitudinal and transverse folds as a result of edema and inflammation has been described as an early finding in reflux esophagitis and may occur in other forms of esophagitis as well. Esophageal varices may appear as thickened folds but are differentiated by their tortuosity and changeability with position and esophageal distention.

Varicoid carcinoma is a form of esophageal carcinoma in which submucosal spread of tumor causes esophageal folds to appear thickened (Fig. 1-36).

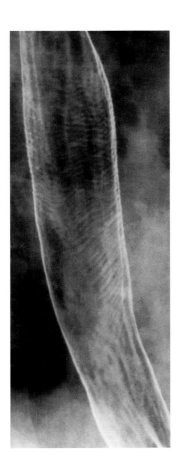

Fig. 1-35   Thin transverse folds (feline esophagus).

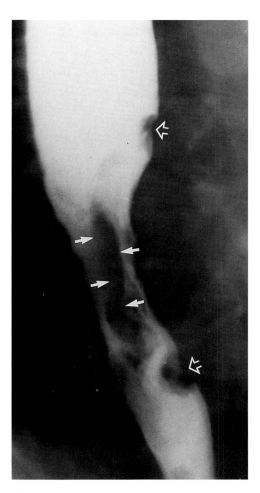

Fig. 1-36   Thickened longitudinal fold *(arrows)* and mural masses *(open arrows)* in the distal esophagus represent varicoid carcinoma.

Esophageal lymphoma is a rare neoplasm that may also produce thickening of esophageal folds because of submucosal spread of tumor. Unlike varices, the deformity seen in varicoid carcinoma and esophageal lymphoma is fixed.

WEBS, HERNIAS, AND RINGS

Webs
  Cervical
  Distal
Hernias
  Axial (sliding)
  Paraesophageal
  Mixed
Rings
  Muscular
  Mucosal
  Schatzki

Webs

Webs are incomplete membranes that appear as thin, transverse filling defects on contrast studies. These most often occur at the anterior aspect of the proximal cervical esophagus and are less often circumferential. Webs can occur spontaneously or secondary to scarring from benign mucous membrane pemphigoid and epidermolysis bullosa. They can also develop in graft-versus-host disease, a complication of bone marrow transplantation in which host tissues are attacked by donor lymphocytes. In Plummer-Vinson syndrome, cervical esophageal webs are associated with iron-deficiency anemia and dysphagia (Fig. 1-37). Distal esophageal webs may result from reflux esophagitis.

Hernias

A hiatal hernia represents an extension of the stomach into the chest through the esophageal hiatus. In the more common axial or sliding hiatal hernia, the gastroesophageal junction lies more than 2 cm above the diaphragm. This type of hernia is frequently associated with gastroesophageal reflux.

Although hiatal hernias usually involve only the proximal portion of the stomach, the entire stomach may herniate into the chest resulting in an intrathoracic stomach (Fig. 1-38). The stomach assumes an inverted position in the chest with the greater curvature located superiorly and the lesser curvature inferiorly. Subsequently, the proximal portion of the stomach

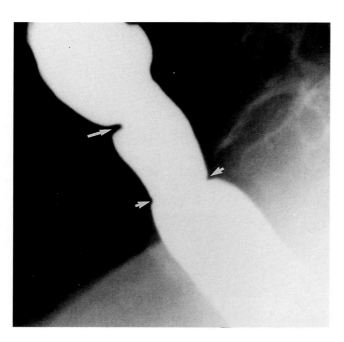

Fig. 1-37 Lateral view of the cervical esophagus demonstrates an anterior web *(arrow)* and a circumferential web *(short arrows)* in a patient with dysphagia and microcytic anemia.

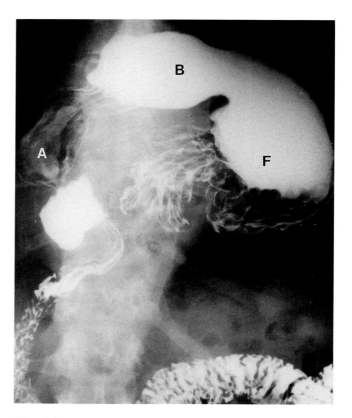

Fig. 1-38 Large hiatal hernia contains the fundus *(F)*, body *(B)*, and antrum *(A)* of the stomach.

may return through the esophageal hiatus to its normal position below the diaphragm, leaving the distal portion within the chest. Complications of intrathoracic stomach include obstruction, volvulus, and perforation.

Paraesophageal hernias account for less than 5% of all hiatal hernias and are not associated with gastroesophageal reflux. In this type of hernia, the gastroesophageal junction is located below the diaphragm but the gastric fundus partially extends upward through the esophageal hiatus to the left of the distal esophagus (Fig. 1-39).

A mixed or combined hiatal hernia demonstrates features of both the axial and paraesophageal types, with the gastroesophageal junction located above the diaphragm and the gastric fundus lying alongside the distal esophagus.

Rings

Rings represent areas of narrowing in the region of the esophageal vestibule, which is the distal end of the esophagus that normally appears slightly distended (Fig. 1-40). The muscular ring (A-ring) is a variable smooth, broad narrowing at the superior aspect of the vestibule. This rarely causes dysphagia and most likely results from transient muscle contractions.

The more commonly noted mucosal ring (B-ring) is a persistent thin, transverse constriction at the inferior aspect of the esophageal vestibule in the region of the gastroesophageal junction. The mucosal ring is smooth, symmetrical, and rarely causes dysphagia unless measuring less than 13 mm in diameter. A narrowed mucosal ring that causes dysphagia is known as a Schatzki ring. Mucosal rings are commonly associated with hiatal hernias and are most easily visualized when the esophagogastric junction is distended during contrast examination in the horizontal position (Fig. 1-41). The maximal diameter of the ring can best be determined by having the patient swallow a 13-mm barium tablet while standing. The tablet will lodge above a Schatzki ring but will pass through a nonstenotic mucosal ring into the stomach.

Although the mucosal ring occurs at the gastroesophageal junction, it does not necessarily correspond to the histological squamocolumnar junction (Z line). This is true in Barrett's esophagus, where metaplasia of the distal esophageal epithelium may cause the Z line to be located proximal to the esophagogastric junction. The Z line is sometimes visualized on double-contrast films as a thin, serrated line in the distal esophagus.

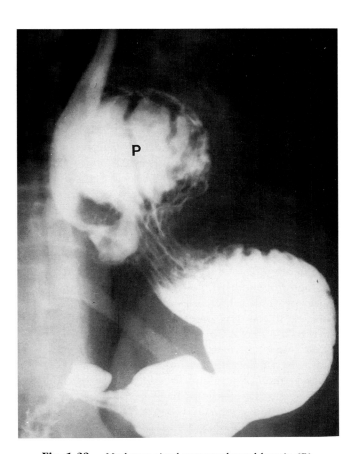

Fig. 1-39   Moderate-sized paraesophageal hernia *(P)*.

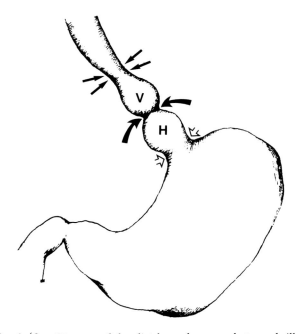

Fig. 1-40   Diagram of the distal esophagus and stomach illustrates esophageal vestibule *(V)*, axial hiatal hernia *(H)*, A-ring *(arrows)*, B-ring *(curved arrows)*, and diaphragmatic impressions *(open arrows)*.

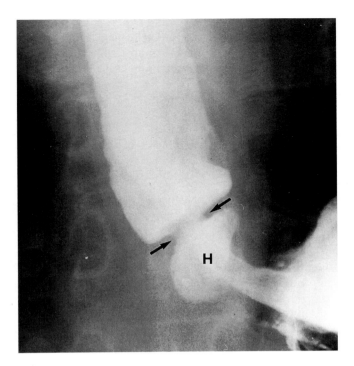

Fig. 1-41 Small axial hiatal hernia *(H)* and B-ring *(arrows)*.

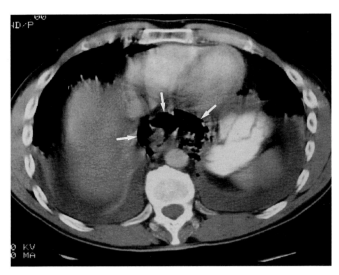

Fig. 1-42 CT shows a large amorphous air collection *(arrows)* in the posterior mediastinum in a patient with esophageal rupture.

TRAUMA AND FOREIGN BODIES

Mallory-Weiss tear
Intramural hematoma
Perforation
    Boerhaave's syndrome
    Instrumentation
    Foreign bodies
Food impaction

Mallory-Weiss tear represents a mucosal disruption in the distal esophagus, usually resulting from prolonged or severe vomiting. This causes hematemesis and is sometimes identified on double-contrast films as a thin linear collection of barium in the distal esophagus. Mallory-Weiss tear usually heals spontaneously within several days.

Esophageal intramural hematoma represents hemorrhage in the submucosal layer of the esophageal wall. This usually occurs by extension of a mucosal tear and appears on contrast examination as a smooth submucosal mass.

Boerhaave's syndrome is also usually caused by persistent or severe vomiting but represents transmural perforation of the distal esophagus. This causes mediastinitis and requires immediate surgical repair of the esophageal perforation. Delay in surgical treatment of

Boerhaave's syndrome is associated with a high mortality rate. Chest films show mediastinal emphysema, and water-soluble contrast examination of the esophagus demonstrates extravasation of contrast material into the mediastinum (Fig. 1-42).

Traumatic perforation of the esophagus may also result from penetrating injuries (e.g., knife or bullet wounds) and instrumentation, either surgical (inadvertent laceration during intrathoracic surgery) or nonsurgical (routine endoscopy, dilatation procedures, and stent placements) (Figs. 1-43 and 1-44).

Ingested foreign bodies, such as chicken bones or fish bones, may lodge in the cervical or thoracic portions of the esophagus and cause focal irritation or perforation. Taco chips and corn chips have been reported to cause mucosal laceration of the esophagus. Ingestion of sharp metallic objects, such as pins or nails, may also cause laceration or perforation of the esophagus.

Food impaction usually occurs when a poorly chewed piece of meat lodges in the esophagus. Although the underlying esophagus may be normal, strictures or other causes of esophageal narrowing can predispose to the development of a food impaction proximal to the narrowed area. Contrast studies in cases of food impaction usually demonstrate a completely or partially obstructing intraluminal mass (Fig. 1-45). Glucagon, anticholinergic medications, and ingestion of effervescent granules have been used with varying success to dislodge impacted food boluses from the esophagus. Ingestion of enzymes or other meat tenderizers is no longer recommended because of complications including esophageal perforation.

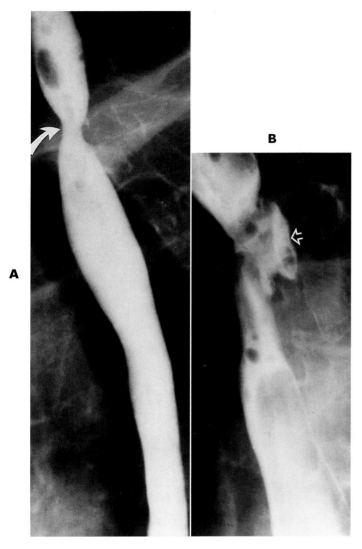

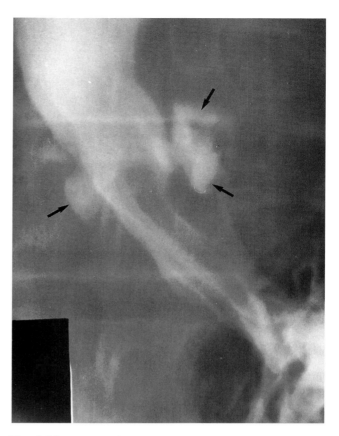

Fig. 1-44   Water-soluble contrast examination shows two focal collections of contrast material *(arrows)* adjacent to the distal esophagus. These represent perforations following endoscopic dilatation for achalasia.

Fig. 1-43   **A,** Short stricture *(curved arrow)* following radiation and chemotherapy for squamous cell carcinoma of the lower cervical esophagus. **B,** Focal collection of contrast material *(open arrow)* at the site of previous stricture represents perforation secondary to endoscopic dilatation procedure.

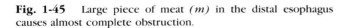

Fig. 1-45   Large piece of meat *(m)* in the distal esophagus causes almost complete obstruction.

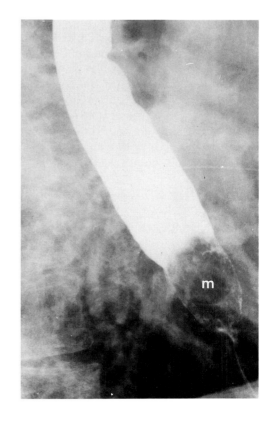

POSTOPERATIVE ESOPHAGUS

Nonsurgical Procedures
  Bougienage
  Balloon dilatation
  Stent placement
  Laser therapy
  Sclerotherapy
  Gastric balloon
Surgical Procedures
  Myotomy
  Interposition
  Fundoplication
  Sugiura procedure

Nonsurgical Procedures

A variety of surgical and nonsurgical procedures have been developed for treatment of esophageal diseases. Bougienage consists of passage of a graded series of dilators into the esophagus to distend a stricture or other narrowed area. Balloon or pneumatic dilators contain a segment that can be placed at the site of narrowing and then inflated. In achalasia, pneumatic dilatation is used to tear the contracted muscle fibers of the lower esophageal sphincter, similar to the effect of a surgical myotomy. The most important complication of these procedures is esophageal perforation.

Endoscopically guided stent placement is often used to maintain patency of the esophagus in patients with esophageal carcinoma (Fig. 1-46). Obstruction and migration of the tube and esophageal perforation are recognized complications of this palliative procedure.

Laser therapy is another endoscopic palliative procedure in which a laser beam (Nd:YAG laser) is used to destroy tumor tissue and thereby widen an obstructed esophageal lumen. This can lead to esophageal perforation or esophagorespiratory fistula.

Sclerotherapy is sometimes used in the treatment of esophageal varices. Sclerosing agents are injected directly into the varices, causing fibrosis and obliteration of the varices. Complications of sclerotherapy include inflammation, ulceration, stricturing, fistula formation, and perforation.

Placement of a balloon into the gastric fundus (Sengstaken-Blakemore tube) is used to control variceal bleeding through a tamponading effect. However, incorrect placement of the tube with inflation of the balloon in the distal esophagus may cause esophageal perforation.

Surgical Procedures

Surgical esophageal myotomy has been used to treat both idiopathic achalasia (Heller's myotomy) and in-

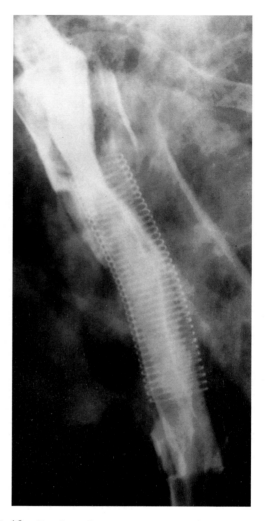

Fig. 1-46 Esophageal stent in a patient with advanced esophageal carcinoma.

complete cricopharyngeal relaxation (cricopharyngeal myotomy). Extensive myotomy of the thoracic esophagus is sometimes performed in severe diffuse esophageal spasm (DES) that is unresponsive to other treatments and in idiopathic muscular hypertrophy of the esophagus, a rare condition characterized by diffuse marked thickening of the esophageal musculature. In these procedures, the abnormally contracted or thickened muscle is surgically incised.

Various types of surgical interpositions can be performed in conjunction with esophageal resection or bypass in the management of esophageal carcinoma or extensive stricture formation. Stomach, colon, or jejunum can be used for this purpose. Contrast studies and CT are useful for demonstrating postoperative complications, both early (anastomotic leak, perforation, ob-

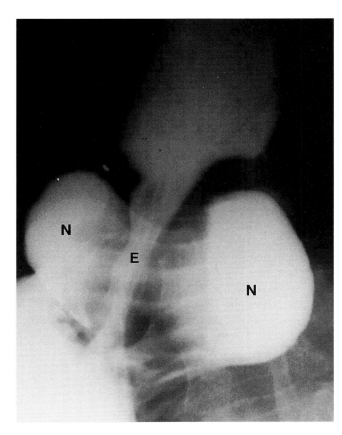

Fig. 1-47   Distal esophagus *(E)* is compressed by Nissen's fundoplication *(N)*.

struction as a result of edema) and late (anastomotic stricture and recurrent tumor).

Fundoplication and related surgical procedures can be used to reduce hiatal hernias and prevent associated gastroesophageal reflux. In fundoplication (Nissen, Mark IV [Belsey], and Hill types), a portion of the gastric fundus is wrapped around the distal esophagus (Fig. 1-47). This fundal wrap prevents reflux by compressing the distal esophagus and may appear as a pseudotumor on routine contrast studies and CT. Complications include obstruction if the wrap is too tight and persistent reflux if it is too loose. The Angelchik device, a ringlike structure filled with silicon, can be used in place of a fundal wrap but is associated with additional complications including migration of the device into the abdominal or thoracic cavity and erosion into the gastric lumen.

The Sugiura procedure is a complex surgical procedure used for treating esophageal varices. This extensive operation includes esophageal transection with

devascularization of the distal esophagus and proximal stomach. Postoperative contrast studies typically reveal indentation at the distal esophageal suture line.

SUGGESTED READINGS
Esophagus

Balthazar EJ, Megibow AJ, Hulnick D, et al: Cytomegalovirus esophagitis in AIDS: radiographic features in 16 patients, *AJR* 149:919-923, 1987.

Balthazar EJ, Naidich DP, Megibow AJ, et al: CT evaluation of esophageal varices, *AJR* 148:131-135, 1987.

Bleshman MH, Banner MP, Johnson RC, et al: The inflammatory esophagogastric polyp and fold, *Radiology* 128:589-593, 1978.

Bova JG, Dutton NE, Goldstein HM, et al: Medication-induced esophagitis: diagnosis by double-contrast esophagography, *AJR* 148:731-732, 1987.

Buchholz D: Neurologic causes of dysphagia, *Dysphagia* 1:152-156, 1987.

Calenoff L, Rogers LF: Radiologic manifestations of iatrogenic changes of the esophagus, *Gastrointest Radiol* 2:229-237, 1977.

Carter MM, Kulkarni MV: Giant fibrovascular polyp of the esophagus, *Gastrointest Radiol* 9:301-303, 1984.

Chasen MH, Rugh KS, Shelton DK: Mediastinal impressions on the dilated esophagus, *Radiol Clin North Am* 22:591-605, 1984.

Curtis DJ: Radiographic anatomy of the pharynx, *Dysphagia* 1:51-62, 1986.

Donner MW, Bosma JF, Robertson DL: Anatomy and physiology of the pharynx, *Gastrointest Radiol* 10:196-212, 1985.

Donner MW, Saba GP, Martinez CR: Diffuse diseases of the esophagus: a practical approach, *Semin Roentgenol* 16:198-213, 1981.

Ekberg O, Nylander G: Dysfunction of the cricopharyngeal muscle: a cineradiographic study of patients with dysphagia, *Radiology* 143:481-486, 1982.

Fisher MS: Metastasis to the esophagus, *Gastrointest Radiol* 1:249-251, 1976.

Freeny PC, Marks WM: Adenocarcinoma of the gastroesophageal junction: barium and CT examination, *AJR* 138:1077-1084, 1982.

Gedgaudas-McClees RK, Torres WE, Colvin RS, et al: Thoracic findings in gastrointestinal pathology, *Radiol Clin North Am* 22:563-589, 1984.

Gelfand DW, Ott DJ: Anatomy and technique in evaluating the esophagus, *Semin Roentgenol* 16:168-182, 1981.

Ghahremani GG, Rushovich AM: Glycogenic acanthosis of the esophagus: radiographic and pathologic features, *Gastrointest Radiol* 9:93-98, 1984.

Gilchrist AM, Levine MS, Carr RF, et al: Barrett's esophagus: diagnosis by double-contrast esophagography, *AJR* 150:97-102, 1988.

Goldstein HM, Zornoza J, Hopens T: Intrinsic diseases of the adult esophagus: benign and malignant tumors, *Semin Roentgenol* 16:183-197, 1981.

Halber MD, Daffner RH, Thompson WM: CT of the esophagus: I. normal appearance, *AJR* 133:1047-1050, 1979.

Halvorsen RA, Thompson WM: Computed tomography of the gastroesophageal junction, *Crit Rev Diagn Imaging* 21:183-228, 1984.

Halvorsen Jr RA, Thompson WM: CT of esophageal neoplasms, *Radiol Clin North Am* 27:667-685, 1989.

Heiken JP, Balfe DM, Roper CL: CT evaluation after esophagogastrectomy, *AJR* 143:555-560, 1984.

Jones B, Kramer SS, Donner MW: Dynamic imaging of the pharynx, *Gastrointest Radiol* 10:213-224, 1985.

Laufer I: Radiology of esophagitis, *Radiol Clin North Am* 20:687-699, 1982.

Lepke RA, Libshitz HI: Radiation-induced injury of the esophagus, *Radiology* 148:375-378, 1983.

Levine MS, Caroline DF, Thompson JJ, et al: Adenocarcinoma of the esophagus: relationship to Barrett mucosa, *Radiology* 150:305-309, 1984.

Levine MS, Loevner LA, Saul SH, et al: Herpes esophagitis: sensitivity of double-contrast esophagography, *AJR* 151:57-62, 1988.

Levine MS, Moolten DN, Herlinger H, et al: Esophageal intramural pseudodiverticulosis: a reevaluation, *AJR* 147:1165-1170, 1986.

Levine MS, Rubesin SE, Herlinger H, et al: Double-contrast upper gastrointestinal examination: technique and interpretation, *Radiology* 168:593-602, 1988.

Love L, Berkow AE: Trauma to the esophagus, *Gastrointest Radiol* 2:305-321, 1978.

Marx MV, Balfe DM: Computed tomography of the esophagus, *Semin US CT MR* 8:316-348, 1987.

Mauro MA, Parker LA, Hartley WS, et al: Epidermolysis bullosa: radiographic findings in 16 cases, *AJR* 149:925-927, 1987.

Olmsted WW, Lichtenstein JE, Hyams VJ: Polypoid epithelial malignancies of the esophagus, *AJR* 140:921-925, 1983.

Olmsted WW, Madewell JE: The esophageal and small-bowel manifestations of progressive systemic sclerosis, *Gastrointest Radiol* 1:33-36, 1976.

Ott DJ, Gelfand DW, Wu WC, et al: Esophagogastric region and its rings, *AJR* 142:281-287, 1984.

Owen JW, Balfe DM, Koehler RE, et al: Radiologic evaluation of complications after esophagogastrectomy, *AJR* 140:1163-1169, 1983.

Phillips LG, Cunningham J: Esophageal perforation, *Radiol Clin North Am* 22:607-613, 1984.

Rubesin SE, Glick SN: The tailored double-contrast pharyngogram, *Crit Rev Diagn Imaging* 28:133-179, 1988.

Rubesin S, Herlinger H, Sigal H: Granular cell tumors of the esophagus, *Gastrointest Radiol* 10:11-15, 1985.

Schneider R: Tuberculous esophagitis, *Gastrointest Radiol* 1:143-145, 1976.

Seaman WB: Pathophysiology of the esophagus, *Semin Roentgenol* 16:214-227, 1981.

Zboralske FF, Dodds WJ: Roentgenographic diagnosis of primary disorders of esophageal motility, *Radiol Clin North Am* 7:147-162, 1969.

Stomach and Duodenum

EXAMINATION TECHNIQUES

The biphasic-contrast examination of the stomach is considered to be the radiological examination of choice at present. This technique consists of examining the stomach, utilizing both double-contrast and single-contrast technique.

In most cases, the stomach examination is combined with the esophagus study. Following the ingestion of effervescent granules and high-density barium and the double-contrast evaluation of the esophagus in the upright position, the patient is quickly lowered into a supine recumbent position. To avoid excessive spillage of the contrast into the small bowel, this should be done promptly after the last esophageal film has been obtained. With the patient in the supine position, a quick fluoroscopic evaluation of the stomach will indicate to the fluoroscopist whether gastric distention is adequate, and if a sufficient amount of barium is retained within the stomach to continue with the examination or whether remedial measures may be necessary at this time.

If the stomach is adequately distended and sufficient barium is in the stomach, the patient is then rotated one to two times to achieve gastric coating. By rotating patients to the left, it is felt that less barium is spilled into the small bowel. The gastric mucosa is covered by a surface layer of mucus that must be washed away by the barium to achieve optimum mucosal coating and detail. Inadequate washing of the barium over the mucosal surface or residual food and secretions will degrade mucosal coating and cause the examination to be limited. Following rotation of the patient, the stomach is again fluoroscopically evaluated for the quality of the mucosal coating.

The menu of spot radiographs obtained varies from institution to institution. Generally, a supine film of the stomach is obtained when adequate coating has been achieved. The patient is turned sharply to the right into a steep right posterior oblique (RPO) or right lateral position, where air-contrast views of the cardia and fundus are obtained. Under fluoroscopic control, the patient is then turned back into the supine position and slightly to the left to thin out the barium pool in the antrum. As the barium flows from the antrum into the proximal stomach, a thin layer of barium is left in the antrum, achieving the *flow technique,* which is an excellent method for demonstrating subtle mucosal findings, such as tiny nodules and linear or punctate erosions (Fig. 2-1). A spot film is obtained at this point. The patient is again turned to the left and air-contrast views of the antrum and duodenum are obtained. This series of maneuvers, basically, represents the double-contrast portion of the stomach examination. Additional films and maneuvers may be necessary to completely demonstrate all areas within the stomach and the duodenal bulb and sweep.

At this point the patient is turned to a recumbent RAO position and ingests low-density barium. A limited evaluation of oropharyngeal function may be obtained during this phase. Esophageal dynamics are also studied, and barium distended views of the gastroesophageal junction obtained. The latter constitutes an important part of the stomach evaluation. With sufficient barium within the stomach and antrum and duodenal bulb, RAO or prone compression views of the antrum and duodenal bulb are obtained. This maneuver is as important in the upper gastrointestinal (UGI) series today as it was 50 years ago. Occasionally, ulcers that are either unfilled during the earlier part of the examination or not well demonstrated can be easily seen with compression views of the antrum and duodenal bulb.

Occasionally, the duodenal bulb and, possibly, the distal antrum will be in a posterior position. In some cases, the bulb will lie almost directly behind the distal antrum. This makes compression of the area somewhat

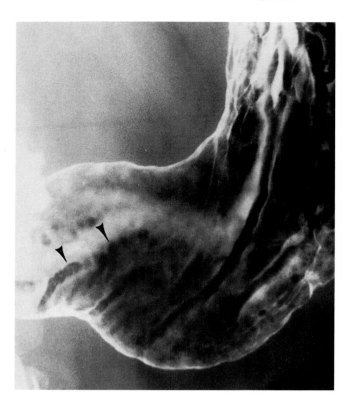

Fig. 2-1   Utilizing flow technique, tiny superficial erosions are seen along one of the folds of the distal stomach. Edema around the erosions results in a beaded appearance of the fold *(arrows)*.

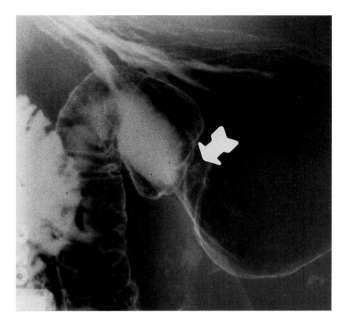

Fig. 2-2   LAO view with compression demonstrates the profiled pyloric channel and duodenal bulb. A small pyloric channel ulcer, not seen on other views, is demonstrated *(arrow)*.

difficult. It also makes air-contrast views of the bulb and antropyloric region difficult as well. In such an instance, the fluoroscopist may utilize angulation of the tube, if this facility is available. However, most fluoroscopic suites have table-side type of fluoroscopy. In such a situation, the fluoroscopist can turn the patient on the left side and firmly position a bolster, which may represent an inflated compression paddle or a balloon against the left costochondral margin. The patient, under fluoroscopy, is then moved down into a left anterior oblique (LAO) position, compressing the bulb as the patient rolls to the left and toward the table. This is often sufficient compression to push away the antrum of the stomach and allow the duodenal bulb and pyloric channel to be demonstrated (Fig. 2-2).

The use of glucagon in UGI studies has been advocated and practiced for over a decade. Small doses of glucagon have been shown to be effective in improving the demonstration of the antrum and duodenal bulb. However, many centers have now ceased this practice, and no intravenous (IV) injection is given before the examination. No objective evidence shows that this results in any decreased sensitivity in the detection of disease in these areas. Without the use of an antiperi-

staltic agent, such as glucagon, gastric contractions may be observed and evaluated.

The last part of the examination consists of rotating the patient again to evaluate for the possibility of spontaneous gastroesophageal reflux. We tend not to use any extraordinary methods for inducing reflux. Valsalva maneuvers, abdominal compression, or bolstering have all been described. Virtually any patient can be made to reflux with sufficient effort. The significance of this reflux is doubtful. However, the rotation of a patient that results in a spontaneous and significant amount of reflux is probably important. This often simulates what happens when the patient rolls over in bed at night and experiences gastric reflux and associated symptoms. It should be remembered that the lack of demonstrated reflux may not necessarily rule out gastroesophageal reflux as the cause of the patient's symptoms.

In many instances instead of the standard biphasic examination, a single-contrast study using low-density barium will be performed. Although this should represent a minority of cases, there are acceptable indications for a single-contrast examination. In elderly or debilitated patients who are unable to stand or who cannot roll or provide the compliance necessary for a double-contrast evaluation of the stomach, a single-contrast examination would be an alternative. In patients with suspected gastric outlet obstruction, single-contrast examination will suffice. In patients who are postoperative or postinstrumentation and in whom

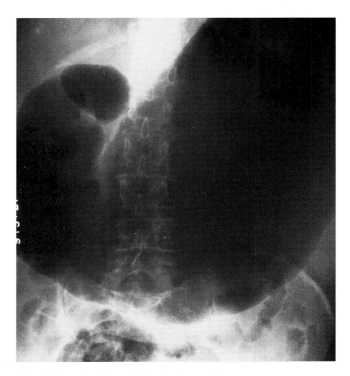

Fig. 2-3 Plain film of the abdomen demonstrates massive air distention of the stomach and duodenal bulb.

there is any question of perforation or leakage, a water-soluble single-contrast examination is indicated.

When faced with the decision as to whether a single or biphasic examination should be undertaken, the radiologist should be guided by the same axiom that applies to the radiological evaluation of the colon—a limited single-contrast evaluation is better than a limited double-contrast evaluation of the organ.

Computed tomography (CT) is extremely useful in evaluating for known or suspected malignant lesions of the stomach. The extent of perigastric involvement and spread to adjacent organs can usually be demonstrated with this type of imaging. Magnetic resonance imaging (MRI) has been extremely limited in evaluation of the stomach at this point and plays little or no role in the diagnostic imaging work-up of patients with gastric disease. Endoscopic ultrasound with a rotating transducer placed on the tip of a specially prepared endoscope has proved to be useful in the evaluation of malignant diseases of the stomach. It is shown to be superior to CT in evaluating the extent of gastric wall involvement and limited perigastric spread and adenopathy, which may not be evident on CT. For evaluation of liver metastatic involvement, however, CT of the liver with pre-IV and post-IV contrast remains the examination of choice.

The following sections approach the differential di-agnosis of gastric disease, based on the dominant radiological problems seen on barium examinations. It closely reflects the way cases are actually encountered in a daily clinical practice. However, it should be kept in mind that the same condition may be discussed under several categories reflecting the different manifestations or stages of the same disease process.

GASTRIC OUTLET OBSTRUCTION RESULTING IN GASTRIC DISTENTION

Peptic Ulcer Disease
Other Inflammatory Causes
    Crohn's disease
    Pancreatitis
    Corrosive materials
    Radiation gastritis
    Tuberculosis
    Syphilis
Malignancy
Gastric Bezoars
Antral Diaphrams
Pyloric Stenosis
Gastric Volvulus

Peptic Ulcer Disease

The most common cause of gastric outlet obstruction in adults is peptic ulcer disease involving the antrum, pyloric channel of the stomach, and the first portion of the duodenum. This complication, however, is seen in only 5% of patients with peptic ulcer disease. Duodenal bulb and pyloric channel ulcers are responsible for over 80% of the cases in which it does occur. Luminal narrowing usually results from the combined changes of chronic and acute inflammation and ulceration. These patients commonly have a long history of peptic ulcer disease and recurrent peptic ulcers. It is unusual for gastric outlet obstruction to be the presenting complaint in a patient with peptic ulcer disease. In such an instance, other possibilities, particularly malignancy, should be considered.

The most common presenting symptoms are vomiting, abdominal pain, and upper abdominal distention. Less prominent findings may include weight loss and anorexia.

The distention of the stomach in patients with chronic peptic ulcer disease is a gradual process in which symptoms can be present for several months or years before diagnosis. As a result, the size of the stomach, when seen on plain films of the abdomen, can be surprisingly large. Over a period of time, the capability of the stomach to distend is remarkable (Fig. 2-3). It

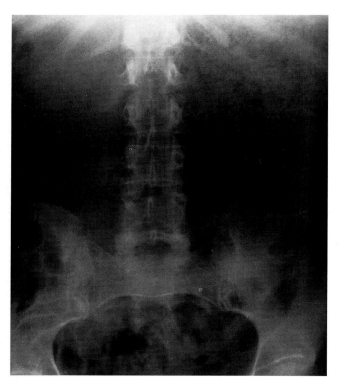

Fig. 2-4   A large, mottled mass occupying the entire upper abdomen and displacing air-filled loops of bowel laterally and inferiorly represents a grossly distended stomach filled with food debris and secretions.

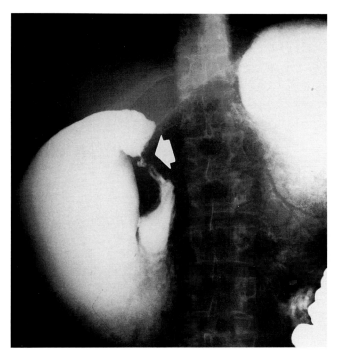

Fig. 2-5   UGI examination in a patient presenting with chronic abdominal pain and distention demonstrates a grossly distended stomach with ulceration in the pyloric channel *(arrow)* and the duodenal bulb.

may appear on plain films as a huge, confusing, mottled or soft tissue mass in the upper abdomen. At other times, the amount of distention can be less and a discernible dilated stomach can be identified. The mottled appearance of the dilated stomach is the result of the accumulation of secretions and the residue of numerous meals (Fig. 2-4). There may be diminished gas distally, although complete obstruction is unusual and air is generally seen in the small bowel and colon. In fact, they may have a normal appearance, except for depression of the transverse colon. Upright films will demonstrate an air-fluid level within the stomach. The presence of an air-fluid level within the duodenum is helpful in distinguishing between delayed outflow of gastric content secondary to gastric or duodenal obstruction.

The plain films are often diagnostic, and barium studies can be undertaken, not necessarily to confirm outlet obstruction, but rather to attempt to identify the site (duodenal or gastric) and the nature of the obstructing process (Fig. 2-5). Gastric dilatation and delayed flow into the small bowel will be the major findings. Ulcers may or may not be seen. Residual food will, generally, make the examination limited. The contrast of choice in the absence of free intraperitoneal air is barium. The large amount of residual fluid within the stomach of most of these patients, along with the pro-

pensity for frequent vomiting, makes the use of water-soluble contrast relatively contraindicated.

Other Inflammatory Causes

Gastric involvement with Crohn's disease has been identified in various studies ranging between 0.5% to 10% of patients. The most common pattern of severe gastric involvement with Crohn's disease is a narrowed, somewhat rigid stomach (Fig. 2-6). On rare occasions, involvement of the distal antrum, in particular the pyloric channel, can result in gastric obstruction.

Patients with severe pancreatitis may present with degrees of gastric outlet obstruction. This is generally secondary to contiguous involvement of the adjacent structures with the inflammatory changes. In the stomach, wall thickening, edema, and spasm can lead to luminal compromise.

Patients ingesting corrosive materials, particularly acids, can present with severe inflammatory changes in the distal antrum, especially along the lesser curvature, and luminal stricturing can occur, either acutely or chronically. The radiological features of such a lesion may be indistinguishable from malignancy.

Other unusual inflammatory causes of gastric outlet obstruction include radiation gastritis, tuberculosis,

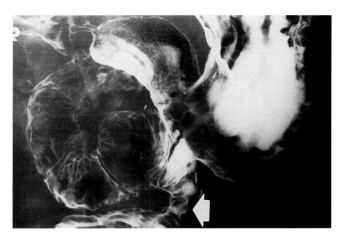

Fig. 2-6 UGI examination demonstrates a contracted stomach and a gastrojejunostomy. There is also fold thickening and narrowing of the efferent loop below the anastomosis *(arrow)*. All the observed inflammatory changes both in the stomach and adjacent small bowel are due to Crohn's disease.

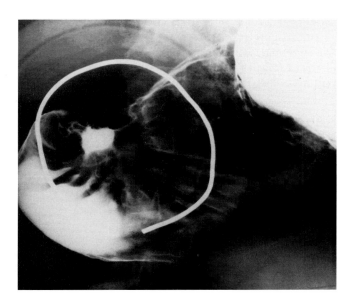

Fig. 2-7 Ulcerating mass with a central barium collection occupies the distal prepyloric region of the stomach resulting in gastric outlet obstruction. The lesion was found to be adenocarcinoma of the stomach.

and syphilis. The changing pattern of disease prevalence and the increased incidence of both of these latter diseases in the population could conceivably result in an increased incidence of gastric involvement. However, because modern treatment regimens usually limit the severity of these diseases commonly seen in previous decades, the number of cases with severe involvement of the stomach and potential gastric outlet ob-

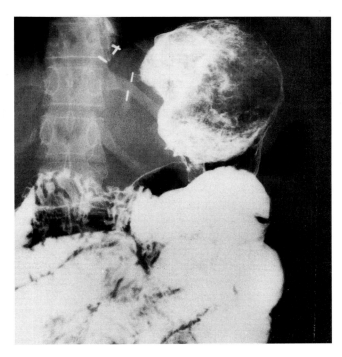

Fig. 2-8 Gastric bezoar is demonstrated in a postoperative stomach.

struction will probably not increase and will remain extremely rare.

Malignancy

Carcinoma, especially of the scirrhous variety, involving the antrum or pyloric region commonly results in gastric outlet obstruction (Fig. 2-7). In addition, carcinoma of the head of the pancreas with adjacent spread involving the gastric antrum can compromise gastric outflow. These two tumors are probably the most common causes of gastric outlet obstruction resulting from neoplastic diseases. On rare occasions, lymphoma can result in outlet obstruction. However, lymphomas, especially the non-Hodgkin's lymphomas, tend to be somewhat pliable tumors, and infrequently cause obstruction, even when the tumor trasverses the pyloric channel and involves the duodenal bulb. However, on rare occasions, a polypoid mass involving the distal stomach and pyloric channel can result in mechanical obstruction by the presence of its sheer bulk in the most anatomically narrowed region of the stomach.

Gastric Bezoars

Generally, gastric bezoars do not obstruct. Indeed, they may be asymptomatic for long periods of time (Fig. 2-8). However, on occasion, the bezoar may act as an occluding agent in a ball-valve type of obstructive process within the stomach. Postgastrectomy patients are most susceptible to bezoar formation and gastric distention. Although a small number of patients may demonstrate degrees of outlet obstruction, distention of the stomach or gastric remnant is often a result of the increasing size of the bezoar. The most common bezoar encountered is the phytobezoar, composed of fiber, plant matter, leaves, and roots. These are usually smaller and more compact than hair bezoars (trichobezoars). They are also more abrasive and the incidence of associated peptic ulcer is higher with phytobezoars. They are the most common type of bezoar encountered following gastric surgery. Occasionally, a bezoar representing an overgrowth of fungi and yeast is also encountered in postoperative patients. The susceptibility of postoperative patients to bezoar formation probably relates to the accompanying vagotomy and diminished ability of the stomach to empty.

Trichobezoars or hairballs are the second most common occurring gastric bezoar. They represent a congealed collection of hair enmeshed with mucus and decaying food material. They are always black in their appearance and have a characteristic odor. They can be asymptomatic and can attain great size with resultant gastric dilatation. They tend to be found in younger female patients. Incidences are higher in institutionalized patients and those with psychiatric disturbances.

A type of bezoar commonly encountered in the medical literature is the persimmon bezoar. This is generally unrelated to gastric surgery and is named for the native American persimmon tree. The fruit of the persimmon tree, although possessing little fiber, has considerable pulp quantity. Unripe persimmon fruit has a well-known astringent property. The interaction of the astringent and the stomach acid results in a coagulum or gelatinous pulpy mass within the stomach and can occasionally result in acute gastric outlet obstruction. Other uncommon types of bezoars that have been reported include food bezoars, actually representing forms of phytobezoars. Some cases of bezoar formation in the stomach relating to the ingestion of vegetable fiber powder and psyllium have been reported. This, no doubt, is related to postoperative stomachs, abnormal gastric emptying, or inadequate amounts of ingested fluids along with the vegetable powders.

Foreign body bezoars, although previously uncommon and almost exclusively seen in children or emotionally disturbed individuals, are being brought to the public's notice as individuals attempting to smuggle illegal drugs into the country have discovered new and lucrative uses for condoms. However, in such individuals, the problem of gastric outlet obstruction fades into insignificance in the light of the relatively high incidence of condom leakage or rupture.

Antral Diaphragms

Antral diaphragms are thin, well-defined symmetrical mucosal webs seen in the distal portion of the antrum compromising the antral lumen to varying degrees. Many feel that this is congenital because of the lack of histological evidence of scarring in some patients. However, the origins of the antral web or diaphragm still remain unclear. Not all diaphragms are congenital in nature. The history of chronic peptic inflammatory disease in many of these patients seriously suggests the possibility that some of these antral diaphragms may in reality be narrowed, well-defined bands of scarring. The circumferential healing of gastric ulcers is well-known.

Most antral diaphragms are not associated with obstruction. However, where the lumen is sufficiently compromised, degrees of gastric obstruction may be encountered. Generally, luminal narrowing of 1.5 cm or less will be symptomatic. Careful fluoroscopic evaluation of the motility through this region, as well as the use of a 12.5-mm barium tablet, is helpful in establishing the degree of luminal compromise.

Fluoroscopically, these must be demonstrated as fixed weblike areas of narrowing in the antral portion of the stomach (Fig. 2-9). The degree of circumferential involvement may be complete or incomplete.

Pyloric Stenosis

In the adult, pyloric stenosis is a confusing entity. Whether it represents a true congenital pyloric stenosis or is an unusual sequela of peptic inflammatory disease is unclear. Most of the patients with the radiological findings of adult hypertrophic pyloric stenosis have concomitant peptic inflammatory disease. Presentation with significant gastric outlet obstruction is, however, unusual. The radiological findings have been described as mass effect in the pyloric region with an elongated pyloric channel measuring two to three times its normal length. A bulging mass in the base of the duodenum or antrum is commonly seen with this process (Fig. 2-10). This should not be confused with prolapsed gastric mucosa, which is a transient finding in patients with antral gastritis. Prolapsing gastric mucosa is, rarely, if ever, associated with gastric outlet obstruction.

A small number of patients will demonstrate a small triangular outpouching of the antrum along the greater curvature, just proximal to the pyloric channel, called Twining's recess. This outpouching represents a protrusion of mucosa between the hypertrophied circular torus muscles of the distal antrum. Twining's recess has been frequently associated with adult hypertrophic pyloric stenosis.

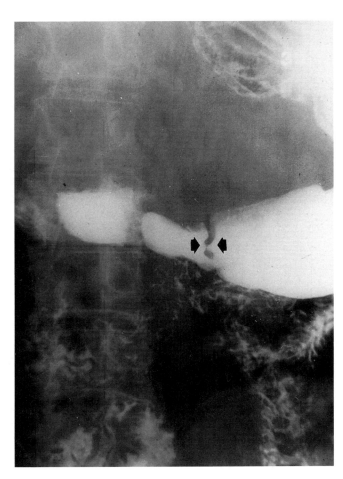

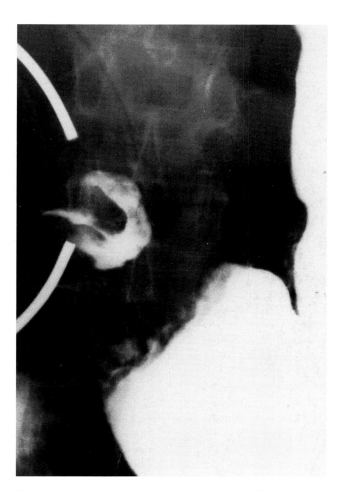

Fig. 2-9   UGI study demonstrates a thin incomplete weblike structure in the antrum of the stomach representing an antral web *(arrows)*.

Fig. 2-10   UGI examination from a patient with gastric outlet obstruction demonstrates mass effect in the pyloric region with elongated pyloric channel and possible ulceration along the course of the channel.

Gastric Volvulus

Gastric volvulus is an unusual condition in which the stomach undergoes a torsion abnormality as a result of twisting on itself. This twisting can occur around the luminal axis of the stomach (organoaxial) or around its mesentery on a plane perpendicular to its luminal axis (mesenteroaxial). These configurations almost always occur as a result of large hiatal hernias with migration of a large amount, if not all, of the stomach into an intrathoracic location (Fig. 2-11).

Surprisingly, unless the degree of torsion is significant enough to result in luminal obstruction, these patients exhibit few symptoms. When obstruction does occur, it becomes a surgical emergency as a result of compromise of the blood supply. Patients will present with severe upper abdominal pain, severe chest pain, constant vomiting, and obstructive interference in attempts to pass a nasogastric tube.

Plain films of the abdomen and chest will reveal typical findings of dilated air-filled proximal segments of the stomach either in the chest or upper abdomen. Barium studies will demonstrate the abnormal positioning of the stomach as a result of the torsion abnormality. Attempts should be made to identify the relative positions of the lesser and greater curvature.

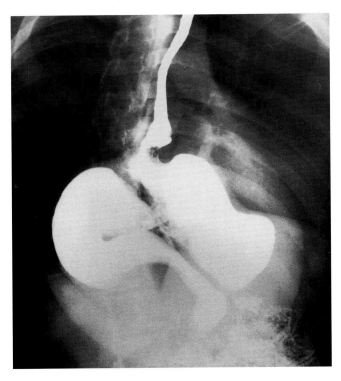

Fig. 2-11 Patient with virtually the entire stomach in an intrathoracic position. There is an organoaxial configuration, although the stomach is not obstructed at this time.

DUODENAL OBSTRUCTION RESULTING IN GASTRIC DISTENTION

Peptic ulcer disease
Pancreatitis
Pseudocysts
Other processes

Gastric distention and impaired outflow resulting from obstructive disease in the proximal duodenum is probably more common than that resulting from primary gastric disease. The most common of the duodenal processes resulting in a gastric outlet obstruction is peptic ulcer disease. Severe pancreatitis and pseudocysts with secondary involvement of the duodenum can also result in obstruction. In addition, pancreatic malignancy commonly invades the duodenum. Primary duodenal malignancy is rare but does commonly present as obstruction with gastric distention. Other processes, such as lymphoma, duodenal adenoma, annular pancreas, superior mesenteric artery syndrome, as well as intraluminal diverticulum, can also result in obstruction. These entities are covered in more detail in the duodenal section of this chapter.

GASTRIC ATONY WITHOUT OBSTRUCTION

Neuromuscular Abnormalities
Chronic Idiopathic Intestinal Pseudoobstruction
Central Nervous System and Electrolyte Abnormalities
Drug-induced Atony
Agonal
Other

Neuromuscular Abnormalities

In scleroderma (progressive systemic sclerosis), the entire bowel can be involved with the neuromuscular degenerative processes resulting in diminished gut motility and subsequent stasis. As a result, it is possible for gastric distention to be observed in some of these patients. More commonly, distention of the esophagus, colon, and duodenum is encountered.

Chronic Idiopathic Intestinal Pseudoobstruction

For similar reasons, thought to relate to diffuse neuromuscular dysfunction throughout the gut, chronic idiopathic intestinal pseudoobstruction can also result in an abnormal gut motility, stasis, and distended portions of the gut. Although the small bowel and colon would predominate in this disorder, a small number of patients may manifest gastric distention as well.

Central Nervous System and Electrolyte Abnormalities

Patients with more central neurological abnormalities, such as tabes dorsalis or bulbar poliomyelitis, may develop degrees of gastric distention.

Significant electrolyte and acid-base imbalances can commonly produce a transient distention of the colon and stomach with the impairment of contractibility of the smooth muscle of the gut, probably secondary to hypokalemia.

Drug-induced Atony

Gastric atony can also be drug-induced, often associated with atropine-like anticholinergic medications. Elderly and bedridden patients are particularly susceptible to drug-induced gastric atony. The use of glucagon may, on rare occasion, induce acute gastric atony. This has been reported in a few patients receiving glucagon for routine UGI examinations. Patients with diabetes mellitus and significant degrees of diabetic peripheral neuropathy may manifest prominent gastric atony as a result of diminished neuromuscular function.

Agonal

Acute massive gastric distention can be seen on abdominal radiographs of patients who are preterminal. The presence of this finding carries a bleak prognosis for survival beyond the next 48 hours. The exact cause of this finding is unclear. It may relate to severe and irreversible electrolyte imbalances or may be associated with major cardiovascular collapse. These patients are severely ill and almost always unconscious. Clinical findings will be limited to a distended tympanic upper abdomen. Nasogastric decompression will not alter the outcome. The radiological finding is but a reflection of the catastrophic systemic events that are occurring simultaneously.

Other

Other diagnostic considerations when faced with the radiological finding of gastric atony include aerophagia, not an unusual occurrence in patients undergoing acute severe emotional stress. Patients who have recently ingested large amounts of carbonated drinks may demonstrate gas in a distended stomach on plain films of the abdomen. The gas, however, should also be well-distributed throughout the remainder of the gut as well. Other considerations include porphyria and lead poisoning, both of which can result in degrees of gastic distention. In addition, degrees of gastric atony may be encountered in pregnant patients.

In patients with severe spinal deformity, chronic gastric distention has been described. The exact cause of this is not clear.

CONTRACTED OR NARROWED STOMACH

Scirrhous Carcinoma
Metastatic Disease
Corrosive Gastritis
Extrinsic Compression of the Stomach
Lymphoma
Crohn's Disease
Zollinger-Ellison Syndrome
Eosinophilic Gastritis
Postradiation
Sarcoidosis
Hepatic Artery Infusion Chemotherapy
Phlegmonous Gastritis
Tuberculosis
Syphilis

A contracted narrow stomach has been historically referred to as the linitis plastica (leather bottle) stomach. This generally implies that all, or a large part of the stomach is involved by the pathological process, which results in a rigid, narrowed, contracted lumen. When the entire stomach is not involved, it is the proximal portion of the stomach that is generally spared.

The problem of a contracted, narrowed stomach gives rise to the consideration of diffuse infiltrative changes in which the normal pliability and peristaltic activity of the stomach wall are impaired or absent. Any process that can excite desmoplastic or fibrotic reaction within the gastric tissues, whether it be neoplastic or inflammatory in nature, can result in such a radiological appearance.

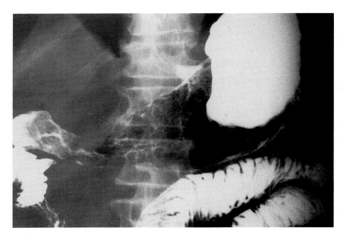

Fig. 2-12   Gastric carcinoma involving the distal half of the stomach with narrowing, irregularity, and rigidity as a result of the desmoplastic changes induced by the neoplasm.

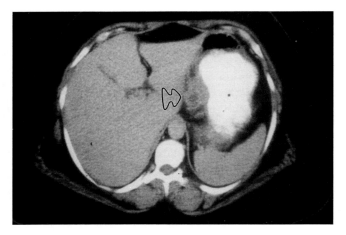

Fig. 2-13   CT image obtained at the level of the gastric cardia demonstrates mass lesion involving the posterior stomach wall, as well as a involvement of the medial wall and gastrohepatic ligament *(arrow).*

Scirrhous Carcinoma

The original description of the linitis plastica stomach was associated with an infiltrating scirrhous (desmoplastic) type of primary malignancy of the stomach. Although there are varied presentations of gastric carcinoma, the most common appears to be focal gastric wall thickening with or without ulceration. However, diffuse infiltrative wall thickening, which will result in a contracted, narrow stomach, is not uncommon and generally has been identified in patients with less-differentiated tumors and poorer prognosis (Fig. 2-12). There is also some evidence to suggest that this form may be more common in younger patients.

The mortality rate and incidence of gastric cancer has been steadily in decline in the United States since 1940. Environmental factors that have been implicated in an increased incidence of gastric carcinoma in some parts of the world include an increase in salt consumption, increased ingestion of smoked meat and fish products, as well as nitrosamines, and a questionable increase in the incidence in patients on long-term cimetidine therapy. Some possible precancerous situations include pernicious anemia, chronic atrophic gastritis, gastric adenomas, and possibly long-term postgastrectomy patients.

The infiltrative form of gastric carcinoma results in diffuse thickening and rigidity of the stomach wall. The involved stomach has a tubular appearance, and a normal fold pattern is not discernible. At fluoroscopy, no peristaltic activity can be detected in the involved area. The infiltrating process usually starts in the pyloric antral region and extends proximally. It is unusual for the

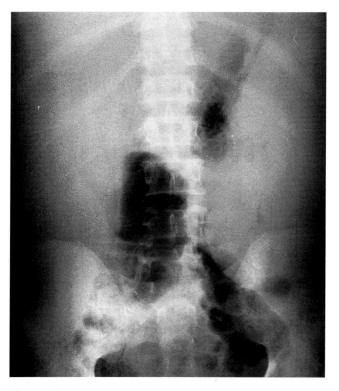

Fig. 2-14   Patient with massive hepatosplenomegaly demonstrates central compression of air-filled stomach on plain film of the abdomen.

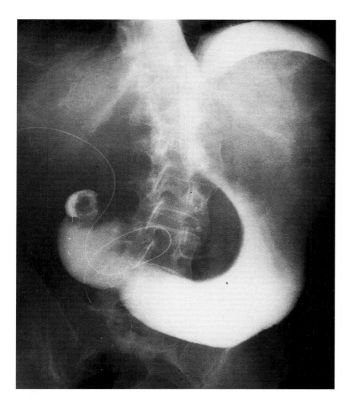

Fig. 2-15   UGI examination demonstrates large extrinsic impression on the fundus and proximal body of the stomach from huge pancreatic pseudocyst.

tumor to cross the pyloric channel into the duodenum.

Barium studies reveal the expected narrow, tubular, rigid, aperistaltic appearance of the involved portion of the stomach. Ulcerations may be present. A fold pattern is either absent or clearly abnormal. CT is particularly helpful in evaluation of gastric carcinoma and will demonstrate extension beyond the gastric wall, involvement of the adjacent perigastric, peripancreatic, and retroperitoneal lymph nodes, in addition to evaluating for liver metastatic lesions (Fig. 2-13).

Metastatic Disease

Metastatic lesions to the stomach will have a varied appearance. However, a common appearance is diffuse infiltrative scirrhous involvement of the stomach that is indistinguishable from primary scirrhous carcinoma. The two major primary sites are breast and lung. Metastatic disease from the breast involving the stomach has been described in 10% to 15% of patients. In over half of these patients, the appearance of gastric involvement is of linitis plastica.

Involvement of the stomach by carcinoma of the pancreas as a result of contiguous spread, especially when it involves the distal stomach, can also give an appearance of a narrow, rigid antrum. These changes are usually regional and not widespread throughout the stomach, such as may be found in the primary or secondary hematogenous scirrhous lesions of the stomach.

Corrosive Gastritis

Patients who ingest strong corrosive materials, such as alkaline caustic agents, tend to have more esophageal damage than stomach damage. On the other hand, the ingestion of strong acids appears to involve the stomach to a greater extent. This is particularly the case in the distal antrum and along the lesser curvature. However, the antrum and body can be involved circumferentially, giving a narrowed, rigid appearance. This can be seen both in the acute and the chronic stage with accompanying ulceration and mass effect. Following healing, permanent stricturing and rigidity of the distal stomach is a common finding, indistinguishable from infiltrating gastric carcinoma.

Extrinsic Compression of the Stomach

A retrogastric or retroperitoneal process resulting in sufficient compression or invasion of the stomach to result in a narrowed or contracted stomach is unusual.

However, a large retroperitoneal tumor, such as leiomyosarcomas or liposarcomas, could result in such an appearance. In addition, significant splenomegaly associated with hepatomegaly could sufficiently compress the stomach to give a very narrowed appearance (Fig. 2-14). A large, left upper quadrant mass, such as a subphrenic abscess, could result in a similar appearance with the gastric spasm resulting from adjacent inflammation. A large pancreatic mass, such as a pseudocyst, can compress the stomach posteriorly and give the impression of a narrowed lumen (Fig. 2-15). Other pancreatic lesions that could result in such an appearance include nonfunctioning islet cell tumors of the pancreas, which can grow to great size; acute or chronic pancreatitis; or cystadenomas of the pancreas.

Lymphoma

Although the common appearance of lymphoma is generally wall thickening, mass effect, and ulceration, the occasional lymphomatous lesion of the stomach can be diffusely infiltrative and result in severe desmoplastic reaction so that the radiological appearance is identical to scirrhous adenocarcinoma (Fig. 2-16). This is especially seen in the Hodgkin's-type lesion. CT evaluation for lymphoma has become the imaging mainstay for this lesion and is particularly useful for evaluation of wall thickening, perigastric nodal disease, liver, spleen, or renal involvement (Fig. 2-17). Recently, there is some evidence that intraluminal endoscopic ultrasound may be more sensitive in detecting both intramural and perigastric disease.

Crohn's Disease

Severe involvement of the stomach with Crohn's disease causing narrowing and rigidity of the stomach is unusual. The classical appearance of the narrow distal stomach and widened normal proximal stomach has given rise to the historical description of the "ram's horn" stomach of Crohn's disease. This stenotic involvement of severe disease in the distal stomach may or may not result in gastric outlet obstruction. The presence of Crohn's disease in the stomach is almost always associated with involvement of the small bowel or colon. Involvement of the stomach in patients with Crohn's disease should be differentiated from peptic ulcer disease, which has been shown to be increased in patients with Crohn's disease.

Zollinger-Ellison Syndrome

This syndrome results from the presence of a non-beta islet cell tumor of the pancreas that continuously secretes gastrin. The high levels of this hormone result in an increased stimulus of the gastric parietal cells to form and secrete hydrochloric acid, resulting in marked hyperacidity of the stomach and proximal small bowel. The severe inflammatory changes involving the stomach are usually manifest by multiple ulcerations, thickened folds, and hypersecretion. However, the presence of chronic inflammation throughout the stomach, particularly in the distal stomach, can result in a narrowed, contracted appearance. Additional radiological findings that may suggest the diagnosis include proximal small bowel ulcerations and history of recurrent intractable ulcer disease.

Up to 50% of the islet cell lesions are malignant with metastatic disease present within the liver. In addition, the primary neoplasms are generally small with 90% of them being less than 2 cm, and many of these not detectable on routine CT scanning. In approximately 60% of cases, the lesions are multiple. The lesions may be detected on angiographic studies of the pancreaticoduodenal region as a result of their hypervascularity. For the same reason, they may be detected during bolus injection of this area on CT scanning using thin (2 to 4 mm) contiguous sections through the pancreas. The operation of choice has been to remove the entire target organ that is represented by the parietal cell-containing portions of the stomach.

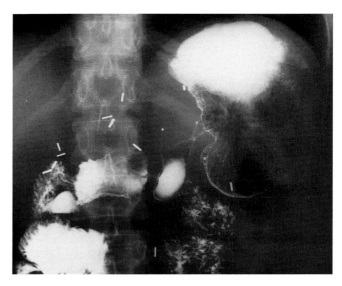

Fig. 2-16 UGI of patient with Hodgkin's disease of the stomach. Note the marked narrowing and irregularity of the distal stomach.

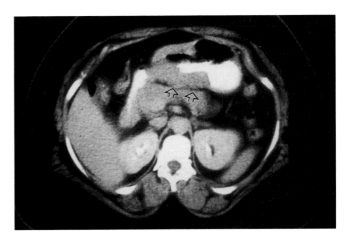

Fig. 2-17 CT image through the distal stomach demonstrates marked focal wall thickening *(arrow)* as a result of lymphomatous infiltration of the stomach.

Eosinophilic Gastritis

Eosinophilic infiltration of the muscular layers of the distal stomach can result in a narrowed, contracted antrum and body (Fig. 2-18). The appearance can be similar to that of malignancy. Patients usually have an associated peripheral eosinophilia and a history of food allergies. The infiltration can result in erosions, ulceration, and subsequent anemia. Affected patients may also demonstrate elevated immunoglobulin E (IgE) levels. Involvement of the proximal small bowel may be

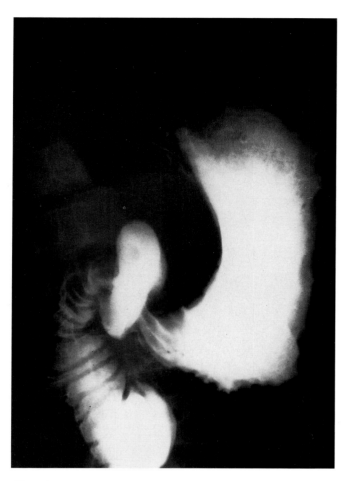

Fig. 2-18   UGI of patient with eosinophilic gastroenteritis demonstrates a contracted and rigid stomach with some irregularity along the greater curvature. The findings could easily be interpreted as malignant infiltration.

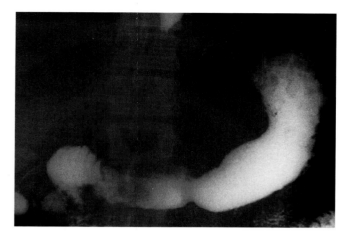

Fig. 2-19   UGI of patient with diffuse involvement of the stomach with sarcoidosis, resulting in a tubular, narrowed stomach.

present, although isolated gastric involvement is not unusual. The disorder usually responds well to daily doses of steroids.

Postradiation

A narrowed, contracted stomach may also be the sequela of radiation injury to the stomach. Radiation doses involving the stomach usually greater than 4000 rad results in an acute inflammatory response with resultant healing that may include extensive fibrosis.

Sarcoidosis

Although involvement of the GI tract in sarcoidosis is unusual, the stomach is the most commonly affected site. Often the patients are asymptomatic. In chronic severe involvement, the possibility of contracture and narrowing of the stomach increases (Fig. 2-19).

Hepatic Artery Infusion Chemotherapy

The increasing use of hepatic artery infusion of chemotherapeutic and cytotoxic agents has resulted in increased incidence of resultant inflammatory changes within the stomach. Despite attempts to control the flow of the chemotherapeutic agents and to reduce deleterious flow to the stomach, the vascular arterial anatomy in the region of the celiac axis can be quite variable, and on occasion some of the agent is delivered to the gastric wall with resultant marked inflammatory changes. The inflammatory changes tend to regress with the termination of the therapy.

Phlegmonous Gastritis

This entity, although common in the early part of the century, is very unusual today. It is a bacterial infection and invasion of the stomach that results in marked thickening of the stomach wall and mucosa. Most reported cases are associated with alpha-hemolytic streptococci, although other organisms including staphylococci and pneumococci, as well as some of the more common gram-negative organisms, have also been demonstrated. Often, when there is associated emphysematous gastritis, clostridial organisms or gram-negative bacteria have been implicated. The exact underlying cause of this condition is unclear, although many have been suggested, including ischemia, ulceration, gastric malignancy, or ingestion of corrosive material. The treatment consists of vigorous antibiotic therapy and prompt surgical intervention.

Tuberculosis

Involvement of the stomach with tuberculosis is rare but can occur, particularly in the pyloric antral region. Wall thickening, rigidity, and a contracted lumen may be demonstrated.

Syphilis

Involvement of the stomach with syphilis is rare, although this manifestation is seen from time to time. Involvement may be identical to that of peptic ulcer disease with erosive changes, ulceration, and thickened folds. Additionally, a contracted, narrowed, deformed stomach has been described in chronic involvement.

THICKENED GASTRIC FOLDS

Focal Thickening
  Peptic gastritis
  Aspirin/NSAID-induced gastritis
  Corrosive gastritis
  Hypertrophic gastritis
  Helicobacter gastritis
  Carcinoma
  Lymphoma
  Pseudolymphoma
  Metastatic disease
  Crohn's disease
  Pancreatitis
  Ménétrier's disease
  Gastric varices
  Eosinophilic gastritis
  Partial gastrectomy
Diffuse Thickening
  Gastritis
  Pancreatitis
  Eosinophilic gastritis
  Ménétrier's disease
  Amyloidosis

In the normal, adequately distended stomach, the folds in the fundal region usually measure approximately 1 cm or less in thickness. As they descend toward the body and antrum of the stomach, the folds become increasingly narrow and ribbonlike until the prepyloric antral folds are found to be 5 mm or less in diameter. The folds should be symmetrical in appearance without nodularity, focal thickening, or areas of discontinuity. The fold pattern in the region of the gastric cardia and along the greater curvature of the body can be complex and at times difficult to evaluate.

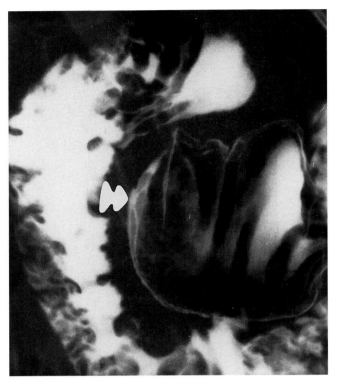

Fig. 2-20   Spot film from gastric antrum demonstrates transverse thickened gastric folds representing peptic gastritis. A tiny shallow ulcer is seen along the greater curvature *(arrow)*.

Focal Thickening

Peptic gastritis   Peptic gastritis can present as widespread diffuse thickening of the gastric folds, although the much more common presentation is fold thickening in the antrum and possibly the distal body (Fig. 2-20). The folds can be nodular. There may or may not be ulceration or evidence of erosions. However, folds that are beaded in appearance generally will have small erosions along their course (Fig. 2-21). The beading process is secondary to the focal edematous changes around the erosions. These erosions may commonly be seen on double-contrast study. Meticulous attention to detail and use of flow technique will often demonstrate them.

When the involvement is throughout the stomach, some consideration should be given to Zollinger-Ellison syndrome, particularly if there is duodenal and proximal small bowel involvement (Fig. 2-22).

Aspirin and nonsteroidal antiinflammatory drug-induced gastritis   The increasing use of aspirin and

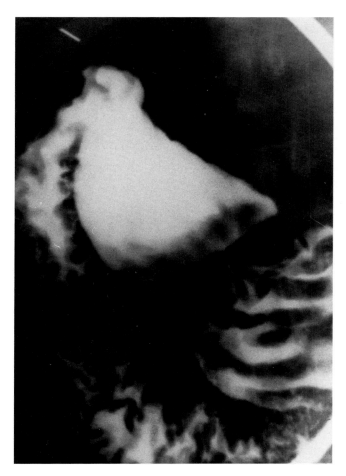

Fig. 2-21   Spot film from the gastric antrum and duodenum demonstrates thickened, beaded appearance of the folds in the gastric antrum, almost always associated with tiny erosions along the folds.

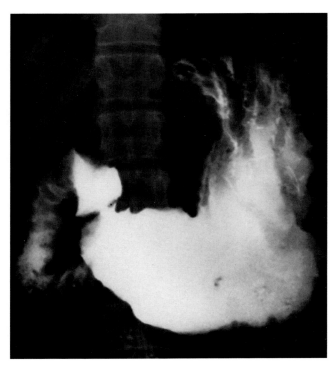

Fig. 2-22   Patient with Zollinger-Ellison syndrome shows abnormalities of the stomach on UGI study with diffuse fold thickening, hypersecretion, and multiple small ulcers.

the availability of over-the-counter nonsteroidal antiinflammatory drugs (NSAID) will increase the frequency of aspirin and NSAID-induced gastritis (Fig. 2-23). These changes tend to be localized in the antral and body region, although diffuse involvement is possible. Although most of the damage caused by these drugs relates to local mucosal irritation and erosions, the process appears to be more complicated. Alterations, as a result of aspirin-induced changes in the gastric mucosal barrier, have been described along with loss of blood across the barrier unrelated to ulcer or erosion formation. There also appear to be higher incidences of peptic ulcer disease. Patients with chronic rheumatic disease taking significant doses of aspirin have a 50% in-

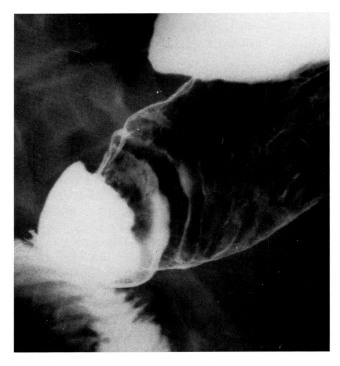

Fig. 2-23   Patient on high doses of NSAID, complaining of abdominal pain. UGI demonstrates transverse thickened folds in the antrum of the stomach.

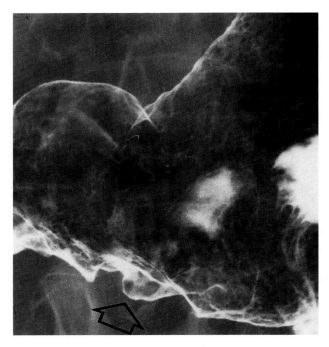

Fig. 2-24 UGI of patient with abdominal pain and bleeding being treated with high doses of aspirin for arthritic disease. An area of mass, with irregularity and ulceration, is seen along the greater curvature of the stomach *(arrow)*. The ulcer does not project beyond the confines and is extremely suspicious. Biopsy was entirely benign. Patient improved rapidly with withdrawal of the medication.

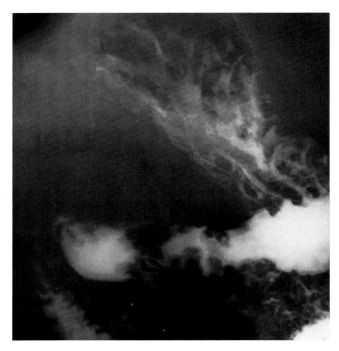

Fig. 2-25 UGI of patient with history of chronic abdominal pain demonstrating diffuse fold thickening throughout the stomach. Biopsy showed epithelial hyperplastic changes of hypertrophic gastritis.

creased incidence of gastric erosions and a 20% increase in gastric ulcers (Fig. 2-24). The use of enteric-coated forms of aspirin is helpful in dealing with the local and erosive effects. However, it probably has little impact on the systemic effect of the drug on the stomach wall.

Corrosive gastritis Ingestion of acid-corrosive materials can give rise to focal inflammatory changes within the distal stomach. The appearance can be varied, but focal fold thickening would be one manifestation. This is often associated with ulceration.

Hypertrophic gastritis Hypertrophic gastritis is thought to represent a widening of the folds secondary to mucosal hyperplastic changes of the epithelial cells (Fig. 2-25). The etiology and prevalence of this entity is controversial, and the changes are thought to relate to chronic inflammation. It may be focal or diffuse and tends to be chronic in nature. In a patient with thickened gastric folds, possibly associated with hyperacidity and without a significant history of alcohol ingestion, hypertrophic gastritis would be a differential consideration. Other types of gastritis can present with fo-

cal thickening of the fold pattern and include such things as herpetic gastritis and gastric candidiasis.

***Helicobactor* gastritis** Within the last decade there has been increasing interest in the possibility of association between the presence of a chronic gastric inflammation, ulceration, and *Helicobacter pylori.* By the use of special silver staining, the presence of this bacteria has been detected in large numbers of patients with gastric and duodenal inflammatory disease. Various studies have been undertaken in which asymptomatic volunteers have undergone endoscopy and gastric mucosal biopsy and have also demonstrated a relatively high incidence of nonsymptomatic gastritis representing approximately half of the volunteers. The presence of *Helicobacter* is often found in conjunction with gastritis.

The question, however, is still unanswered as to whether the gastritis is a result of the presence of the bacteria or if the bacterial presence is secondary to the underlying inflammatory process.

The treatment of *Helicobacter* gastritis has consisted of bismuth compounds and antimicrobial agents. H_2-blockers, as well as antacids, appear to have little effect on the presence of these organisms. Unfortunately,

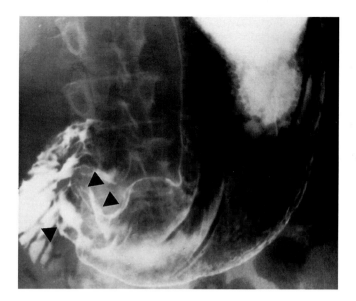

Fig. 2-26 UGI of patient with abdominal pain and weight loss demonstrates some slight narrowing of the distal stomach with thickened nodular folds through the area *(arrowheads)*. Biopsy confirmed the diagnosis of gastric carcinoma.

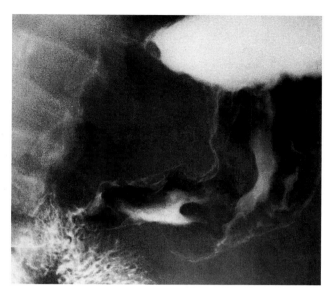

Fig. 2-27 Patient with diffuse lymphomatous involvement of the stomach demonstrates marked thickening and nodularity and distortion of the folds throughout the distal two thirds of the stomach.

symptomatic patients with gastritis and known presence of the bacteria in the stomach do not necessarily respond to the prescribed treatment. However, there is much interest in the *Helicobacter*-associated gastritis. There is also considerable interest in the possibility of some association between the bacteria and the presence of duodenal or gastric ulcers. However, considerable questions remain to be answered with respect to this relationship and the therapeutic approach suggested by the presence of the bacteria.

Carcinoma Irregular focal thickening is an unusual presentation of carcinoma of the stomach. The most common presentation tends to be a mass with ulceration. However, thickened irregular folds, usually limited to one portion of the stomach and indistinguishable from gastric lymphoma, are not a rare finding in gastric carcinoma (Fig. 2-26).

Lymphoma The most common presentation of lymphoma is a thickened, distorted, nodular gastric fold pattern (Fig. 2-27). This may or may not be associated with a mass effect or ulceration. There may be a degree of residual distensibility and pliability that may help distinguish lymphoma from carcinoma. However, the definitive diagnosis will require biopsy. Extension across the pyloric channel into the duodenal bulb tends to be more common with lymphoma, although one should bear in mind that lymphoma represents 5%

or less of gastric malignancies. Associated findings that may be seen with lymphoma include extrinsic masses associated with aggregates of lymphomatous nodes or an enlarged spleen.

Pseudolymphoma Lymphoreticular hyperplasia of the stomach (pseudolymphoma or lymphoreticular gastritis) can present with findings of focal fold thickening. These benign lesions almost always have the radiological appearance of malignancy with most common findings being mass and ulceration. However, cases of infiltrative lesions with associated focal fold thickening have been reported. Anemia is a common finding, and the average age is slightly younger than that seen in gastric carcinoma.

Metastatic disease Metastatic disease presenting with focal fold thickening is unusual but does occur (Fig. 2-28). This may be seen in the early metastatic involvement of the stomach with breast or lung lesions. Leukemic involvement of the stomach may result in a focal or diffuse thickening of gastric folds. Direct contiguous spread of carcinoma of the pancreas to the stomach can also produce a radiological pattern of focal gastric fold thickening along the greater curvature.

Crohn's disease Crohn's involvement of the stomach may manifest in fold thickening in the antral region. Superficial erosions may also be detected.

Pancreatitis A relatively common cause of fold thickening within the distal stomach relates to inflammatory disease in the adjacent pancreas. Folds along the greater curvature of the body and in the antrum may be enlarged and nodular, as a result of contiguous inflammatory changes. More severe disease may result in more widespread gastric changes.

Ménétrier's disease Ménétrier's disease is a relatively rare condition of unknown etiology. It is characterized by prominence and tortuosity of the gastric mucosal fold pattern. At one time, this was thought to be an antral sparing process, although recently degrees of antral involvement have been demonstrated. The preponderance of changes, however, appears to be in the proximal stomach. The process is associated with increased protein loss from the stomach and diminished gastric acid production. The disease is generally detected between 30 to 60 years of age and tends to be more common in men. Presenting complaints include epigastric pain, anorexia, and weight loss. The radiological pattern will demonstrate a large tortuous fold pattern predominantly proximally and, in most cases, with sparing of the antrum. There will also be some evidence of hypersecretion within the stomach.

Gastric varices Gastric varices can readily cause apparent thickening of the gastric folds, particularly in the proximal fundal region of the stomach (Fig. 2-29). These are commonly seen in association with signifi-cant portal hypertension and in patients with splenic vein thrombosis. The radiological findings usually are those of a smooth, thickened, proximal fold pattern most prominent in the fundus, but they can be seen more distally. Esophageal varices can be demonstrated by increasing the venous distention of the varices through various techniques associated with patient positioning and respiration. These tend to be less useful in gastric varices, and this is particularly the case in those patients with splenic vein thrombosis.

Eosinophilic gastritis The stomach is commonly involved in this relatively rare disorder. The predilection appears to be for the gastric antrum, although the entire stomach may be involved. The disease results in eosinophilic infiltrates of the mucosal and muscular layers of the stomach. Radiological manifestations are generally those of thickened rugal fold pattern predominantly distally. Clinical features are nonspecific, and the patients may present with early satiety, nausea, or vomiting. Involvement of the small bowel is helpful in making the diagnosis, and thickened folds will be demonstrated in the proximal small bowel wall. However, isolated gastric involvement is relatively common. In patients with thickened gastric folds, small bowel involvement, peripheral eosinophilia, abdominal pain, history of food allergies, and no evidence of parasitic GI infestation, the diagnosis of eosinophilic gastritis should be considered.

Partial gastrectomy In patients with long-term gastric resection, particularly Billroth II procedure, the presence of thickened folds within the gastric remnant is common. The exact etiology of this is unclear. It is felt by some to represent the sequela of chronic bile reflux. The long-term significance is also not absolutely

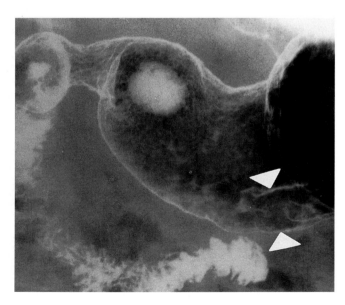

Fig. 2-28 UGI examination on patient with history of breast cancer. There are chronic changes seen in the distal stomach. However, there is an area of focal fold thickening and nodularity *(arrowheads)* that proved to be a focal metastatic lesion.

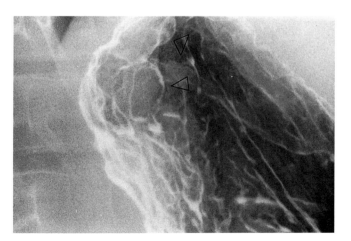

Fig. 2-29 Patient with gastric varices demonstrates area of focal fold thickening and nodularity. Note the smooth mucosal surface over the affected area *(arrowheads)*.

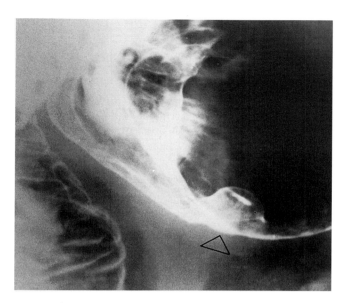

Fig. 2-34 A patient with a solitary eosinophilic granuloma of the stomach *(arrowhead)* located along the greater curvature of the antrum. The lesion is smooth and mucosal in appearance. A small, linear ulceration is seen on the surface.

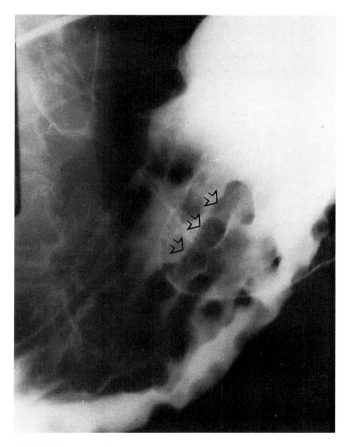

Fig. 2-35 UGI demonstrates numerous, rounded filling defects throughout the body and antrum of the stomach *(arrows)* that on endoscopic evaluation proved to be multiple hyperplastic polyps.

ently are unrelated to eosinophilic gastroenteritis. There is no history of food allergies nor is there peripheral eosinophilia. The lesion is usually solitary and less than 2 cm in size. It has no distinctive appearance radiologically and is seen as a smooth, sessile polypoid filling defect in the distal stomach (Fig. 2-34). Patients are usually asymptomatic, and these lesions are rarely associated with any significant symptoms. The possibility of erosions on the surface of the lesion and subsequent bleeding does exist.

Carcinoids

These lesions usually do not involve the stomach and are seen in this organ in less than 3% of cases. They may be seen as small mucosal polypoid lesions in the antrum, often solitary. A more common appearance is that of a larger fungating lesion involving the antral portion of the stomach, which may radiologically be indistinguishable from an ulcerating carcinoma. Approximately 25% of gastric carcinoids will have associated metastatic disease.

MULTIPLE SMALL MASSES

Hyperplastic Polyps
Adenomas
   Familial polyposis coli
   Gardner's syndrome
Hamartomas
   Peutz-Jeghers syndrome
   Cronkhite-Canada syndrome
   Cowden's disease
Hemangiomas
Peptic Erosions
Candidiasis

Hyperplastic Polyps

The hyperplastic polyp is the most common cause of small polypoid filling defects within the stomach. They are also referred to as regenerative and sometimes inflammatory polyps and are felt to represent the sequelae of chronic inflammation. They are small and sessile, commonly multiple in nature, although they can be solitary. They tend to be seen predominantly in the antral region (Fig. 2-35).

The hyperplastic polyp is not a neoplastic lesion. Malignant degeneration is virtually unheard of. Despite this, there is a well-documented increase in the incidence of coexisting hyperplastic polyps found in stomachs harboring gastric carcinoma.

Adenomas

The finding of multiple gastric adenomas not related to one of the polyposis syndromes is rare. Gastric polyps are reported in most of polyposis syndromes. More commonly they are seen in familial polyposis coli and Gardner's syndrome. Although these adenomatous polyps have a high malignant potential within the colon, malignant degeneration of adenomatous gastric polyps in patients with either Gardner's or familial polyposis syndrome is exceedingly rare.

Hamartomas

Hamartomatous gastric polyps develop in the stomach almost exclusively in patients with Peutz-Jeghers or Cronkhite-Canada syndromes. They are multiple, generally small and are seen in conjunction with the more common presentation of small bowel polyps and mucocutaneous pigmentation changes. There is relatively little malignant potential related to hamartoma formation. Although a slight increase in small bowel cancer has been reported in patients with Peutz-Jeghers syndrome there is no known increase in gastric cancer.

Multiple hamartoma syndrome (Cowden's disease) is a rare condition manifested by hamartomatous polyps within the stomach and elsewhere within the GI tract, along with associated thyroid and breast lesions. The GI polyps are almost always hamartomatous, although simple hyperplastic polyps have been reported.

Hemangiomas

Rarely, multiple hemangiomas are seen within the stomach, occasionally associated with typical calcification. The blue rubber bleb nevus syndrome (Bean syndrome) is rare. This is inherited as a sporadic, autosomal dominant trait in some families. It is manifested by mucosal hemangiomas, mostly reported in the stomach and associated with GI bleeding. These are always seen as multiple, small filling defects.

Peptic Erosions

Multiple, small filling defects may be identified in patients with multiple gastric erosions. This finding relates to the edematous raised mucosa around the site of the punctate ulceration (Fig. 2-36). On single-contrast examination, this may appear as multiple, small filling defects predominantly in the distal stomach. Good quality double-contrast examination will almost always demonstrate the punctate ulceration present in the center of the filling defect. Quite often these erosions line up on the folds of the body and antrum of the stomach.

Candidiasis

With the increasing pool of immunocompromised patients in the health care system today, there is an increasing incidence of gastric candidiasis. This may present, as in the esophagus, with multiple, rounded filling defects throughout the stomach, which if untreated, can go on to the ulcerative hemorrhagic stage commonly seen in the esophagus.

LARGE SOLITARY MASSES

Adenomas
Leiomyomas
Metastatic Lesions
Duplication Cysts
Polypoid Carcinomas
Jejunal Gastric Intussusception
Gastric Bezoars

Adenomas

Solitary gastric adenomas greater than 2 cm are extremely uncommon but occur and carry a high risk of malignancy. Larger adenomatous polyps within the stomach have more likelihood of being pedunculated (i.e., on a stalk).

Leiomyomas

Although multiple leiomyomas of the stomach have been reported, the solitary lesion is more common. These lesions can be quite large and the patients often asymptomatic (Fig. 2-37). Occasionally, leiomyomas can continue to grow within the gastric wall and reach sizable proportions. The leiomyoma greater than 5 cm in diameter is quite likely to be a leiomyosarcoma. These tumors often outgrow their blood supply and undergo central necrosis, often leading to large barium-filled cavities within the tumor mass. The ulcerations are usually centrally located in the tumor mass. Although leiomyomas appear to have a predilection for the proximal stomach, leiomyosarcomas have been described throughout the stomach. Leiomyosarcomas carry a relatively good prognosis, and distal metastasis is rare. Direct extension to the adjacent spleen, liver, and pancreas does occur. Lymph node spread is unusual. Symptoms are produced usually when the lesions are quite large, and patients most commonly present with bleeding. Occasionally, obstruction or even perforation may be presenting features.

Because of the tendency for these lesions to grow in an exophytic manner, CT is helpful in identifying the

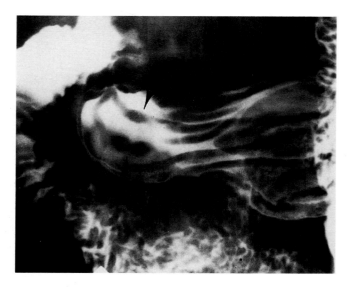

Fig. 2-36 Focal swelling and beaded appearance *(arrow-heads)* are demonstrated in the distal stomach of this patient as a result of tiny superficial erosions and the associated edema surrounding each erosion.

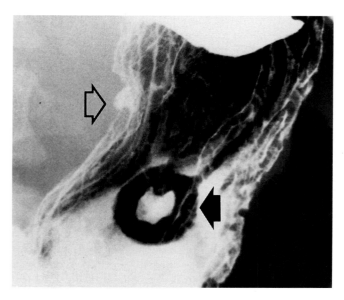

Fig. 2-38 UGI of patient with known lung cancer in which at least two bull's eye metastatic lesions to the stomach are demonstrated. The classical appearance of a mass with an ulcerated, barium-filled center is seen en face *(closed arrow)*, while the same type of lesion is seen profiled *(open arrow)*.

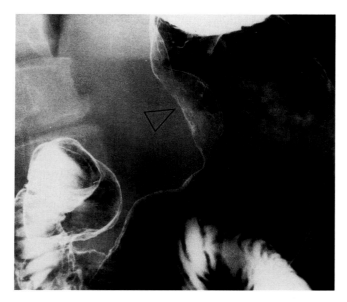

Fig. 2-37 Large, smooth submucosal mass *(arrowhead)* is seen arising from the lesser curvature of the body of the stomach. This represents a large gastric leiomyoma.

limits of the tumor mass. Barium studies may demonstrate wall abnormalities and possibily evidence of extrinsic mass relating to the exophytic component of the lesion.

Metastatic Lesions

Again, the usual presentation of metastatic lesions is multiple polypoid or infiltrative lesions within the stomach. Occasionally, a larger, isolated metastatic lesion will be encountered. This is most likely to occur in metastatic melanoma (Fig. 2-38).

Duplication Cysts

Gastric duplications are rare and may present in various sizes and configurations. A solitary filling defect within the stomach, usually along the greater curvature, is one presentation. Alternatively, the cyst may communicate with the lumen and present as a large diverticulum-like barium collection along the margin of the stomach.

Polypoid Carcinomas

Approximately a quarter of gastric carcinomas present as polypoid mass lesions growing into the gastric lumen. These polypoid lesions may or may not be ulcerated on their surface (Fig. 2-39). In addition, there may be an adjacent spread along the wall. It is thought that about a third of all malignant gastric carcinomas will manifest all of the characteristics of polypoid, ulcerative, and infiltrating types.

Discrete isolated polypoid lesions tend to carry the best prognosis. The most common sites tend to be in the distal portion of the stomach, although in patients with gastric atrophy, proximal regions are more involved.

Jejunal Gastric Intussusception

This complication is occasionally encountered after the Billroth II partial gastrectomy. Intussusceptive changes occur within the adjacent jejunum, and retrograde progression of the intussusception results in a large filling defect within the gastric remnant. This has a typical radiographic appearance on barium studies of a large intragastric mass with evidence of a fold pattern within it that may or may not have the typical "coil spring" appearance. There is usually a significant degree of obstruction to the distal flow of barium.

Gastric Bezoars

Small, asymptomatic bezoars can be seen as a filling defect within the stomach. These are usually less than 2 cm and mobile.

MULTIPLE LARGE MASSES

Metastatic Disease
Leiomyoma
Neurogenic Tumors
Kaposi's Sarcoma
Lymphoma

Metastatic Disease

As already suggested, metastatic disease to the stomach can be eclectic in appearance. Multiple, large nodular lesions can be seen in metastatic melanoma. On occasion, metastatic lesions arising from breast and lung lesions may present in such a fashion. Quite often these types of metastatic lesions are sharply circumscribed and have the typical "bull's-eye" or "target lesion" appearance when associated with central ulceration. The lesions, particularly melanoma, may remain silent for some time and increase in size. Bleeding will usually be the first manifestation of gastric involvement.

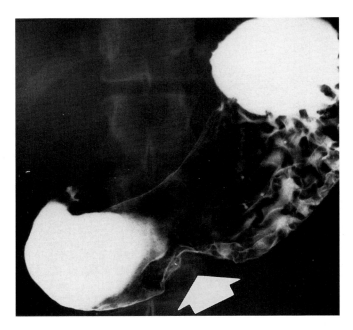

Fig. 2-39   A polypoid carcinoma is seen arising from the greater curvature of the stomach at the junction of the antrum and body *(arrow)*.

Leiomyoma

Leiomyoma can, on rare occasion, occur in the stomach as multiple, large submucosal masses. These lesions can grow to large sizes, and the patient can be entirely asymptomatic. The usual presentation is bleeding associated with ulceration on the surface of one of the leiomyomas.

Neurogenic Tumors

Neurofibromas occur as isolated tumors of the stomach. However, they can be multiple, and in a patient with generalized neurofibromatosis, there may be involvement of the stomach with multiple neurofibromata. Apart from the possibility of ulceration and bleeding, these are generally asymptomatic.

Kaposi's Sarcoma

Kaposi's sarcoma is a vascular endothelial tumor that was described approximately 100 years ago. There has been significant resurgence in the incidence with the advent of the acquired immune deficiency syndrome (AIDS) epidemic. Involvement of the GI tract is common and probably the most frequent site of involve-

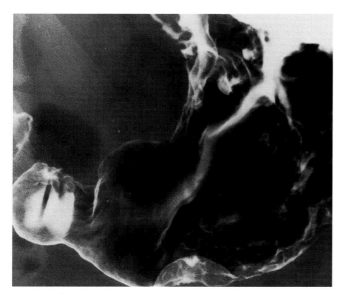

Fig. 2-40   Patient with Kaposi's sarcoma of the stomach demonstrates numerous rounded, ulcerated masses of the stomach.

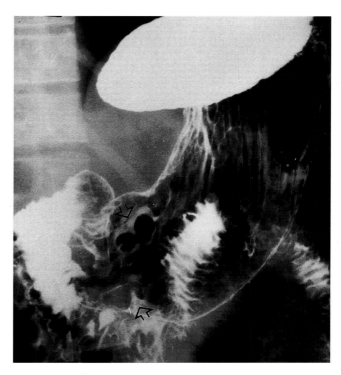

Fig. 2-41   Lymphoma of the stomach presenting as multiple polypoid lesions in the antrum *(arrows).*

ment after the skin. It is estimated that some 40% to 50% of patients with Kaposi's sarcoma lesions of the skin have GI involvement. Nearly any level of the GI tract may be involved, from the pharynx to the rectum, although most are in the upper tract. The GI lesions are almost always seen in homosexual males. Gastric involvement can either be diffuse or in the form of large discrete nodules (Fig. 2-40). The nodules may or may not have central ulceration. CT is helpful in defining the extent of wall involvement and the presence or absence of perigastric disease. The lesions themselves are generally asymptomatic, although they can bleed.

Lymphoma

Primary lymphoma of the stomach is much less common than adenocarcinoma and accounts for about 5% of malignant lesions of the stomach. As with gastric adenocarcinoma, the patients may present with non-specific complaints of abdominal pain, nausea, vomiting, and weight loss. The radiological manifestations of lymphoma can be quite variable. Ulcerating, infiltrating types of lesions are common, as well as multiple polypoid filling defects within the stomach (Fig. 2-41). Unfortunately, lymphoma can imitate numerous conditions, and radiological differentiation can be difficult. When faced with multiple large nodules in the stomach, factors that favor the possibility of lymphoma include relative preservation of the pliability of the stomach, associated fold thickening, and extension of the lesion into the duodenum.

INFILTRATING MASSES
Adenocarcinoma
Lymphoma
Pseudolymphoma
Metastatic Lesions
Leukemic Infiltration

Adenocarcinoma

The incidence of gastric cancer has dropped strikingly during the past 4 decades, and it continues to decrease. However, in the Orient and in particular Japan, gastric cancer is one of the more common carcinomas and causes of mortality. There may be some slight decline in the rate in Japan, possibly associated with intensive screening programs.

Historically, adenocarcinoma, which manifests as a diffuse infiltrative process within the stomach, is described as a scirrhous type of lesion and is the most common cause of the linitis plastica configuration of the stomach seen on UGI studies. The diffuse infiltrative process results in desmoplastic changes in the wall of the stomach, rendering the stomach somewhat tubular, narrow, and rigid (see Fig. 2-12).

Lymphoma

Primary gastric lymphoma may have a multiplicity of presentations in the stomach. A marked increase in the fold pattern and infiltrative changes are the most common presentation (Fig. 2-42). This can be accompanied by ulceration. The stomach may be involved in part or in whole. Evaluation of radiographs may present difficulty in distinguishing between lymphoma and carcinoma. Fluoroscopic examination can be helpful in many cases of lymphoma because of the relative pliability of the stomach despite the apparent extent of disease. In many cases, degrees of peristalsis will also be retained. These findings relate to the overall lack of fibrosis and desmoplastic reaction associated with lymphoma but commonly seen with adenocarcinoma. The exception might be a Hodgkin's-type lymphoma.

Pseudolymphoma

Although pseudolymphoma or lymphoreticular hyperplasia of the stomach is a benign condition, it is virtually impossible to distinguish this benign process from malignant disease of the stomach, such as lymphoma or carcinoma. The spectrum of radiological problems presented by this disease includes gastric masses with associated ulceration and infiltrative disease of the stomach commonly with associated ulceration. The etiological origins of this process, also occasionally referred to as lymphofollicular gastritis, are not clear. It is felt by some to represent an unusual late stage of peptic ulceration of the stomach, while others have suggested that it is the least aggressive of the spectrum of lymphoma types. Focal lymphoreticular hyperplastic changes have been reported elsewhere in the bowel, often associated with ulcers. Microscopic examination of this lesion presents some difficulty to the pathologist in attempting to differentiate it from lymphoma. This is particularly the case on a frozen section.

Metastatic Lesions

As previously discussed, metastatic lesions, particularly breast and lung, can present as both focal or diffuse infiltrative changes in the stomach. A local contiguous spread, such as from adjacent pancreatic malignancy, may on rare occasions give a similar appearance.

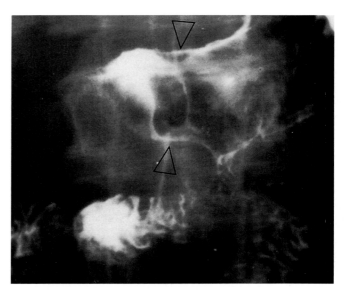

Fig. 2-42 Patient with lymphomatous infiltration of the distal stomach giving a narrow, tubular appearance without obstruction *(arrowheads)*.

Leukemic Infiltration

All types of leukemia may involve the GI tract. Indeed, autopsy studies suggest that virtually all patients have some degree of GI involvement. In the stomach, this generally is an infiltrative, diffuse process resulting in thickened irregular folds and is virtually indistinguishable from adenocarcinoma. There may be associated ulcerations and bleeding.

GASTRIC EROSIONS AND ULCERS

A gastric erosion is a superficial mucosal defect, which unlike a gastric ulcer does not penetrate into the submucosa. These are virtually impossible to see on single-contrast examinations and can be detected relatively frequently utilizing high-quality double-contrast technique. An integral part of the double-contrast technique consists of washing barium over the portions of the stomach most likely to harbor erosions and obtaining a barium pool sufficiently thin to demonstrate the erosions.

These erosions may be seen in any portion of the stomach but are most common within the antrum (Fig. 2-43). The distribution can be asymmetrical. There is a tendency for erosions to line up on folds. A small lucent halo around an erosion is commonly demonstrated and has been referred to as complete erosion. This halo represents a circular area of edema around

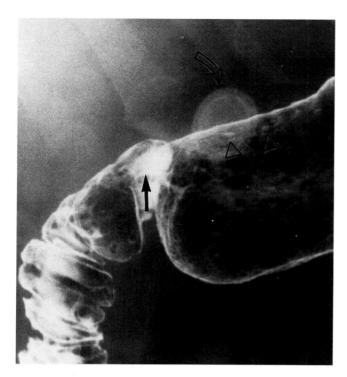

Fig. 2-43 Patient with chronic peptic disease and numerous tiny erosions *(arrowheads)*, as well as a 1.5 cm pyloric channel ulcer *(arrow)* and a laminated gallstone *(curved arrow)*.

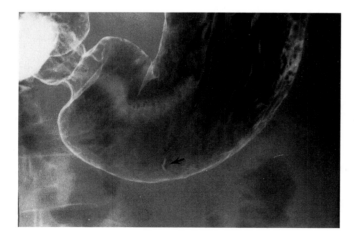

Fig. 2-44 Air-contrast UGI examination demonstrates short, superficial linear ulcer along the greater curvature of the stomach *(arrow)*.

the erosive defect. Erosions lacking this edematous halo have been referred to as incomplete erosions and are often difficult to demonstrate even on high-quality double-contrast studies. Often, these are short, linear erosions (Fig. 2-44).

There is considerable controversy regarding gastric erosions and their etiology and clinical course. High-quality double-contrast evaluations of the stomach show that these lesions are much more common than previously thought.

The gastric mucosa, under normal circumstances, is protected from the acidic environment of the stomach by a surface layer of mucus in which secreted bicarbonate results in a pH gradient near neutral at the cellular level. In addition, prostaglandins within the gastric mucosa appear to play an important part in maintaining and supporting the epithelium in the presence of potentially harmful acid.

Gastric mucosal erosive changes may be acute or chronic. Erosive changes appear to be most common in patients with peptic disease and hyperacidity. It may be a manifestation of peptic ulcer disease in many patients. There is also a higher incidence of gastric erosions associated with excessive ingestion of alcohol or salicylates. Other medications including indomethacin, reserpine, corticosteroids, ibuprofen, and potassium chloride have also been implicated.

Gastric erosive changes can be a common cause of UGI bleeding, and hemorrhagic erosive gastritis is thought to be responsible for between 10% and 20% of upper tract bleeding.

Other causes that may result in gastric mucosal erosions include Crohn's disease and viral gastritis, such as cytomegalovirus or herpesvirus. Such lesions have also been described in Behçet's syndrome. There is also reason to suspect that a significant proportion of erosive gastritis, particularly of the chronic nature, may be idiopathic, thus distinctively different from that induced by peptic ulcer disease, aspirin, alcohol, or other medications.

Another different manifestation of multiple superficial gastric erosions is related to patients undergoing acute, severe physiological or emotional stress. This has been described as a relatively common occurrence in patients with extensive burns in which the superficial ulcers have been referred to as Curling's ulcers. Cushing's ulcers are identical gastric superficial ulcers that have been described as a complication in patients with intracranial disease, severe head trauma, or postcraniotomy. These stress-type ulcers are almost always superficial, virtually never perforate, and in many patients are painless, with an incidence of GI bleeding in the range of 10% to 20%.

MALIGNANT VERSUS BENIGN GASTRIC ULCERATION

The widespread use of high-quality double-contrast technique in evaluation of the stomach has improved the ability of the radiologist to detect and classify ulcers as benign versus malignant. Various distinguishing features of gastric ulceration have been suggested to successfully classify gastric ulcers as benign versus malignant. The features listed in Table 2-1 can be helpful in making this differentiation. Some of the items will be more useful than others but taken all together they can give the radiologist direction as to how to classify gastric ulcerations.

There are three radiological classifications of gastric ulcers—benign, malignant, and indeterminate. In general, it has been found that when ulcers contain well-defined radiological features of benignity they are almost always benign, and ulcerations that blatantly display the features of malignancy are almost always malignant. There is, however, a large category in which there may be features of both benignity and malignancy demonstrated. In such an instance, the disposition to assign the ulcer to one category or another is unclear. Such ulcers are categorized as indeterminate in nature. In patients with radiologically malignant or indeterminate gastric ulcers, follow-up gastroscopy and biopsy is always indicated. In patients in which radiological features of benignity are overwhelming, automatic gastroscopy and biopsy is probably a poor use of medical resources, personnel, and health care dollars.

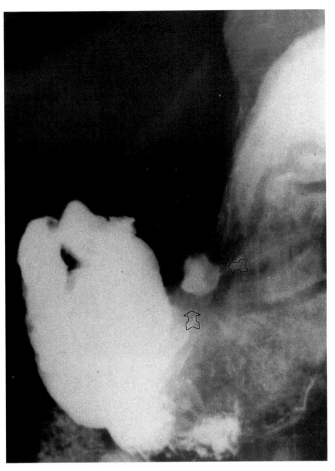

Fig. 2-45   A large benign ulcer is seen along the lesser curvature of the body of the stomach. Note the gastric folds coming up to the edge of the ulcer crater *(arrows)*.

Table 2-1 Malignant versus benign ulceration: radiological distinguishing features		
	Benign	**Malignant**
Location	Mostly antrum, 75% lesser curvature	Most lesions in antrum but can occur anywhere
Convergence of folds	To edge of crater	Stop short of crater edge
Fold shape	Normal or uniformly swollen (edematous)	Amputated, fused, or clubbed folds that may fail to reach crater edge
Projects beyond expected confines of gastric wall	Yes	No
Position of ulcer mound or mass	Central	Eccentric
Ulcer shape	Round or linear	Irregular
Ulcer collar	Yes, well-defined	May be present but shaggy and irregular
Multiplicity	Increased frequency 10%-30%	Less frequent
Associated duodenal ulcer disease	Increased association 50%-60%	Less frequent
Carman's sign and Kirklin complex	No	Yes
Crescent sign	Yes	No
Response to therapy	Reduction of size in 4-6 weeks	No reduction in size, ulcer may enlarge

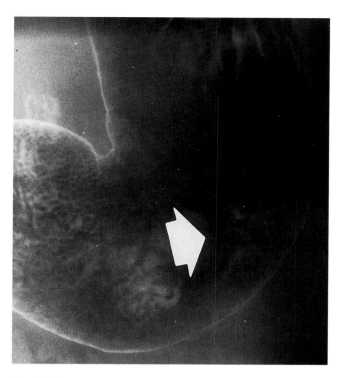

Fig. 2-46   A shallow gastric ulcer *(arrow)* is seen with associated adjacent clubbed and amputated folds indicative of malignant lesion.

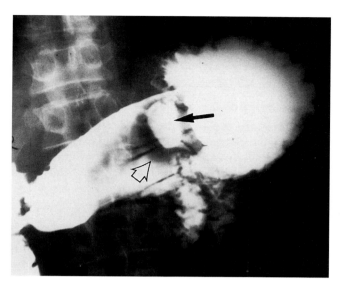

Fig. 2-47   A large, benign gastric ulcer with barium-filled ulcer crater is demonstrated *(arrow)*, as well as an edematous ulcer collar *(open arrow)*.

Location

Ninety percent of all benign gastric ulcers are located in the antrum, and 75% of these are on the lesser curvature. Although most malignant ulcers occur in the antrum, various studies suggest that they occur here with less frequency than benign ulcers, and, in fact, malignant ulcers can be seen anywhere in the stomach. In particular, ulcers seen on the greater curvature or in parts of the stomach other than the antrum should be viewed with greater degrees of suspicion.

Convergence of Folds

In virtually all benign ulcers, gastric folds can be identified up to the edge of the ulcer crater (Fig. 2-45). It is extremely common for the rugal pattern to stop short of the crater margin of a malignant ulcer. This differentiation is one of the more important radiological differences between the types of ulcers.

Fold Shape

In benign ulcers, the adjacent fold pattern can be normal, or it may demonstrate the uniform or beaded widening secondary to edema and swelling. However,

as previously stated, these folds will proceed to the edge of the ulcer crater. The malignant ulcer may demonstrate a variety of abnormal fold patterns in the adjacent mucosal surface. This can include amputated, fused, or clubbed folds, all of which are abnormal and often fail to reach the crater edge (Fig. 2-46). Fold configuration represents an important differentiating factor.

Projects Beyond Expected Confines of Gastric Wall

This has been an acceptable and reliable sign of differentiation for decades. Benign ulcers tend to excavate into the normal mucosal wall, giving a distinct impression of projecting beyond the adjacent mucosal boundaries. On the other hand, a malignant ulcer representing ulceration in a mass will quite frequently give the impression of ulceration that does not extend beyond the adjacent mucosal confines of the stomach. However, some care should be taken with the interpretation of this sign. A chronic gastric ulcer in which some degree of alternating healing and exacerbation has occurred can give a configuration identical to that of a malignant ulcer as a result of fibrosis, cicatrization, and contraction of the adjacent gastric wall.

Position of the Ulcer on the Mound or Mass

Benign ulcers excite inflammatory and edematous changes in the adjacent tissues in a concentric distribution about the ulcer crater (Fig. 2-47). The appearance is therefore that of a centrally located ulcer on a raised mass or mound of edematous tissue. Conversely, the point of ulceration that occurs on a malignant tumor is not predictable and is often eccentric.

Ulcer Shape

Benign ulcers are generally round. Distinct linear ulcers will almost always be benign. Malignant ulcers can be occasionally round and well-defined but more often are found to be irregular with poor definition of the margins.

Ulcer Collar

A uniform ulcer collar about a centrally located ulcer is a good sign for benignity (Fig. 2-48). Undermining of the adjacent soft tissue and subsequent edematous changes result in the appearance of an ulcer collar. When the edematous changes are restricted to the overhanging mucosa about the crater margin, the configuration may, in profile, be that of a thin, well-demarcated lucent ulcer collar, known as Hampton line. Ulcer collars may be present on malignant ulcers but they are generally thick, irregular, and shaggy in appearance.

Multiplicity

Although this cannot be considered a strong sign for either benignity or malignancy, it does apparently have some statistical significance. Literature reports have suggested an increased potential of benignity when multiple ulcers are present (Fig. 2-49).

Associated Duodenal Ulcer Disease

Associated duodenal ulcer disease is a statistically differentiating point that must be correlated with all other distinguishing features. The increased association between benign gastric ulcers and duodenal ulcers has been reported with considerable variance.

Carman's Sign and the Kirklin Complex

First described by Carman in the late 1920s, Carman's sign is thought to be diagnostic of a particular type of ulcerated neoplasm. The ulcer is almost always located on the saddle portion of the stomach on the lesser curvature of the antrum and body. The malignant lesion will lack significant mass effect. The type of ulceration is usually large, flat, and with raised edges.

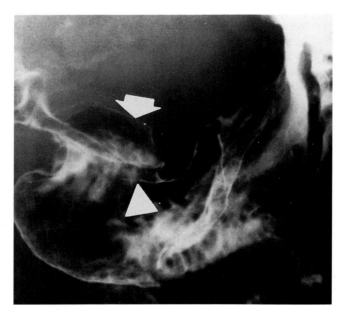

Fig. 2-48   A huge gastric ulcer is seen along the lesser curvature of the stomach *(arrow)*. A well-defined ulcer collar *(arrowhead)* is seen at the margin of the ulcer.

In single-contrast barium-filled examination of the stomach with compression of this saddle region, the heaped up edges of the ulcer will approximate and entrap barium within the flat ulcer bed, giving a meniscoid configuration to the trapped barium within the ulcer in which the inner margin is concave toward the lumen (Fig. 2-50).

Where the heaped-up margins of the ulcer approximate and meet and entrap barium, as a result of compression, the lucent margin that surrounds the concavity of the ulcer represents the approximated heaped-up ulcer edges. This is called the Kirklin complex. Because of the special circumstances regarding the nature of the mass, configuration and location of the ulcer, and the need for the barium-filled stomach and compression views, this sign will rarely be identified on double-contrast views of the stomach.

Crescent Sign

Benign ulcers occurring along the greater curvature of the antrum or body and in which significant mucosal undermining has occurred may demonstrate the configuration of a crescent-shaped ulceration with its concavity directed away from the gastric lumen.

Response to Therapy

With adequate treatment, almost all benign gastric ulcers will undergo a reduction of size in a 4 to 6 week period. Expected deformity changes associated with scarring and cicatrization can also be identified. Alternatively, there will be no change in malignant ulcers or they will increase in size. This differentiating factor is significant, although it has been noted that on rare occasions a malignant ulcer may undergo some degree of decrease in size with peptic ulcer treatment.

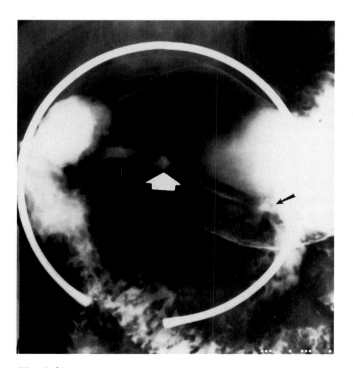

Fig. 2-49 Multiple, small gastric ulcers are demonstrated (*arrows*).

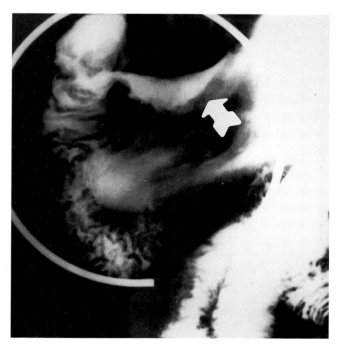

Fig. 2-50 Large ulcer along the lesser curvature of the antrum of the stomach, under compression, demonstrates concavity of the ulcer crater (*arrow*) along its luminal side. This is Carman's meniscus sign of malignancy.

MISCELLANEOUS

Diverticula
    Fundal diverticula
    Antral diverticula
Postoperative Stomach
    Pseudomass
    Postoperative gastric bezoars
    Gastric stump carcinoma
    Chronic gastric remnant gastritis
    Stomal ulceration
    Chronic gastroesophageal reflux
    Jejunal gastric intussusception
Gastric wall emphysema

Diverticula

Fundal diverticula The most common of diverticula encountered in the stomach arise from the cardiofundal region, usually seen on the posterior wall of the stomach. It is a true diverticulum, containing all the layers of the stomach, and can range in size from 1 to 10 cm. These are considered to be congenital and, for the most part, of no clinical significance. Reports of bleeding from gastric diverticula exist in the literature, citing incidences as high as 14%. However, this is probably considerably higher than the experience of most endoscopists and GI radiologists. Additionally, if a diverticulum becomes sufficiently large, impaired emptying and stasis may result, although this is a rare complication.

Antral diverticula Antral diverticula are unusual intramural projections of mucosa in the gastric wall. They are almost always located along the greater curvature of the antrum of the stomach. There has been an association with ectopic pancreatic tissue reported in approximately 10% to 15% of cases (Fig. 2-51).

Radiologically, the partial diverticulum on the greater curvature of the antrum has a "collar-button" appearance and is often misdiagnosed as a benign gastric ulcer. The persistent appearance, lack of inflammatory changes around the partial diverticulum, and lack of tenderness when compressing this region should help the radiologist avoid this mistake.

Postoperative Stomach

The most common types of gastric surgeries are the partial gastrectomy and gastrojejunostomy (Billroth II), antrectomy and gastroduodenostomy (Billroth I), diverting gastrojejunostomy, and gastric partitions for morbid obesity. Radiographic abnormalities seen in complications of gastric resection include the following:

Pseudomass Pseudomass can be seen following

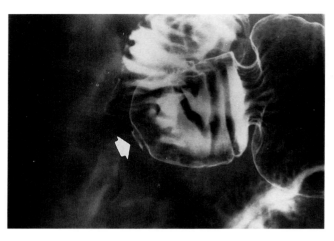

Fig. 2-51 Small, shallow protrusion along the greater curvature of the stomach *(arrow)* was diagnosed at UGI to be a shallow gastric ulcer. Note the absence of inflammatory changes about the area. Endoscopy showed no evidence of inflammation or ulceration and a small antral diverticulum.

Billroth I or Billroth II procedure, although it is more common in the latter. It represents the plication deformity that results when the divided end of the stomach is oversewn to restrict the size of the stoma (Fig. 2-52). The radiological problem presented in this situation is that of a masslike filling defect seen at or near the anastomotic site. It is generally more prominent on immediate postoperative examinations secondary to the edematous changes that persist in the region. On subsequent exams, it may seem less prominent, and over a period of time may appear static in its configuration and size. Without a baseline postoperative examination, the deformity can easily simulate neoplastic recurrence.

Postoperative gastric bezoars As previously discussed, bezoar is not an uncommon complication of gastric surgery (see Fig. 2-8). The bezoars encountered in this setting are almost always phytobezoars and can be asymptomatic. If the bezoar becomes sufficiently large, obstruction of the stoma, distention of the gastric remnant, and irritation and erosion of the mucosa can occur.

Gastric stump carcinoma Although there continues to be some controversy regarding the incidence and occurrence of carcinoma in the gastric remnant, the postoperative stomach is at higher risk for carcinoma than the nonoperated stomach. These lesions are most commonly seen in patients 10 years after partial gastrectomy and, as previously discussed, may be due to chronic gastritis secondary to bile reflux (Fig. 2-53).

Chronic gastric remnant gastritis One of the more common postoperative complications seen in the stomach is chronic gastritis. It is hypothesized that the

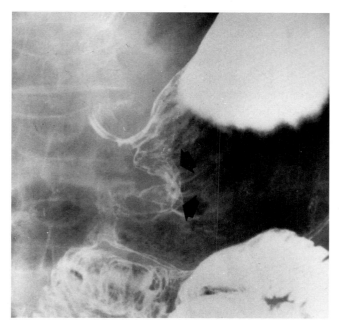

Fig. 2-52   This patient has had a Billroth II gastric resection. UGI examination shows large mass along the margin of the gastric stump *(arrows)*. Ominous as this appears, it represents nothing more than a prominent plication defect.

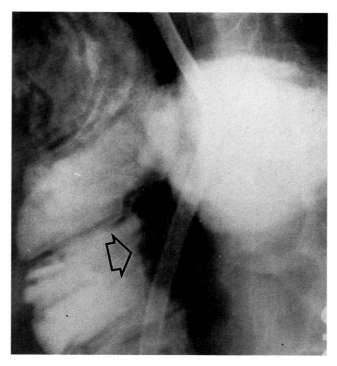

Fig. 2-53   UGI in a patient with previous gastrectomy. The anastomosis is open. Along the margin of the efferent loop there is nodularity *(arrow)* that proved to be a recurrent adenocarcinoma.

lack of pyloric protection results in chronic reflux of bile and pancreatic secretions stimulating inflammatory changes in the gastric remnant. The common radiological appearance is of enlarged gastric rugae, although erosions and even ulcers have been associated with chronic gastritis.

Stomal ulceration   Recurrent ulceration after partial gastrectomy for peptic ulcer disease commonly appears on the jejunal side of the gastrojejunostomy and is known as a stomal or marginal ulcer (Fig. 2-54). When these ulcers are sufficiently large, they are difficult to miss. However, smaller marginal ulcers are readily missed on UGI studies and particularly on single-contrast examinations. The presence of recurrent ulcers on the anastomotic margin is probably unrelated to chronic small bowel reflux and more likely suggests the possibility of inadequate gastric resection, or possibly the existence of an antral remnant inadvertently left behind, or even the presence of a pancreatic islet cell Zollinger-Ellison–type tumor. Additionally, some have suggested that an excessively long afferent loop may predispose to marginal ulcers.

Chronic gastroesophageal reflux   Patients with partial gastric resections will experience an increased incidence of gastroesophageal reflux. Indeed, any pa-

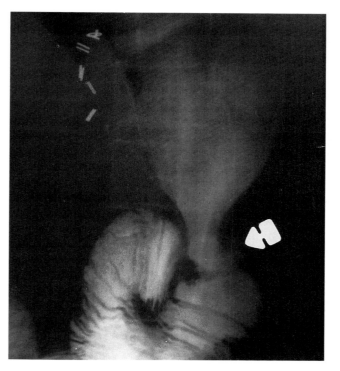

Fig. 2-54   Patient with previous gastrectomy and Billroth II resection presents with recurrent pain. UGI demonstrates large stomal ulcer *(arrow)*.

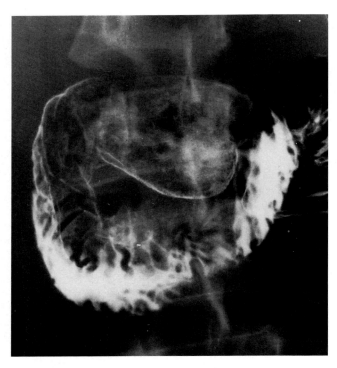

Fig. 2-55   Air-contrast view of normal duodenal bulb utilizing 0.1 mg IV glucagon.

tient undergoing any surgery involving mobilization of the stomach may experience increased reflux and subsequent reflux esophagitis.

Jejunal gastric intussusception   Jejunal gastric intussusception is infrequent, but when it does occur it can occur as an acute or chronic recurrent process. The acute intussusception is often a surgical emergency with compromise of the blood supply in the intussuscepted small bowel loops. These patients will present with severe abdominal pain, nausea and vomiting, and evidence of UGI obstruction. Patients with the chronic recurring type may have no more symptoms than occasional vague upper abdominal discomfort. The intussusception may spontaneously decompress after several minutes.

A large intraremnant filling defect often suggestive of intussusception in its configuration and barium pattern will be seen. In the chronic transient variety, the patient may have vague upper abdominal symptoms, and unless the intussusception is occurring at the time of examination, the diagnosis will probably not be considered.

Gastric Wall Emphysema

Gastric intramural pneumatosis is an unusual finding. The most common cause relates to the ingestion of corrosive acidic material with subsequent necrosis of the mucosa. In addition, it can be seen in phlegmonous type of gastritis where the offending bacterial agent is a gas-producing organism. Air in the gastric wall has also been associated with gastric ulcers and instrumentation of the stomach secondary to endoscopy and placement of tubes.

DUODENUM

Dilated (Nonobstructed) Duodenal Lumen
Scleroderma
Idiopathic intestinal pseudoobstruction
Diabetes mellitus
Drugs
Sprue
Severe acute illness/trauma/burns
Chagas' disease
Anorexia nervosa
Postpartum cachexia
Narrowed Lumen
Peptic ulcer disease
Crohn's disease
Tuberculosis
Annular pancreas
Intraluminal diverticulum
Midgut malrotations
Aorticoduodenal fistula
Adenocarcinoma
Thickened Folds
Peptic ulcer disease
Pancreatitis
Zollinger-Ellison syndrome
Parasites
Sprue
Eosinophilic gastroenteritis
Whipple's disease
Duodenal varices
Intramural hemorrhage
Lymphomas
Amyloidosis

The evaluation of the duodenum is normally included as part of the UGI examination. It should include both air-contrast views and compression views, particularly of the duodenal bulb region. Hypotonic duodenography has also been helpful in evaluating this region. The desired result is usually achieved by 0.1 to 0.5 mg of IV glucagon (Fig. 2-55). Occasionally, the duodenum can be located in a posterior position directly behind the gastric antrum. Under such circumstances, profiling the duodenal bulb, particularly for air-contrast views, can be difficult. In the left lateral position, the air-filled bulb may be overlapped by portions of the an-

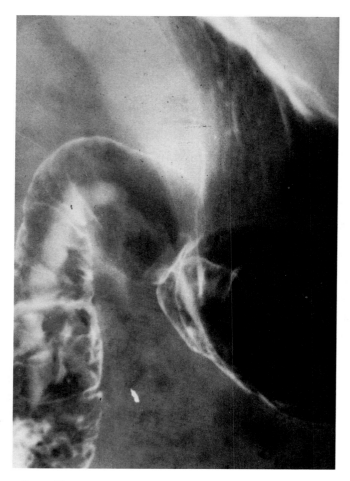

Fig. 2-56 Profiled gastric antrum and duodenal bulb in a posteriorly located duodenum.

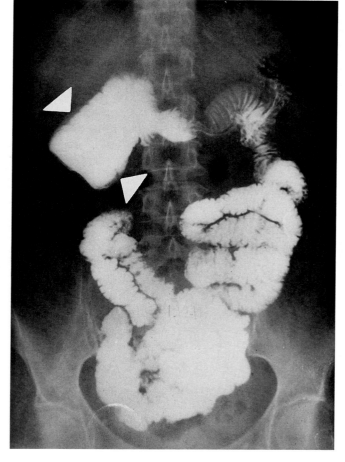

Fig. 2-57 Megaduodenum *(arrowheads)* in a patient with scleroderma.

trum. Angulation of the x-ray tube during fluoroscopy, if this facility is available, may be helpful in separating the duodenal bulb from the antrum. When angulation is not available, a few simple maneuvers may be undertaken. The first is an attempt to evaluate the duodenum in the left oblique position while the patient is upright. The weight of the barium within the stomach may sufficiently pull the gastric antrum downward to allow visualization of the duodenum bulb, which tends to be fixed. Alternatively, with the patient recumbent and in the left lateral position, a bolster (inflated balloon or pillow) is placed in the patient's epigastrium and the patient is asked to roll downward toward the bolster and the table (LAO position). This maneuver will often displace the stomach away from the duodenum, permitting an unobstructed profile view of the air-filled duodenum and pyloric channel (Fig. 2-56).

Most of the radiological problems associated with the duodenum are also common to the remainder of the small bowel. For this reason, discussion of these entitites in this section will be quite limited and more detail will be found in Chapter 3.

Dilated (Nonobstructed) Lumen

Neuromuscular abnormalities account for most of the findings of a dilated flaccid duodenum during UGI examination. These include scleroderma, idiopathic intestinal pseudoobstruction, and diabetes mellitus. Patients on anticholinergic atropine-like medication may exhibit similar findings (Fig. 2-57).

In patients with nontropical sprue, dilatation of the small bowel is a common finding and may be seen within the duodenum as well. Most of the other findings associated with sprue tend to be confined to the more distal small bowel.

Occasionally, a dilated nonobstructed duodenal

sweep may be seen in patients with severe acute illnesses, trauma, or burns. In these patients, distention of both the stomach and occasionally the duodenum may be encountered. Intraabdominal processes, which result in an adynamic ileus, can also involve the duodenum, causing dilatation.

Although the esophagus is the main GI site of involvement in patients with Chagas' disease, the intramural plexi of the duodenum can also be damaged by the trypanosomes, resulting in diminished peristalsis and dilatation.

Dilated duodenum has been described in eating disorders, such as anorexia nervosa or postpartum cachexia.

Narrowed Lumen

Greater than 90% of peptic ulcer disease involving the duodenum affects the duodenal bulb. It can occur as an acute episode, recurrent disease, or chronic disease. In recurrent and chronic disease, duodenal bulb deformity is common, and a small, contracted narrow duodenal bulb will often be seen in patients with chronic peptic ulcer disease. This can occasionally result in obstruction and a dilated stomach.

Approximately 10% of duodenal ulcers are postbulbar in location. These are radiologically difficult to see. Quite often, the radiological findings are thickened, irregular folds, with an area of focal narrowing. However, Crohn's disease or tuberculosis involving the duodenum, although relatively uncommon, can give an identical appearance (Fig. 2-58). Inflammatory changes affecting adjacent pancreas or, less commonly, the gallbladder can also result in postbulbar stricture. Malignancy arising from the pancreatic head can also invade any portion of the duodenal sweep, resulting in strictured narrowing (Fig. 2-59). This most commonly occurs in the descending and proximal transverse portion of the duodenum.

Annular pancreas is an unusual condition involving the descending duodenum. It represents an embryological abnormality of pancreatic development in which the ventral bud of the pancreas encircles the duodenum. This produces circumferential indentation of the descending duodenum by the surrounding pancreatic tissue. It is often diagnosed in infancy or childhood, although a significant number of these patients will not be identified until adolescence or adulthood. Occasionally, periduodenal fibrosis of the duodenal wall can develop at the site of the long-standing stricture resulting from the annular pancreatic tissue. For this reason, surgical relief of the annular extrinsic compression may not always be curative and, on occasion, a gastroenterostomy bypass may be indicated.

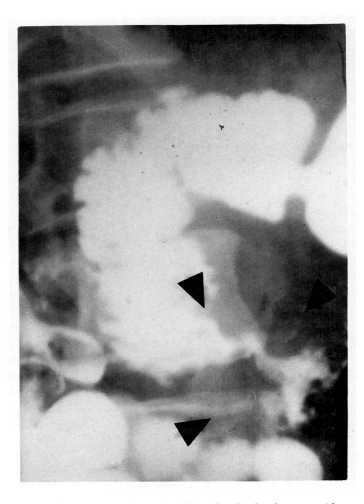

Fig. 2-58   Crohn's disease involving the duodenal sweep with resultant stricture *(arrowheads)*.

The intraluminal diverticulum of the duodenum, or "wind sock deformity," is a thin, intraluminal web or membrane (Fig. 2-60). The "wind sock" configuration occurs as a result of the web being stretched and billowed into the distal lumen by the prolonged and constant effect of peristaltic activity.

Bleeding into the duodenal wall, as a result of either trauma or other causes, such as Henoch-Schönlein purpura, hemophilia, or patients on anticoagulation therapy, can present as discrete intramural mass, diffuse infiltrative changes with thickened fold pattern, or a combination, with associated narrowing.

The superior mesenteric artery syndrome is a condition in which duodenal obstruction occurs as a result of narrowing of the angle between the aorta and the

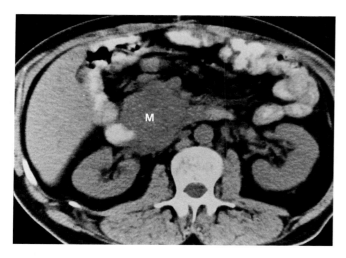

Fig. 2-59 CT through the pancreas demonstrates a large mass *(M)* invading the adjacent contrast-filled duodenal sweep.

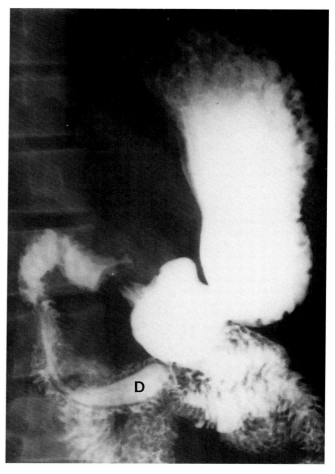

Fig. 2-60 UGI demonstration of intraluminal diverticulum and "wind sock" configuration *(D)*.

superior mesenteric artery at the point where the duodenum passes between them. This is most commonly seen in burn patients, patients in body casts, or patients who have experienced acute severe illness with substantial weight loss. It is thought that the loss of retroperitoneal fat results in a narrowing of the angle between the vessels. Another condition that can result in duodenal narrowing and potential obstruction is midgut volvulus, seen in patients with incomplete rotation of the midgut. The volvulus can occur as a result of fibrous bands overlying the proximal portion of the duodenum, around which the midgut can rotate (Ladd's bands) and twist. Volvulus can also occur as a result of rotation of the midgut about a markedly abbreviated small bowel mesentery that may occur as a result of incomplete rotation.

Aorticoduodenal fistulas are usually complications of prosthetic aortic dacron grafts. However, they originally were described as complications of aortic abdominal aneurysms. The distal portion of the duodenum, in contact with the graft or aneurysm, will break down as a result of focal pressure or erosion of the aorta dissecting into the duodenal wall. The condition is potentially fatal. Contrast examination of the distal duodenum can show several possible findings. These include mass effect, luminal narrowing, ulceration, and even tracking of contrast along the outside of the graft.

Complete obstruction of the intestinal lumen in the neonate (duodenal atresia) results from failure of cannulization of the duodenum during early intrauterine life. The incidence is higher in infants with Down syn-

drome, and quite often these patients present within several hours after birth with the classical "double-bubble" sign, representing an air-filled and distended stomach and duodenal bulb. Another congenital cause of duodenal narrowing is duodenal duplication. Although this is quite rare, it can result in a large periduodenal mass impressing and narrowing the duodenum. The duplicated segment may also be continuous with the main lumen.

Adenocarcinoma of the duodenum, although rare, occurs most commonly in the distal half of the duodenum and, in most instances, has the typical apple-core configuration (Fig. 2-61). Metastatic disease to the duodenum is also uncommon but can occur as an encircling obstructing mass, quite often in the distal portion of the duodenal sweep (Fig. 2-62).

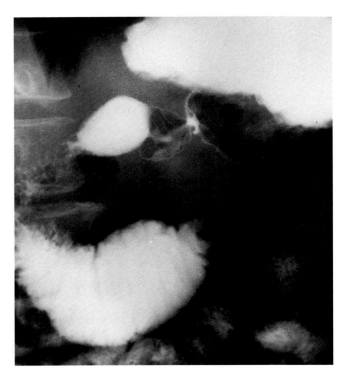

Fig. 2-61   Primary adenocarcinoma of the duodenum with annular narrowing and obstruction *(arrows)*.

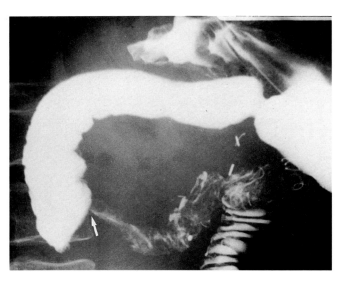

Fig. 2-62   Metastatic disease involving the duodenal sweep *(arrows)*, eccentrically narrowing the lumen.

Thickened Folds

The most common causes of thickened duodenal folds, particularly in the more proximal duodenum, are peptic ulcer disease and pancreatitis. The changes are a result of edema, both from direct inflammatory changes involving the duodenum and indirectly from changes involving the pancreatic head.

In acute pancreatitis, the changes may be limited to the medial inner curve of the duodenal sweep. There may be thickening and tethering of folds that can result in the "reverse figure 3 sign" (also seen with pancreatic carcinoma) described on the UGI examination (Fig. 2-63).

Patients with Zollinger-Ellison syndrome will always have fold prominence within the duodenum as a result of the marked amount of gastric acid secretion stimulated by pancreatic gastrinoma. It should be mentioned that a small number of patients with this uncommon disease will have the offending gastrinoma located within the duodenum.

Crohn's disease of the duodenum most commonly is seen as thickened folds (Fig. 2-64).

Parasitic infection in the small bowel commonly involves the duodenum and results in thick, irregular

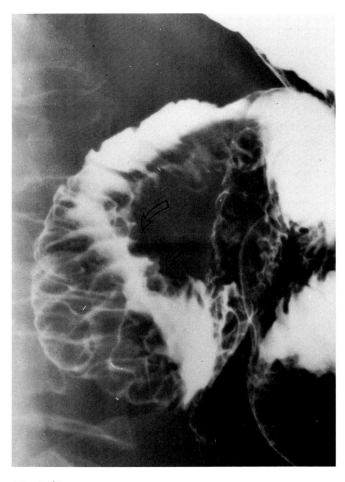

Fig. 2-63   UGI in patient with acute severe pancreatitis resulting in marked thickening of duodenal folds and the "reverse figure 3" configuration on the inner margin *(arrows)*.

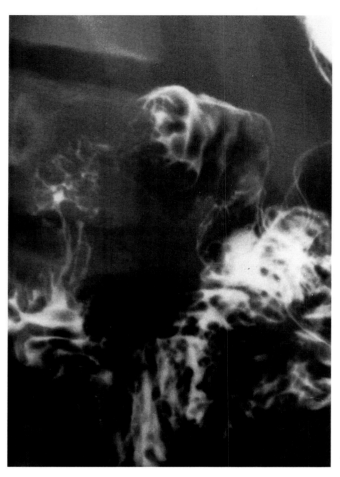

Fig. 2-64   Thickening of folds in the duodenal bulb and postbulbar region secondary to Crohn's disease.

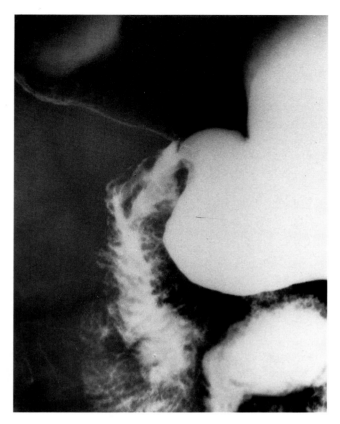

Fig. 2-65   Patient with giardiasis with thickened, irregular folds with fine nodularity.

folds. *Ascaris lumbricoides* commonly involves the distal small bowel. However, both *Strongyloides stercoralis* and intestinal hookworm, *Ancylostoma duodenale,* have a marked preference for the proximal small bowel, particularly the duodenum. *Giardia lamblia* is a relatively common protozoan parasite that involves the duodenum and jejunum with resultant fold thickening and irregularity (Fig. 2-65). Both hypersecretion and hypermotility may also be seen in patients with giardiasis. Additionally, the presence of lymphoid hyperplasia has been observed in some patients with giardiasis.

Fold thickening can also be observed in patients with eosinophilic gastroenteritis. These patients often present with abdominal pain, nausea, vomiting, and eosinophilia on their peripheral blood smear. Fold thickening usually involves the gastric antrum and duodenum. Whipple's disease involves the proximal small bowel with thickened and irregular folds in the duodenum and proximal jejunum.

Occasionally, patients with portal hypertension and esophageal varices may also manifest varicoid formation within the proximal duodenum. This is seen as thickened and smooth serpiginous folds. Frequently, the presence of duodenal varices is an indication of portal vein occlusion. Duodenal intramural bleeding may also manifest as thickened regular folds with the classic "stack of coins" appearance.

Lymphomas may have multiple physical manifestations within the small bowel, among which is diffuse fold thickening. Its presence in the duodenum is very uncommon, and, when present, like lymphomas elsewhere in the gut, it almost never obstructs. Patients in chronic renal failure or on chronic dialysis will commonly demonstrate thickened folds within the duodenum. There is also an increased incidence of peptic ulcer disease within such patients, although the persistent thickened folds are probably not peptic in origin. Uniform thickening of folds within the duodenum, and indeed within both the jejunum and ileum, can occur in both primary and secondary amyloidosis.

FILLING DEFECTS

Flexural pseudotumor
Pancreatic rest
Mesenchymal tumors
Adenoma
Carcinoid/APUDoma
Brunner's gland hyperplasia
Brunner's gland adenoma
Lymphoid hyperplasia
Choledochocele
Kaposi's sarcoma
Papillitis
Hetertophic gastric mucosa

One of the most common and most troublesome of duodenal filling defects is the flexural pseudopolyp (Fig. 2-66). This phenomenon is usually seen in thin patients with a sharp, acute angle between the apex of the duodenal bulb and the descending duodenum. Because of the acuteness of the angle, mucosa can pile up on the medial inner aspect of the duodenum at the level of the apex of the bulb. This results in a filling defect that can easily be diagnosed as a nonexistent polypoid mass. Demonstration of this mass in a thin individual with a sharp bulbar duodenal angle should alert radiologists to the possibility of a flexural pseudotumor. This can be confirmed by evaluating the area in question with the patient in different positions, particularly supine positions that may open the bulbar duodenal angle and change the configuration of the filling defect.

Pancreatic rests or ectopic pancreatic tissue within the duodenum can result in a well-defined filling defect (Fig. 2-67). These are not neoplastic lesions and are of embryonic origin. They are smooth, can be round or lobulated, and usually measure 1 to 2 cm in diameter. They more commonly present as solitary filling defects in the duodenal bulb or second portion of the duodenum. They can also be seen in the gastric antrum. A characteristic radiological finding is the central collection of barium (dimple) that may be confused with a small ulcer on the surface of a neoplastic polypoid lesion.

Mesenchymal benign tumors, such as leiomyomas and lipomas, are the most common benign lesions of the duodenum. They are usually solitary and submucosal in origin and have a smooth surface. These can ulcerate on the surface, although this is uncommon in the duodenum. The duodenal variety are usually smaller than seen elsewhere in the bowel. Neurofibroma and hemangioma

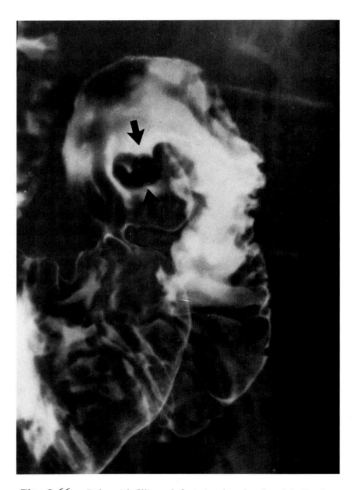

Fig. 2-66   Polypoid filling defect in the duodenal bulb *(arrows)* that proved to be a flexural pseudotumor. No polyps were identified at endoscopy.

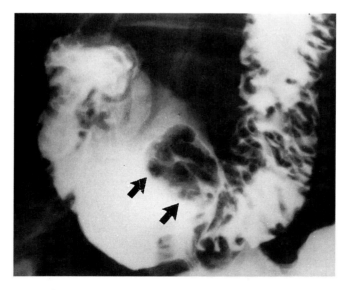

Fig. 2-67   A lobulated filling defect *(arrows)* is seen in the duodenal bulb with a small, central barium collection (dimple) representing a pancreatic rest.

can also occur within the duodenum but are rare.

Duodenal adenomas are uncommon. When present, they are seen radiologically as mucosal polypoid lesions usually no more than 1 cm in diameter. The exception is the villous adenoma, which when symptomatic is commonly 2 to 3 cm in size (Fig. 2-68). Patients may present with either GI bleeding or symptoms related to intussusception. These lesions have a high potential for malignant degeneration.

Similarly, carcinoid tumors arising from argentaffin cells within the mucosa can be seen in the duodenum and particularly in the peripapillary region of the second portion of the duodenum. The radiological appearance is variable and may appear as discrete smooth polyps or as irregular infiltrating processes. A variant of this, the APUDoma, can arise from APUD (amine precursor uptake and decarboxylation) cells. These tumors are histologically similar to ileal carcinoid tumors and are frequently associated with multiple endocrine neoplasia (MEN) syndromes.

Various polypoid syndromes may also have polyps within the duodenum. This includes familial polyposis, Peutz-Jeghers syndrome, and Cronkhite-Canada syndrome, as well as Cowden's disease.

Multiple filling defects in the duodenal bulb are also a presentation of Brunner's gland hyperplasia (Fig. 2-69). This process can also extend into the second portion of the duodenum. The etiology of this condition is unclear. Normal function of the Brunner's glands, which produce alkaline secretion to protect the sensitive duodenal mucosa from damaging effects of gastric acid, does not appear to be impaired. A variation of this is the Brunner's gland adenoma or hamartoma, which is a rare lesion caused by focal overgrowth of the tissue elements of the Brunner's glands

in the proximal duodenum (Fig. 2-70). They are usually seen as smooth polypoid masses, often about 1 cm in size.

Benign lymphoid hyperplasia of the duodenum with multiple small filling defects may be a normal finding in children, although in adults the condition has been associated with hypogammaglobulinemia and the concomitant presence of giardiasis.

Occasionally, a round, smooth defect arising in the region of the papilla is seen and is a result of choledochocele formation. This is a variation of the choledochal cyst (Fig. 2-71).

Kaposi's sarcoma is a relatively common lesion seen in AIDS patients. The major sites of involvement include the stomach and small bowel, although lesions may be demonstrated within the duodenum. The appearance is that of multiple polyploid lesions frequently

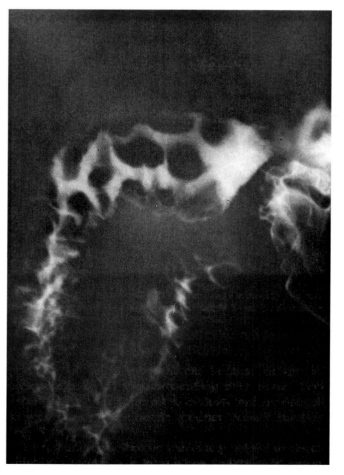

Fig. 2-69   Multiple, large, and rounded nodular filling defects in the duodenal bulb and postbulbar region representing Brunner's gland hyperplasia.

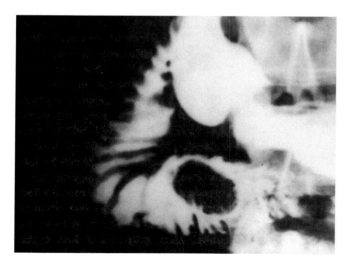

Fig. 2-68   A well-defined, lobulated filling defect in the transverse portion of the duodenum representing a villous adenoma.

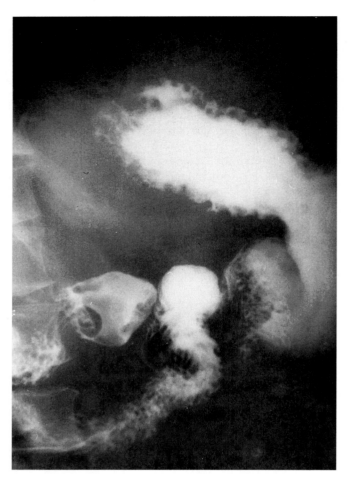

Fig. 2-70 A solitary filling defect near the apex of the duodenal bulb suggests the possibility of a flexural pseudotumor. However, this was found to be a Brunner's gland adenoma.

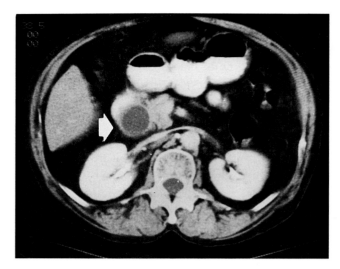

Fig. 2-71 Large cystic dilatation in the common bile duct representing a choledochal cyst *(arrow)* impressing the duodenum.

ulcerated on the surface. Hematogenous metastatic disease, particularly breast or melanoma, may have a similar appearance.

Abnormalities of the papilla of Vater may also manifest as a duodenal filling defect. Most commonly this is papillitis, resulting from inflammation and an enlargement of the major papilla, usually resulting from traumatic stone passage or peripapillary fibrotic changes.

An uncommon cause of multiple plaquelike filling defects in the duodenal bulb is heterotopic gastric mucosa (Fig. 2-72). These filling defects can be of varying size and configuration and form a mosaic pattern usually in the base of the duodenal bulb and can easily be missed on single-contrast examination. The exact clinical significance of this condition is unclear. There appears to be no malignant potential.

EXTRINSIC PROCESSES

Pancreatic Disease
Kidney and Adrenal Gland
Enlarged Common Bile Duct, Gallbladder, and Liver
Choledochal Cysts
Retroperitoneal Lymph Node Masses

The most common extrinsic process involving the duodenal sweep is a result of pancreatic disease in the head of the pancreas. This can be inflammatory, with diffuse enlargement of the pancreas or pseudocyst formation. Also, pancreatic neoplasms, either benign or malignant, can impress the duodenum.

Disease processes arising from the right kidney or adrenal gland, if sufficiently large, can impress the outer aspect of the descending portion of the duodenal sweep.

Abnormalities arising in the liver and biliary system can also, on occasion, result in extrinsic impression of the duodenum. This includes an enlarged gallbladder, whether it be from obstructive causes or passive dilatation. An enlarged common bile duct can occasionally impress the duodenal sweep at the level of the apex of the bulb (Fig. 2-73). Large choledochal cysts can also result in a significant duodenal impression. Retroperitoneal lymph node masses in the peripancreatic region can also lead to an extrinsic impression on the duodenal sweep (Fig. 2-74).

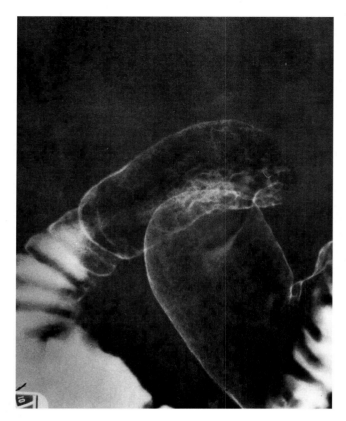

Fig. 2-72 Multiple, irregular, plaquelike filling defects at the base of the duodenal bulb representing heterotopic gastric mucosa.

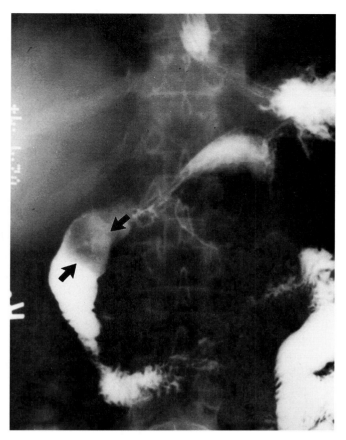

Fig. 2-73 Obstruction of the biliary system and extrinsic impression of the postbulbar duodenum *(arrows)* by a dilated common bile duct.

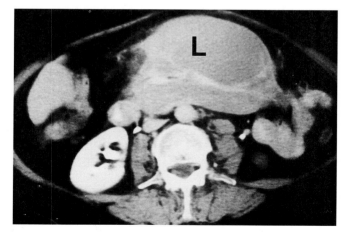

Fig. 2-74 Large, retroperitoneal lymph node mass *(L)* sandwiching and compressing the retroperitoneal portion of the duodenal sweep.

DUODENAL ULCERATION

Peptic ulcer disease
Zollinger-Ellison syndrome
Crohn's disease
Tuberculosis (TB)
Viral diseases

Duodenal peptic ulcer disease is a common entity and accounts for a sizeable portion of the health care costs expended on GI diseases. It is estimated that between 10% and 15% of North American men have suffered from duodenal ulcer disease at some time in their lifetime. The incidence is less for women. The disease is a direct effect of the corrosive effect of gastric acid on the duodenal mucosa and the breakdown of normal protective antiacid mechanisms within the duodenal bulb. Various risk factors are also thought to play an important role in the possible etiological origins of the disease. These include alcohol and certain types of drugs, such as aspirin and other NSAIDs that also have a direct corrosive effect.

The presence of duodenal ulcer disease is probably not an isolated phenomenon and is simply a manifestation of one facet of the spectrum of peptic ulcer disease involving the distal esophagus, gastric antrum, and duodenal bulb. Careful evaluation of the stomach of patients with duodenal ulcer disease will almost always demonstrate gastritis. The incidence of peptic esophagitis in these patients is also increased.

Radiological diagnosis traditionally has been based upon a persistent barium collection seen within the duodenal bulb (Fig. 2-75). However, the advent of widespread use of endoscopy resulted in numerous assertions that the radiological evaluation of the duodenum for peptic ulcer disease was quite insensitive. The ability of the radiologist to demonstrate duodenal ulceration can be significantly improved if the examination of the duodenal bulb includes both good air-contrast views, as well as single-contrast views with compression (Fig. 2-76). Occasionally, a good portion, if not all of the duodenal bulb may be ulcerated, resulting in a "giant duodenal ulcer" (Fig. 2-77). These ulcers may assume triangular configuration of the duodenal bulb and, as a result, be missed during UGI study. Certain factors should alert the radiologist to the possibility of a giant duodenal ulcer. These include the unusual

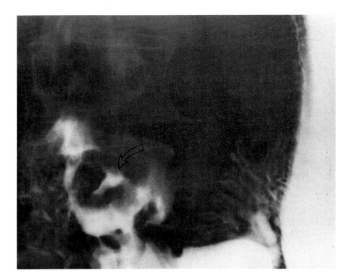

Fig. 2-75   Typical appearance of duodenal bulb ulcer with central ulcer crater *(curved arrow)* and surrounding edema.

persistence of barium within the duodenal bulb, little or no discernible fold pattern within the bulb, and postbulbar narrowing or spasm.

Duodenal ulcerations or erosions may be seen in a variety of other conditions, including the Zollinger-Ellison syndrome, Crohn's disease of the duodenum, tuberculosis of the small bowel, as well as ulceration resulting from viral diseases.

DUODENAL DIVERTICULOSIS

Duodenal diverticula are seen on approximately 5% of routine UGIs. They represent serosal and mucosal herniations through the muscular wall and are not true diverticula (Fig. 2-78). They usually occur in the second portion of the duodenum along the inner margin of the duodenal C-loop within 1 to 2 cm of the major papilla. Duodenal diverticula are usually only incidental findings. Complications, such as hemorrhage, infection, or enterolith formation, have been reported. On occasion, the papilla of Vater may empty directly into a duodenal diverticulum, resulting in the potential of difficult cannulation and possible perforation during endoscopic retrograde cholangiopancreatography (ERCP).

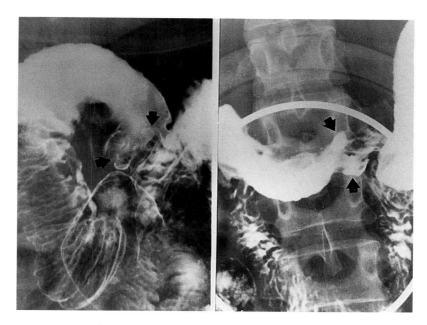

Fig. 2-76 Air-contrast views *(on the left)* suggest possibility of ulcer craters in the form of "ring shadows" *(arrows)*. Single-contrast compression views of the same area *(on the right)* demonstrate two well-defined ulcer craters *(arrows)*.

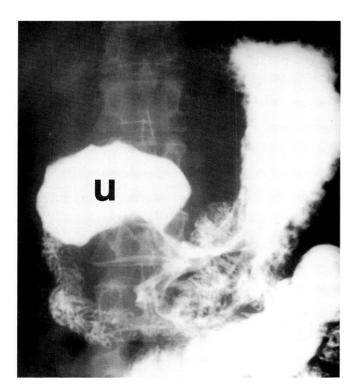

Fig. 2-77 A giant duodenal ulcer *(U)* is demonstrated.

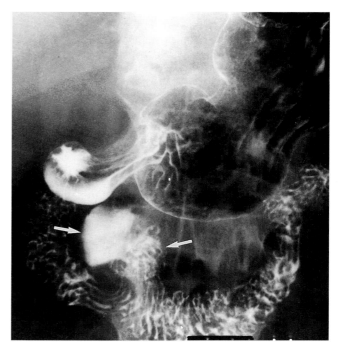

Fig. 2-78 Duodenal diverticulum *(arrows)* arising from the medial aspect of the transverse duodenum.

SELECTED READINGS

Balfe DM, Koehler RE, Karstaedt N, et al: Computed tomography of gastric neoplasms, *Radiology* 140:431-436, 1981.

Balthazar EJ, Rosenberg H, Davidian MM: Scirrhous carcinoma of the pyloric channel and distal antrum, *AJR* 134:669-673, 1980.

Blaser MJ: Gastric campylobacter-like organisms, gastritis, and peptic ulcer disease, *Gastroenterology* 93:371-383, 1987.

Bothen NF, Eklof O: Diverticula and duplications (enterogenous cysts) of the stomach and duodenum, *AJR* 96:375-381, 1966.

Buchholz PR, Haisten AS: Phytobezoars following gastric surgery for duodenal ulcer, *Surg Clin North Am* 52:341-352, 1972.

Butz WC: Giant hypertrophic gastritis, *Gastroenterology* 39:183-190, 1960.

Camblos JF: Acute volvulus of the stomach, *Am Surg* 35:505-509, 1969.

Choi SH, Sheehan FR, Pickren JW: Metastatic involvement of the stomach by breast cancer, *Cancer* 17:791-797, 1964.

Chuang VP, Wallace S, Stroehlein JR, et al: Hepatic artery infusion chemotherapy: gastroduodenal complications, *AJR* 137:347-350, 1981.

Clements JL, Jinkins JR, Torres WE, et al: Antral mucosal diaphrams in adults, *AJR* 113:1105-1111, 1979.

Cohen S, Laufer I, Snape WJ, et al: The gastrointestinal manifestations of scleroderma: pathogenesis and management, *Gastroenterology* 79:155-166, 1980.

Cohen Y, Heun SW: Phytobezoar after gastrectomy, *Br J Surg* 58:236-237, 1971.

Cotton PB, Shorvon PJ: Analysis of endoscopy and radiography in the diagnosis, follow-up and treatment of peptic ulcer disease, *Clin Gastroenterol* 13:383-403, 1984.

Davenport HW: Salicylate damage to the gastric mucosal barrier, *N Engl J Med* 276:1307-1312, 1967.

Delikaris P, Golematis B, Missitzis J, et al: Smooth muscle neoplasms of the stomach, *South Med J* 76:440-442, 1983.

Dodd GD, Sheft D: Diverticulum of the greater curvature of the stomach: a roengenologic curiosity, *AJR* 107:102-104, 1969.

Dooley CP, Cohen H: The clinical significance of *Campylobacter pylori*, *Ann Intern Med* 108:70-79, 1988.

Edelman MJ, March TL: Eosinophilic gastroenteritis, *AJR* 91:773-778, 1964.

Farman J, Faegenburg D, Dallemand S, et al: Crohn's disease of the stomach: the "ram's horn" sign, *AJR* 123:242-251, 1975.

Feczko PJ, Halpert RD, Ackerman LV: Gastric polyps: radiological evaluation and clinical significance, *Radiology* 155:581-584, 1985.

Feliciano DV, Van Heerden JA: Pyloric antral mucosal webs, *Mayo Clin Proc* 52:650-653, 1977.

Felson B, Berkmen YM, Anastacio MH: Gastric mucosal diaphragm, *Radiology* 92:513-517, 1969.

Gelfand DW, Moskowitz M: Massive gastric dilatation complicating hypotonic duodenography, *Radiology* 97:637-639, 1970.

Gerson DE, Lewicki AM: Intrathoracic stomach: when does it obstruct? *Radiology* 119:257-264, 1976.

Ghahremani GG: Nonobstructive mucosal diaphragms or rings of the gastric antrum in adults, *AJR* 121:236-247, 1974.

Goldberg HI: Radiographic evaluation of peptic ulcer disease, *J Clin Gastroenterol* 3(suppl 2):57-65, 1981.

Goldner FH, Boyce HW: Relationship of bile in the stomach to gastritis, *Gastrointest Endosc* 22:197-199, 1976.

Goldstein HM, Cohen LE, Hagen R, et al: Gastric bezoars: a frequent complication in the postoperative ulcer patient, *Radiology* 107:341-344, 1973.

Goldstein SS, Lewis JH, Rothstein R: Intestinal obstruction due to bezoars, *Am J Gastroenterol* 79:313-318, 1984.

Gonzalez G, Kennedy T: Crohn's disease of the stomach, *Radiology* 113:27-29, 1974.

Goodwin CS, Armstrong JA, Marshall BJ: Campylobacter pyloridis, gastritis and peptic ulceration, *J Clin Pathol* 39:353-365, 1986.

Hricak H, Thoeni RF, Margulis AR, et al: Extension of gastric lymphoma into the esophagus and duodenum, *Radiology* 135:309-312, 1980.

Hyson EA, Burrell M, Toffler R: Drug induced gastrointestinal disease, *Gastrointest Radiol* 2:183-212, 1977.

Ishikura H, Sato F, Naka H, et al: Inflammatory fibroid polyp of the stomach, *Acta Pathol Jpn* 36:327-335, 1986.

Ivey KJ: Drugs, gastritis, and peptic ulcer, *J Clin Gastroenterol* 3(suppl 2):29-34, 1981.

Jacobs DS: Primary gastric lymphoma and pseudolymphoma, *Am J Clin Pathol* 40:379-394, 1963.

Joffe N: Some unusual roentgenologic findings associated with marked gastric dilatation, *AJR* 119:291-299, 1973.

Johnson OA, Hoskins DW, Todd J, et al: Crohn's disease of the stomach, *Gastroenterology* 50:571-577, 1966.

Jolobe OM, Montgomery RD: Changing clinical pattern of gastric ulcer: are anti-inflammatory drugs involved? *Digestion* 29:164-170, 1984.

Kilman WJ, Berk RN: The spectrum of radiological features of aberrant pancreatic rests involving the stomach, *Radiology* 123:291-296, 1977.

Kobayashi S, Prolla JC, Kirsner JB: Late gastric carcinoma developing after surgery for benign conditions. Endoscopic and histologic studies of the anastomosis and diagnostic problems. *Am J Dig Dis* 15:905-912, 1970.

Kressel HY: Peptic disease of the stomach and duodenum. In Margulis AR, Burhenne HJ, editors: *Alimentry tract radiology*, ed 3, St Louis, 1983, Mosby—Year Book.

Laufer I, Hamilton J, Mullens JE: Demonstration of superficial gastric erosions by double contrast radiography, *Gastroenterology* 68:387-391, 1975.

Levine MS, Creteur V, Kressel HY, et al: Benign gastric ulcers: diagnosis and follow-up with double contrast radiography, *Radiology* 164:9-13, 1987.

Llaneza PP, Salt WB: Gastric volvulus: more common than previously thought? *Postgrad Med* 80:279-288, 1986.

Loo FD, Palmer DW, Soergel KH, et al: Gastric emptying in patients with diabetes mellitus, *Gastroenterology* 86:485-494, 1984.

Lucas CE, Sugawa C, Riddle J, et al: Natural history and surgical dilemma of "stress" gastric bleeding, *Arch Surg* 102:266-273, 1971.

DILATED SMALL BOWEL

Mechanical Obstruction Resulting in Distention
   Adhesion
   Hernias
   Volvulus
   Intussusception
   Neoplasms
   Nonneoplastic strictures
   Intraluminal masses
   Extrinsic masses
   Colonic lesions
Distention with No Obstruction
   Sprue
   Lactose intolerance, other hypersecretory states
   Neuromuscular and motility abnormalities
   Peritonitis/severe abdominal pain
   Drug-induced
   Electrolyte abnormalities
   Vagotomy, postoperative
   Idiopathic pseudoobstruction
   Ischemia

Mechanical Obstruction Resulting in Distention

Dilatation of the small bowel occurs in a wide variety of conditions, some associated with mechanical obstruction and others in which no obstructing lesion is present. The most common obstructing lesion causing distention of the mesenteric small bowel is an adhesion or band, usually resulting from previous abdominal surgery. Supine plain films typically demonstrate distended air-filled loops of small bowel, identified by the linear folds traversing the circumference of the bowel lumen (valvulae conniventes or plicae circulares) (Fig. 3-4). Distended loops may lie in a tiered or stepladder pattern, and variable amounts of air are present in the colon, depending on the level, grade, and duration of the obstruction. Distended small bowel loops containing mostly fluid (with little or no air) usually appear as a gasless abdomen on supine films.

On erect or lateral decubitus films, the small amounts of air rise within the dilated fluid-filled loops to form a series of bubbles or short air-fluid levels (string of pearls). When more air is present, air-fluid levels are longer and often appear at different heights

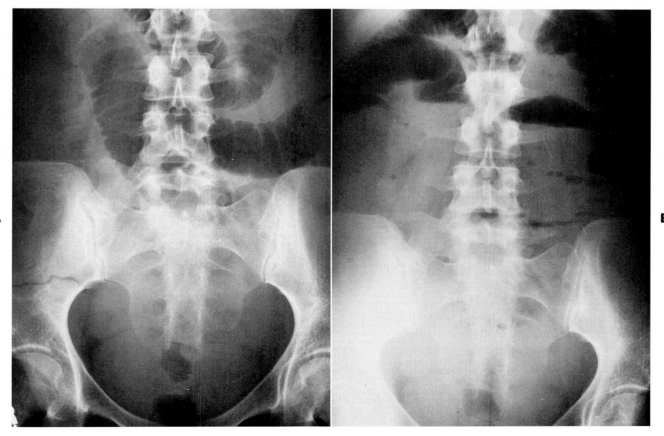

Fig. 3-4   **A,** Supine film demonstrates multiple dilated small bowel loops in a patient with small bowel obstruction secondary to adhesions. **B,** Upright film shows associated air-fluid levels.

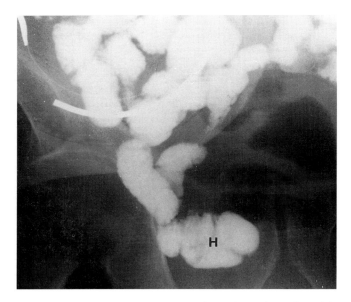

Fig. 3-5 A loop of distal ileum *(H)* overlying the right pubic bone lies in an inguinal hernia.

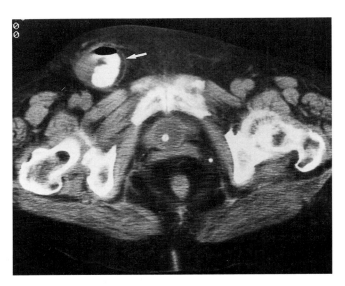

Fig. 3-6 CT shows an opacified loop of bowel in a right inguinal hernia *(arrow)*.

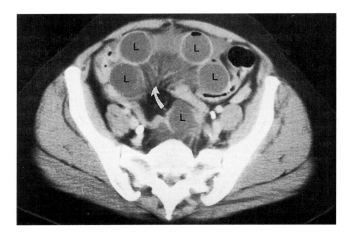

Fig. 3-7 CT demonstrates fluid-filled small bowel loops *(L)* around edematous mesentery *(curved arrow)*. (From Goodman P, Raval B: CT diagnosis of acquired small bowel volvulus, *Am Surg* 56:628-631, 1990.)

within the same bowel loop (differential levels).

Although small bowel obstruction resulting from an adhesion may spontaneously resolve, continued or worsening symptoms may lead to barium studies to delineate the level, cause, and severity of the obstruction. In an incomplete small bowel obstruction, a transition zone can be detected between the dilated loops proximal to the obstruction and the normal caliber loops distal to it. An adhesion appears as a well-defined linear impression crossing the bowel lumen at the site of obstruction. Entrapment of a loop of bowel by one or more adhesions may result in a closed-loop obstruction.

CT is also useful for evaluating suspected small bowel obstruction. In addition to possibly determining the site of obstruction, CT can provide information about intramural and extraintestinal disease, which may indicate the cause of obstruction.

External and internal hernias containing small bowel may be associated with obstruction and proximal distention and, like adhesive bands, sometimes cause closed-loop obstruction. Inguinal hernias are common and may contain a variable length of ileum. Paraumbilical hernias, incisional hernias involving the anterior or lateral abdominal wall, and spigelian hernias (caused by weakness at the lateral aspects of the rectus abdominis muscles) may all contain loops of small bowel. Other unusual external hernias include femoral, obturator, sciatic, peristomal, and lumbar types.

Internal hernias usually represent defects in the mesentery or peritoneum and include paraduodenal, paracecal, and intersigmoid hernias. Small bowel loops rarely extend into the lesser sac through the foramen of Winslow.

On contrast studies, hernias containing small bowel may be indicated by abnormal location or clustering of loops (Fig. 3-5). Smooth extrinsic compression on the loops as they enter and exit the hernia is also a useful finding on contrast studies. Supplementary examination in the lateral position is usually necessary to detect herniation through the anterior abdominal wall because this is easily obscured on frontal films. CT is often useful in displaying the abnormal location of herniated loops of bowel and may also define other hernia contents including colon and omentum (Fig. 3-6).

Small bowel volvulus occurs when a loop of bowel twists around its mesenteric axis. Primary volvulus is seen mostly in children as a result of intestinal malrotation, whereas secondary volvulus occurs in adults and is associated with preexisting factors including adhesions, internal hernias, and tumors. Torsion of a bowel loop causes constriction of its mesenteric vascular supply and often results in ischemia or infarction if not treated promptly. Plain films and barium studies are frequently nonspecific, but CT is useful in demonstrating dilated loops of small bowel radially distributed around the twisted edematous mesentery (Fig. 3-7).

Intussusception represents invagination or telescoping of a bowel loop to form an inner loop (intussusceptum) enclosed within an outer loop (intussuscipiens). The inner loop and its associated mesentery may become edematous and cause a small bowel obstruction. In adults, small bowel intussusception is usually caused by a tumor or other mass acting as a lead point, and symptoms are often sporadic. On barium examination, small bowel intussusception typically demonstrates a coil-spring appearance, denoting barium trapped between the inner and outer loops of bowel (Fig. 3-8). CT shows the inner loop and its mesentery surrounded by the outer loop and may identify the lead mass.

Various intrinsic neoplasms, both primary and metastatic, can occlude the small bowel lumen (Fig. 3-9).

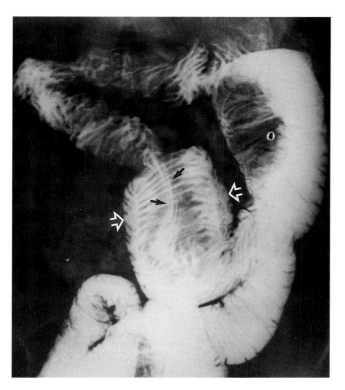

Fig. 3-8 Small bowel intussusception demonstrates intussusceptum *(arrows)* and intussuscipiens *(open arrows).*

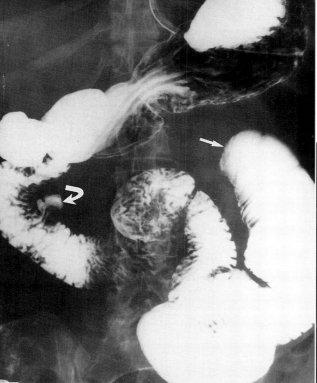

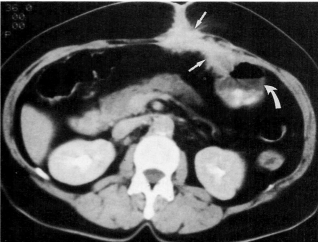

Fig. 3-9 **A,** Complete jejunal obstruction *(arrow)* with proximal dilatation. A duodenal diverticulum is also noted *(curved arrow).* **B,** CT shows an irregular soft tissue mass *(arrows)* in the anterior abdominal wall adjacent to a distended bowel loop *(curved arrow).* This represents metastatic colon carcinoma.

A

B

Intrinsic inflammatory, infectious, and ischemic processes can lead to stricture formation with distention of proximal small bowel loops. Postoperative anastomotic strictures may also cause proximal obstruction.

Intraluminal masses may cause small bowel obstruction by occluding the lumen. These masses most commonly lodge at the ileocecal valve and include impacted foreign bodies and gallstones (gallstone ileus).

In meconium ileus equivalent, inspissated fecal material obstructs the distal ileum in children or adults with cystic fibrosis. This complication may be prevented by routine ingestion of pancreatic enzyme supplements.

Likewise, extrinsic inflammatory and neoplastic masses can compress and obstruct adjacent small bowel loops. This is less important in the mesenteric small bowel than in the duodenum, which is fixed and in close proximity to many organs including the pancreas, right kidney, gallbladder, and liver.

Colonic lesions, particularly carcinoma of the proximal colon, may produce distended loops of small bowel with little or no air in the colon. This mimics a distal small bowel obstruction but is easily evaluated with a barium enema.

Distention with No Obstruction

Small bowel distention can also occur in the absence of a mechanical obstruction. Nontropical sprue (celiac disease), a reversible condition caused by malabsorption of dietary gluten, typically produces dilatation of proximal small bowel loops due to hypersecretion of fluid. Flocculation, segmentation, and a moulage (featureless or castlike) appearance of the barium column were once considered classic features of sprue but are less often demonstrated with the improved barium suspensions now widely available. An increase in separation of jejunal folds is suggestive of sprue and is best demonstrated with enteroclysis technique. Sprue is associated with an increased incidence of small bowel intussusception, which occurs without a lead mass and is typically transitory and asymptomatic. Other complications of sprue include small bowel ulcerations or strictures (ulcerative enteritis), lymphoma, adenocarcinoma of the proximal small bowel, squamous cell carcinoma of the esophagus, hyposplenism, and a rare condition known as cavitating lymph node syndrome.

Tropical sprue occurs in certain tropical locations and appears radiographically similar to nontropical sprue. However, unlike nontropical sprue, the tropical form is associated with severe vitamin B_{12} and folic acid deficiencies and megaloblastic anemia. Tropical sprue responds to folic acid or antibiotic therapy but not to a gluten-free diet.

Lactose intolerance is a common cause of malabsorption in adults that results from acquired deficiency of the enzyme lactase in the small bowel. Following a lactose-containing meal, hypersecretion of fluid into the small bowel causes luminal distention and symptoms of bloating and cramps. Lactose intolerance is easily treated by either eliminating dairy products from the diet or supplementing the diet with commercially available lactase enzymes. Other hypersecretory states including Zollinger-Ellison syndrome and cryptosporidial enteritis may likewise cause small bowel distention as a result of increased fluid content.

Various neuromuscular and motility abnormalities can affect the small bowel and lead to luminal distention. The best known of these is scleroderma (progressive systemic sclerosis), in which smooth muscle atrophies and is replaced by fibrous tissue. In the mesenteric small bowel, smooth asymmetric sacculations (pseudodiverticula) are sometimes seen. Crowding of folds (hidebound bowel) is a characteristic finding of scleroderma involving the small bowel.

Chagas' disease, a parasitic infection common in Brazil, can cause distention of the duodenum and mesenteric small bowel by destroying the neural plexus. Associated abnormalities are often seen in the esophagus, colon, and heart.

Peritonitis, severe abdominal pain, and recent abdominal surgery are important causes of adynamic ileus, a condition characterized by decreased peristalsis of the bowel. Supine abdominal films reveal distention of small bowel, colon, or both, and upright films typically show air-fluid levels to be at equal heights within the same bowel loop (nondifferential levels). Localized abdominal pain caused by conditions such as appendicitis, cholecystitis, or pancreatitis may be associated with focal bowel dilatation and air-fluid levels (sentinel loops).

Other causes of adynamic ileus include drugs (anticholinergics, morphine), metabolic disorders resulting in electrolyte imbalance, and previous vagotomy. Idiopathic pseudoobstruction is a chronic form of adynamic ileus of unknown etiology.

Ischemia resulting from thromboembolic disease, vasculitis, or low-flow states may decrease small bowel motility and increase distention. Associated fold thickening caused by intramural edema or hemorrhage may also be present.

NARROWED SMALL BOWEL

Narrowing Resulting from Intrinsic Abnormality
    Crohn's disease
    Infectious
    Zollinger-Ellison syndrome
    Graft-versus-host disease
    Ischemia
    Radiation
    Drug-induced
    Postoperative
    Volvulus
    Intussusception
    Neoplasms
Small Bowel Narrowing Resulting from Extrinsic Abnormality
    Adhesion
    Hernia
    Extrinsic masses

Narrowing Resulting from Intrinsic Abnormality

Narrowing of the small bowel lumen can result from numerous intrinsic and extrinsic processes.

Crohn's disease (regional enteritis) is usually confined to the terminal ileum but may involve any portion of the small bowel. Early in the disease, spasm and edema associated with ulcerations can cause luminal narrowing, and later in the disease, continued inflammation and fibrosis often lead to stricture formation (Figs. 3-10 and 3-11). Skip lesions consisting of narrowed segments of small bowel separated by normal or dilated segments are sometimes noted.

Several infectious agents can cause small bowel narrowing. The protozoan *Giardia lamblia* may cause narrowing secondary to thickening of folds in the duodenum and proximal jejunum. The roundworm *Strongyloides stercoralis* causes similar findings and also may cause tubular narrowing of the bowel lumen resulting from spasm or stricture formation.

Tuberculosis of the small bowel caused by *Mycobacterium tuberculosis* may result from drinking unpasteurized milk or swallowing infected sputum. The ileocecal region is most often involved, with narrowing sometimes causing marked distortion of this area. Small intestinal tuberculosis may be difficult to distinguish from Crohn's disease. Other infections in which fold thickening and luminal narrowing are usually localized to the distal ileum include *Campylobacter fetus jejuni,* *Yersinia enterocolitica,* and *Salmonella typhi* (ty-

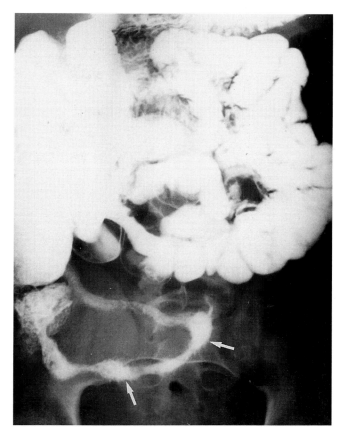

Fig. 3-10   Narrowing and mucosal irregularity of the distal ileum *(arrows)* associated with separation of bowel loops in a patient with Crohn's disease.

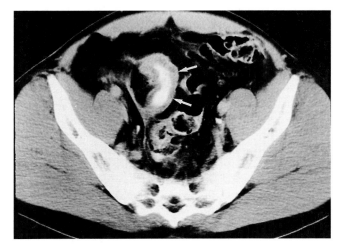

Fig. 3-11   CT shows thickened wall *(arrows)* of distal ileum in a patient with Crohn's disease.

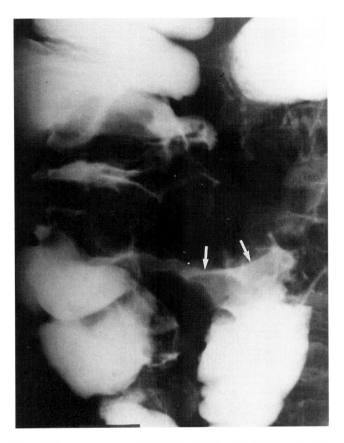

Fig. 3-12   Large polypoid mass in the ileocecal region causing narrowing of the terminal ileum *(arrows)* represents non-Hodgkin's lymphoma.

phoid fever). *Anisakis,* a small roundworm transmitted by eating raw fish, has been reported to cause narrowing of the jejunum or ileum secondary to spasm and ulceration.

Cytomegalovirus (CMV) enteritis occurs with increased frequency in immunocompromised patients, especially those with acquired immune deficiency syndrome (AIDS). This can cause diffuse small bowel narrowing, ulcerations, and effacement of folds. Associated esophagitis, gastritis, or colitis may also be present in patients with disseminated CMV infection.

Involvement of the distal duodenum and proximal jejunum is uncommon in peptic ulcer disease but sometimes occurs in severe ulcer diathesis, as seen in Zollinger-Ellison syndrome.

Graft-versus-host disease is a potential complication of bone marrow transplantation in immunocompromised patients and represents rejection of the patient's own tissues by the donor bone marrow lymphocytes. Diffuse narrowing of the small bowel with effacement of folds has been compared with the appearance of ribbon or toothpaste.

Small bowel ischemia can cause luminal narrowing secondary to spasm, intramural edema or hemorrhage, or stricture formation. Similar findings are sometimes seen following radiation and are caused by endarteritis and subsequent small bowel ischemia.

Various drugs have been associated with small bowel narrowing because of their local toxic effects. These include potassium chloride tablets and floxuridine (FUDR) and other related chemotherapeutic agents.

Narrowing at surgical anastomoses is usually related to edema in the immediate postoperative period and stricture formation later on. In small bowel volvulus, narrowing results from torsion of a loop of bowel, whereas in intussusception, edema of the intussuscepted loop and its mesentery causes narrowing.

Primary neoplasms of the small bowel including adenocarcinoma, lymphoma, leiomyosarcoma, and carcinoid tumor can cause focal narrowing of the lumen (Fig. 3-12). Metastatic spread to the small bowel through contiguous, peritoneal, or hematogenous routes can also lead to one or more areas of narrowing.

Narrowing Resulting From Extrinsic Abnormality

Extrinsic narrowing of the small bowel is usually related to an adhesion or hernia. Various extrinsic masses can also compress and narrow the small bowel lumen.

THICKENED FOLDS

Uniformly Thickened
    Intramural hemorrhage
    Edema
      Ischemia
      Congestive heart failure
      Hypoproteinemia
      Angioneurotic edema
    Radiation
    Eosinophilic enteritis
    Abetalipoproteinemia
Nodular Thickened (Focal)
    Whipple's disease
    Edema
      Zollinger-Ellison syndrome
      Adjacent inflammatory mass
    Infections
    Eosinophilic enteritis
    Abetalipoproteinemia
    Crohn's disease
    Lymphoma
Nodular Thickened (Diffuse)
    Mastocytosis
    Lymphangiectasia
    Infections
    Eosinophilic enteritis
    Graft-versus-host disease
    Amyloidosis
    Waldenström's macroglobulinemia
    Lymphoma

Fold thickening is characteristic of a variety of abnormalities affecting the small bowel. In some conditions, folds appear uniformly or regularly thickened, whereas in other conditions, thickening is nodular or irregular. Fold thickening can also be focal or diffuse, depending on the underlying disease. These features provide a pattern-based approach to the differential diagnosis of thickened small bowel folds.

Uniformly Thickened

Uniformly thickened small bowel folds are typical of intramural hemorrhage or edema. In these conditions, blood or transudate infiltrates into the submucosal

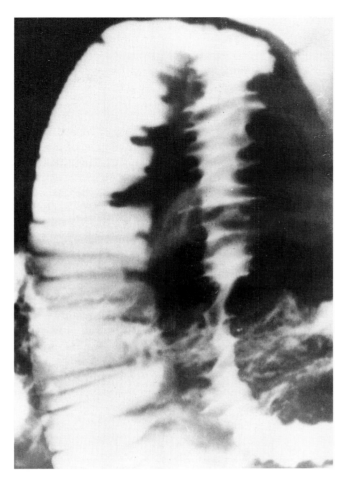

Fig. 3-13 Thickened folds and luminal narrowing represent segmental small bowel ischemia secondary to oral contraceptive medication.

layer of the bowel wall. As the folds become thicker, the space between adjacent folds becomes shorter, with the overall appearance likened to a stack of coins (Fig. 3-13).

Small bowel hemorrhage is caused by various insults including mesenteric ischemia or infarction, vasculitis, coagulopathy, anticoagulant medications, and trauma. Edema of the small bowel may complicate mesenteric ischemia or infarction, congestive heart failure, and hypoproteinemia (resulting from hepatic, renal, or GI disease). Angioneurotic edema is an unusual cause of small bowel edema. In this disease, a genetic defect in the complement inactivation system can trigger episodes of small bowel edema, as well as hives and life-threatening laryngeal edema. Between attacks of angioneurotic edema, patients are asymptomatic and the small bowel folds appear normal. Other causes of small bowel edema that are associated with nonuniform or nodular fold thickening are discussed later in this section.

Radiation to the abdomen or pelvis can lead to end-arteritis in small bowel loops within the radiation port. Like other forms of ischemia, radiation enteritis causes uniform thickening of small bowel folds.

Eosinophilic enteritis is characterized by eosinophilic infiltration of the GI tract. This disease most often affects the stomach or small bowel and may be transmural or confined to the mucosa, muscularis, or serosa. With primary mucosal involvement of the small bowel, folds often appear thickened. The thickening may be uniform or nodular, focal or diffuse. Associated fold thickening or luminal narrowing of the gastric antrum and proximal duodenum may also occur. Although peripheral eosinophilia and a history of allergy suggests the diagnosis of eosinophilic enteritis, these factors are absent in approximately 25% and 50% of patients, respectively.

Abetalipoproteinemia is a rare genetic disease in which abnormal lipid metabolism leads to fat malabsorption, cerebellar degeneration, and acanthocytosis (pointed-shaped red blood cells). Deposits of fat in epithelial cells of the duodenum and jejunum produce uniform or nodular thickening of folds. Similar findings have been noted in small bowel xanthomatosis, an extremely rare condition in which lipid-laden macrophages infiltrate the bowel wall.

Nodular Thickened (Focal)

In contrast to the straight thickened folds typical of intramural hemorrhage, nodular or nonuniform fold thickening is featured in numerous diseases affecting the small bowel. In some, involvement is primarily focal or segmental, whereas in others, the small bowel is diffusely abnormal.

Whipple's disease causes nodular thickened folds in the duodenum and proximal jejunum (Fig. 3-14). Macrophages containing abundant periodic acid-Schiff (PAS) positive material are found throughout the lamina propria layer of the bowel wall, and characteristic rod-shaped gram-positive bacilli have been identified within these cells. Whipple's disease occurs mostly in middle-aged men and presents with diarrhea, arthralgias, fever, and adenopathy. The pleura, pericardium, and central nervous system may also be involved. Although long-term treatment with antibiotics is often curative, an infectious etiology for this disease remains controversial.

Small bowel edema, though typically causing uniform fold thickening, is sometimes associated with coarsened or nodular thickened folds. In Zollinger-Ellison syndrome, the markedly elevated levels of gastric acid result in severe inflammation and edema of the proximal duodenum and may even cause similar findings in the distal duodenum and proximal jejunum.

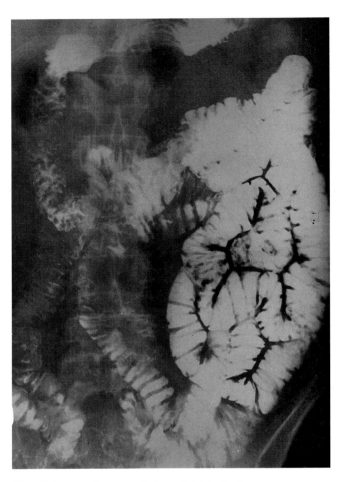

Fig. 3-14 Diffuse small bowel fold thickening represents Whipple's disease.

Nodular thickened folds are also seen in edematous small bowel adjacent to an inflammatory mass. This can involve the jejunum (pancreatitis) or ileum (appendicitis, tubo-ovarian abscess).

Numerous organisms can affect the small bowel and many cause nodular fold thickening. The parasites *Strongyloides* and *Giardia* usually are localized to the duodenum and proximal jejunum (Fig. 3-15). A similar appearance has been described in hookworm infestation (ancylostomiasis). Focal involvement of the distal ileum is suggestive of tuberculosis, typhoid fever, and *Yersinia* or *Campylobacter* enteritis.

In AIDS, otherwise unusual types of small bowel infections occur frequently, with most causing focal or diffuse thickening and nodularity of folds. Etiologies include CMV, *Mycobacterium avium intracellulare* (MAI), *Cryptosporidium,* and *Isospora belli* (Fig. 3-16).

Thickened folds in eosinophilic enteritis and abetalipoproteinemia can appear straight or nodular. In-

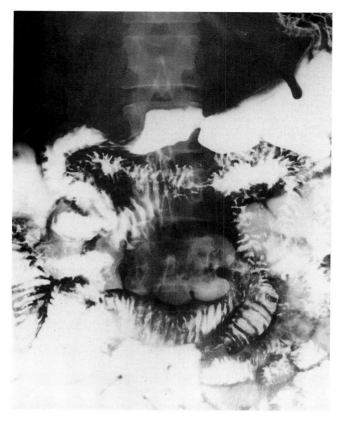

Fig. 3-15   Diffuse, irregular small bowel fold thickening in a patient with giardiasis.

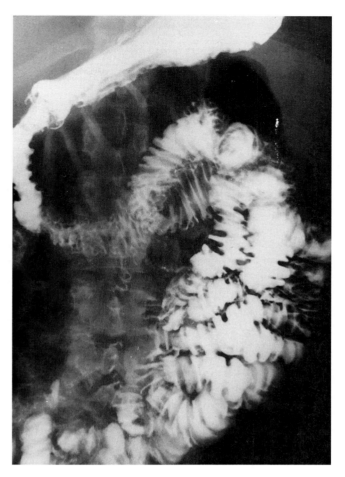

Fig. 3-16   Diffuse small bowel fold thickening caused by MAI in a patient with AIDS.

volvement in eosinophilic enteritis may be focal or diffuse, whereas in abetalipoproteinemia, the ileum is usually spared.

Crohn's disease of the small bowel may demonstrate coarsely thickened folds. This represents edema or inflammation and is usually localized to the distal ileum. Associated findings include ulcerations, eccentric involvement, and skip lesions.

Nodular thickened folds are an uncommon manifestation of small bowel lymphoma. The infiltration of malignant lymphocytes into the mucosal and submucosal layers of the bowel wall may be focal or diffuse.

Nodular Thickened (Diffuse)

Mastocytosis is an uncommon disease characterized by the proliferation of histamine-secreting mast cells. Although often localized to the skin (urticaria pigmentosa), the disease may also involve lymph nodes, liver, spleen, and bone (osteoblastic lesions). GI tract involvement produces fold thickening and nodularity throughout the small bowel and occasionally in the dis-

tal stomach. Episodes of flushing, pruritus, headache, and diarrhea may occur following the release of histamine from the mast cells.

Lymphangiectasia represents dilatation of intestinal lymphatic channels caused by inadequate lymph drainage. The disease may be congenital or acquired and typically demonstrates diffuse nodular thickening of small bowel folds.

Disseminated histoplasmosis involving the small bowel is a rare cause of diffuse nodular fold thickening. As noted in the previous section, patients with AIDS may harbor otherwise unusual types of small bowel infections that typically produce nodular thickened folds.

Both eosinophilic enteritis and graft-versus-host disease can cause a similar alteration of the small bowel fold pattern.

Amyloidosis is a systemic disease in which extracellular deposits of amyloid occur throughout the body, including the GI tract. Small bowel folds may appear

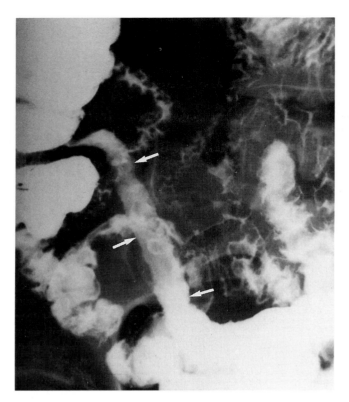

Fig. 3-17   Tubular distal ileum *(arrows)* resulting from CMV enteritis in a patient with AIDS.

diffusely thickened and nodular. This disease most often occurs in patients with underlying multiple myeloma or chronic inflammatory conditions.

Waldenström's macroglobulinemia, a rare disease caused by proliferation of immunoglobulin M (IgM)-producing plasma cells, may involve the small bowel. This results in diffuse fold thickening and tiny mucosal nodules.

Lymphoma can cause either focal or diffuse small bowel fold thickening and nodularity.

DIMINISHED FOLDS

Infections
Graft-versus-host disease
Sprue
Crohn's disease
Ischemia
Radiation
Chemical toxicity
Amyloidosis
Lymphoma
Backwash ileitis
Cathartic colon

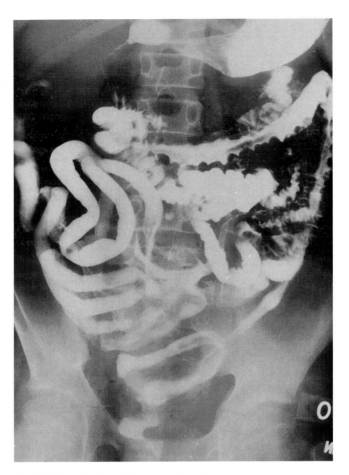

Fig. 3-18   Diffuse effacement of small and large bowel folds in a child with graft-versus-host disease.

Loss of the normal small bowel fold pattern results in a tubular appearance that may be focal or diffuse. This is often associated with thickening and rigidity of the bowel wall and may be preceded by focal or diffuse fold thickening.

Several infectious agents can cause effacement of small bowel folds and narrowing of the lumen. In CMV enteritis and cryptosporidiosis, small bowel involvement is typically diffuse, whereas in strongyloidiasis, disease is localized to the duodenum and proximal jejunum (Fig. 3-17).

In graft-versus-host disease, donor lymphocytes from a bone marrow transplant attack host tissues. The GI tract is usually affected, and a tubular appearance of the small bowel is frequently noted (Fig. 3-18).

Sprue (celiac disease) is associated with a decrease in the number of folds per inch in the duodenum and proximal jejunum. Occasionally, folds may be absent, resulting in a tubular-shaped lumen. However, unlike most other causes of diminished small bowel folds,

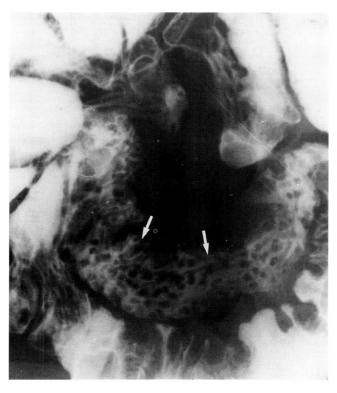

Fig. 3-19   Multiple small uniform nodules *(arrows)* in the terminal ileum of a 17-year-old patient represent nodular lymphoid hyperplasia.

sprue produces luminal dilatation rather than narrowing.

In Crohn's disease, small bowel loops may appear featureless and narrowed secondary to edema or fibrosis.

Small bowel ischemia or infarction sometimes causes effacement of the fold pattern. Dilatation or narrowing of the lumen and scalloping of the bowel wall (thumbprinting) may also be noted. Similar findings in radiation enteritis reflect the underlying endarteritis and subsequent ischemia.

Toxic chemicals, introduced either by direct ingestion (potassium chloride tablets) or by vascular infusion (floxuridine and related chemotherapeutic agents), can reduce or eliminate small bowel folds.

A tubular-appearing small bowel may result from infiltration of the bowel wall. This has been described in amyloidosis, lymphoma, and other infiltrative diseases.

Featureless dilatation of the terminal ileum (backwash ileitis) sometimes occurs in patients with chronic ulcerative pancolitis. A similar finding can also result from long-term cathartic abuse (cathartic colon). In both conditions, the ileocecal valve is patulous.

TINY NODULES

Lymphangiectasia
Whipple's disease
Mastocytosis
Waldenström's macroglobulinemia
Infection
Nodular lymphoid hyperplasia

Discrete tiny nodules in the small bowel are usually associated with thickened folds. This pattern is seen in lymphangiectasia, Whipple's disease, mastocytosis, Waldenström's macroglobulinemia, and small bowel infection (*Yersinia* enteritis, MAI, disseminated histoplasmosis).

Tiny nodules can also be seen in the absence of fold thickening. In nodular lymphoid hyperplasia, prominent lymphoid follicles in the small bowel wall appear as tiny round uniform nodules (Fig. 3-19). This is a normal finding in children and young adults, especially in the terminal ileum where lymphoid tissue is most abundant. The small bowel folds appear normal in these patients. However, fold thickening is often present in older patients with diffuse nodular lymphoid hyperplasia associated with immunoglobulin deficiency or giardiasis of the small bowel.

SOLITARY MURAL MASSES

Malignant Tumors
    Adenocarcinoma
    Leiomyosarcoma
    Lymphoma
    Metastasis
    Kaposi's sarcoma
    Carcinoid
Benign Tumors
    Mesenchymal tumor
    Adenomas
    Carcinoid
    Inflammatory fibroid polyp
Other Masses
    Endometrioma
    Duplication cyst
    Hematoma
    Inverted Meckel's diverticulum

Malignant Tumors

Adenocarcinoma, though the most common primary malignant neoplasm of the duodenum, occurs with decreasing frequency from proximal jejunum to distal ileum. It arises in the mucosal layer and typically infiltrates the bowel wall to cause a short annular narrowing with mucosal destruction, circumferential wall thickening, and overhanging margins. Less commonly, small bowel adenocarcinoma appears as a polypoid intraluminal mass.

Clinical symptoms associated with adenocarcinoma include bleeding, abdominal pain, and obstruction. An increased incidence of adenocarcinoma has been noted in the duodenum and proximal jejunum in patients with celiac disease and in the ileum in patients with Crohn's disease.

Leiomyosarcoma of the small bowel arises in the muscular or submucosal layer and grows either away from the lumen (exoenteric) or toward it (endoenteric). Leiomyosarcomas are more common in the jejunum and ileum than in the duodenum and account for approximately 9% of primary malignant neoplasms of the small bowel.

Exoenteric lesions often produce few symptoms until they have attained a large size and have outgrown their blood supply. Central necrosis and cavitation of the tumor lead to ulceration and hemorrhage into the adjacent bowel lumen. Contrast studies may show either extrinsic compression of bowel loops by the large

intramural mass or an irregular collection of barium within the necrotic portion of the tumor itself. CT is useful in demonstrating both the enhancing peripheral component and the necrotic or gas-containing central component of the lesion.

The endoenteric form of small bowel leiomyosarcoma usually appears as a compressible intraluminal mass. This may cause bleeding, intussusception, or obstruction. Leiomyosarcomas may be difficult to distinguish from leiomyomas both radiographically and histologically. Metastases usually occur through hematogenous spread to the liver or lungs.

Lymphoma affects the small bowel more often than any other portion of the GI tract. This usually represents secondary involvement by non-Hodgkin's lymphoma and occurs with greatest frequency in the distal ileum because of the predominance of lymphoid tissue there.

Small bowel lymphoma has a variety of radiographic appearances including fold thickening or effacement, luminal narrowing, aneurysmal dilatation, diffuse nodularity, and extrinsic compression by mesenteric masses (Fig. 3-20). Solitary or multiple focal mural masses can

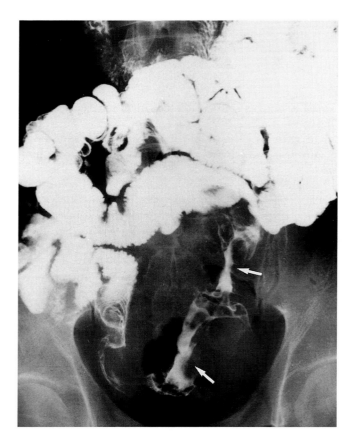

Fig. 3-20 Distorted, irregular ileal loop *(arrows)* represents non-Hodgkin's lymphoma.

also be seen. With continued enlargement, these masses may become exoenteric, undergoing excavation and ulceration, or endoenteric, producing an intraluminal polypoid mass with the potential for intussusception.

Non-Hodgkin's lymphoma of the small bowel is a recognized complication of celiac disease. It also occurs with increased frequency in patients with immunodeficiency as a result of AIDS or immunosuppresion resulting from antirejection medications following organ transplantation. In Mediterranean lymphoma, diffuse small bowel involvement results in severe intestinal malabsorption.

Metastatic disease to the small bowel occurs through hematogenous, peritoneal, contiguous, or lymphatic spread and can cause a variety of radiographic findings. Although metastases are often multiple, solitary lesions are sometimes demonstrated.

Hematogenous dissemination can affect any segment of the small bowel. This occurs most frequently in malignant melanoma and less often in breast or lung carcinoma. Metastatic melanoma typically produces submucosal nodules that may contain a central ulceration (target lesions). With further growth, these lesions may become primarily exoenteric (with subsequent necrosis and ulceration) or endoenteric (with subsequent intussusception). Small bowel metastases from breast carcinoma often result in focal scirrhous-type narrow-

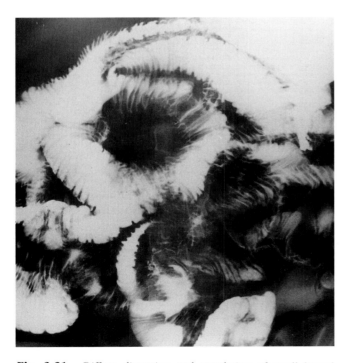

Fig. 3-21 Diffuse distortion and angulation of small bowel loops caused by peritoneal spread of colon carcinoma.

ing similar to that seen more commonly in the stomach.

Peritoneal spread through ascitic fluid leads to seeding of tumor on the serosal surface of the small bowel. Peritoneal fluid accumulates in the mesenteric reflections of the small bowel, especially at the ileocecal region because of its relatively dependent position. Serosal metastases most often occur secondary to GI or gynecological malignancies, particularly ovarian carcinoma. In addition to the nodular masses representing serosal tumor implants, associated fibrous reaction may cause tethering of folds and angulation of bowel loops (Fig. 3-21). CT is useful for demonstrating associated findings of peritoneal tumor spread including ascites, peritoneal implants, mesenteric infiltration, and omental cakes.

Direct or contiguous spread of tumor may involve the mesenteric small bowel, as seen in invasion of the distal ileum by pelvic or cecal tumors. Lymphatic spread has been reported to involve the distal ileum following ileocolic anastomosis for colon carcinoma.

Kaposi's sarcoma is a vascular tumor of the skin that can also affect visceral organs including the GI and respiratory tracts. Although once a rare disease, Kaposi's sarcoma is a common neoplasm in AIDS, particularly in homosexual men with AIDS. Submucosal nodules of Kaposi's sarcoma in the small bowel often resemble hematogenous metastases. Like metastatic malignant melanoma, Kaposi's sarcoma nodules may contain a central ulceration and at times act as a lead point for small bowel intussusception.

Carcinoid tumor is the most common primary neoplasm of the small bowel. It arises from argentaffin cells in the crypts of Lieberkühn and occurs most commonly in the distal ileum. Carcinoid tumors less than 1 cm in diameter usually cause no symptoms and rarely metastasize. A carcinoid tumor may be noted incidentally on contrast studies as a smooth, round submucosal mass.

As the tumor enlarges, it may extend into the overlying mucosa and lead to ulceration or intussusception. Outward extension into the muscular and serosal layers may induce a local desmoplastic reaction consisting of angulation, tethering of folds, and partial obstruction. This represents the local effects of serotonin, which is produced by the tumor from the dietary amino acid tryptophan.

Carcinoid tumors measuring 1 to 2 cm in diameter metastasize in about 50% of cases, and those larger than 2 cm metastasize in about 90% of cases. Regional metastases are usually located in the mesentery or lymph nodes and are commonly larger than the primary tumor. On CT, these lesions may demonstrate a stellate appearance or dystrophic calcifications.

Liver metastases from carcinoid tumor are usually

hypervascular and may cause carcinoid syndrome, characterized by episodic cutaneous flushing, wheezing, and diarrhea. The liver normally degrades serotonin into 5-hydroxyindoleacetic acid (5-HIAA) and thereby prevents it from entering the systemic circulation. However, in the presence of liver metastases, serotonin may pass through the right heart into the lungs, producing carcinoid syndrome and damaging the right heart valves before being broken down in the lungs to 5-HIAA. Bone metastases from carcinoid tumor are typically osteoblastic.

Benign Tumors

Benign tumors arising in mesenchymal tissues of the small bowel wall include leiomyoma, lipoma, hemangioma, and neurofibroma. The most common of these is leiomyoma, a hypervascular nonencapsulated smooth muscle tumor (Fig. 3-22). Leiomyoma, like its malignant counterpart leiomyosarcoma, can undergo endoenteric or exoenteric growth with resultant complications of intussusception or tumor necrosis and ulceration, respectively.

Lipoma, an encapsulated fatty tumor, is characterized fluoroscopically by its softness and compressibility during palpation. Continued stretching of the tumor by bowel peristalsis may form a pedunculated intraluminal mass that can ulcerate or act as a lead point for intussusception (Fig. 3-23).

Hemangioma represents a focal proliferation of vascular channels. Though phleboliths are uncommonly demonstrated, their presence in association with a submucosal mass is indicative of a hemangioma.

Neurofibroma and other neural tumors are unusual solitary mural masses in the small bowel.

Adenomas, benign mucosal tumors arising in glandular epithelium, may appear sessile or pedunculated.

Carcinoid tumor of the small bowel demonstrates variable malignant potential.

Inflammatory fibroid polyp (eosinophilic granuloma) is composed primarily of connective tissue and appears as a smooth submucosal mass in the small bowel, stomach, or colon. Although eosinophilic infiltration of the mass is characteristic, the focal nature of the mass and the absence of associated peripheral eosinophilia differentiate it from eosinophilic gastroenteritis. Complications of inflammatory fibroid polyp include ulceration and intussusception.

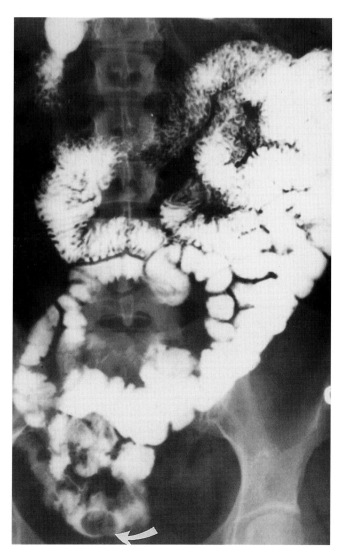

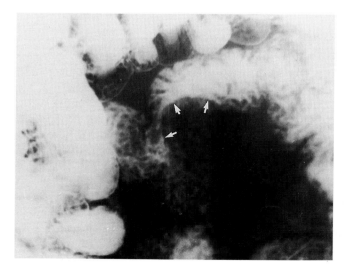

Fig. 3-22 Submucosal mass *(arrows)* represents a jejunal leiomyoma.

Fig. 3-23 Ovoid mass *(curved arrow)* in the distal ileum represents a lipoma.

Other Masses

Endometrioma of the small bowel represents a focal deposit of ectopic endometrial tissue on the serosal surface of the distal ileum. The etiology of endometriosis is uncertain, and proposed theories include reflux of endometrial tissue through the fallopian tubes, hematogenous or lymphatic spread, and metaplasia of celomic epithelium. Small bowel involvement is uncommon and may appear as a focal mass with associated serosal tethering resulting from repeated episodes of intramural hemorrhage and subsequent fibrosis.

Duplication cyst is an embryologic abnormality that can occur anywhere in the small bowel. These cysts are tubular or round and may communicate with the adjacent bowel lumen. Although often discovered in childhood, duplication cysts are occasionally recognized incidentally in adults as a smooth intramural mass seen on contrast examination.

Unlike duodenal hematoma, focal hematoma of the mesenteric small bowel rarely causes a focal masslike appearance, possibly because of the tamponading effect of the circumferential serosal layer there.

An inverted Meckel's diverticulum can also appear as a smooth, round or oval-shaped mass on contrast studies.

MULTIPLE MURAL MASSES

Malignant Tumors
  Metastases
  Lymphoma
  Kaposi's sarcoma
  Carcinoid
Benign Tumors
  Hamartomas
  Adenomas
  Mesenchymal tumors
  Carcinoid
Other Masses
  Postinflammatory polyps
  Pneumatosis cystoides intestinalis
  Varices

Many of the lesions that can occur as solitary mural masses can also occur as multiple mural masses. These lesions were described in greater detail in the previous section.

Malignant Tumors

Metastasis to the small bowel can occur through peritoneal, hematogenous, lymphatic, or contiguous spread. Lesions are often multiple and may show variability in size secondary to repeated episodes of seeding.

Non-Hodgkin's lymphoma of the small bowel can produce multiple, discrete mural masses or diffuse nodularity. This most often involves the ileum as a result of the normal abundance of lymphoid tissue there (Fig. 3-24).

Kaposi's sarcoma of the GI tract often produces multiple submucosal masses. Ulceration or transient intussusception of the masses may cause hemorrhage or abdominal pain, respectively.

Carcinoid tumors of the small bowel are multiple in approximately one third of cases.

Benign Tumors

Multiple hamartomas of the small bowel occur in several polyposis syndromes including Peutz-Jeghers, Cronkhite-Canada, and Cowden's syndromes. Peutz-Jeghers syndrome is an autosomal dominant disease characterized by mucocutaneous pigmentation and multiple small bowel polyps that may cause transient

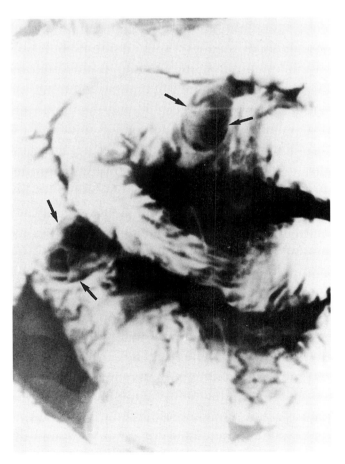

Fig. 3-24 Submucosal masses *(arrows)* represent non-Hodgkin's lymphoma in a patient with AIDS.

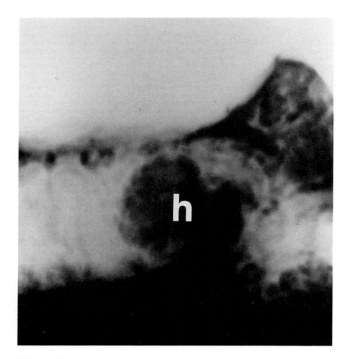

Fig. 3-25 Polypoid mass *(h)* in the jejunum represents a hamartoma in a patient with Peutz-Jeghers disease.

intussusception (Fig. 3-25). Cronkhite-Canada syndrome consists of multiple GI polyps, ectodermal abnormalities, and intestinal malabsorption. In Cowden's syndrome, GI polyps are associated with tumors of the breast, thyroid, and skin.

Multiple small bowel adenomas can occur in Gardner's syndrome. This autosomal dominant disease is characterized by diffuse adenomatous polyps of the colon and subsequent development of colon carcinoma. Extraintestinal tumors including osteomas of the facial bones, sebaceous cysts, and desmoid tumors of the mesentery also occur. Patients with Gardner's syndrome have an increased incidence of ampullary carcinoma.

Benign mesenchymal tumors of the small bowel, though usually solitary, may be multiple. This is especially true in neurofibromatosis, a genetic disease in which neural tumors can involve the skin, visceral organs, or central nervous system. Multiple neurofibromas of the small bowel in neurofibromatosis typically occur along the antimesenteric border. Small bowel lipomatosis is a rare condition characterized by multiple lipomas of the small bowel.

Carcinoid tumors exhibit variable malignant potential and are multiple in approximately one third of cases.

Other Masses

Postinflammatory polyps of the small bowel are similar to those seen in the colon in the healing stages of inflammatory bowel disease. In the small bowel, these well-defined round or branching (filiform) polyps most often involve the terminal ileum and may be secondary to Crohn's disease or, rarely, ulcerative pancolitis with backwash ileitis.

Pneumatosis cystoides intestinalis is a disorder of uncertain etiology in which multiple subserosal cystic collections of gas indent the lumen of the small bowel or colon. The radiolucent appearance of the mural masses on plain films or CT is characteristic of this benign form of intestinal pneumatosis.

Varices of the mesenteric small bowel are unusual but can produce smooth submucosal masses similar to those seen in esophageal or gastric varices.

INTRALUMINAL MASSES

Worms
Bezoars
Other foreign bodies
  Ingested
  Iatrogenic
Gallstone
Air bubbles/stool
Lipoma
Inverted diverticulum

Intraluminal masses in the small bowel include worms, bezoars, tubes, ingested foreign bodies, and calculi. Other lesions, such as pedunculated tumors and inverted diverticula, may simulate intraluminal masses.

The most common worm encountered in the small bowel is *Ascaris lumbricoides.* This roundworm is seen frequently, especially in tropical areas of the world. On contrast studies, ascaris appears as a long tubular intraluminal filling defect. A thin white line sometimes shown to bisect the length of the worm represents ingested barium in the worm's own GI tract (Fig. 3-26). Ascaris worms can be solitary or multiple, and when especially numerous, may cause a small bowel obstruction.

Tapeworms also can produce linear intraluminal filling defects on contrast exams. These flatworms are usually much longer than ascaris worms and never demonstrate a thin white line bisecting their length because they do not have a continuous GI tract.

Bezoars are uncommon in the small bowel. Phytobezoars (concretions of vegetable matter) usually result from ingestion of a large amount of high-fiber foods, such as citrus fruit. An increased incidence of

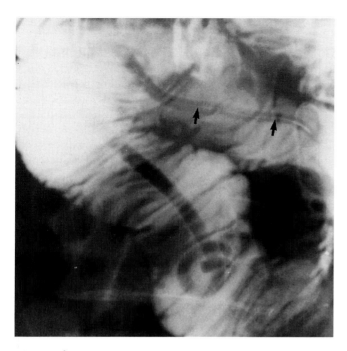

Fig. 3-26   Tubular intraluminal filling defect in the jejunum represents an ascaris worm. The thin white line bisecting part of the length of the worm *(arrows)* indicates barium in the worm's GI tract. (From Goodman P: Diagnostic radiology case number 16, Intern Med 12(7):46,55, 1991.)

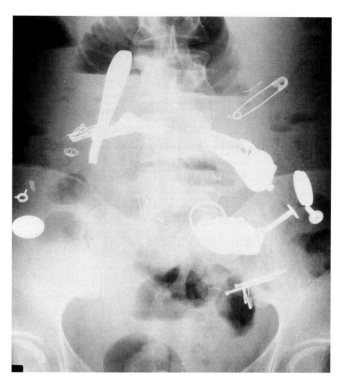

Fig. 3-27   Small bowel obstruction in a psychiatric patient who has ingested multiple metallic objects.

small bowel phytobezoars has also been reported in patients with previous gastric outlet surgery and recent ingestion of persimmons. Phytobezoars can cause an obstruction anywhere in the jejunum or ileum and may resemble a villous tumor on contrast studies as a result of barium filling numerous interstices.

Ingested foreign bodies sometimes become obstructed at the ileocecal valve because of physiological narrowing there. Prune pits have a characteristic biconvex shape. Radiopaque objects, such as coins, keys, and screws, are sometimes seen in the small bowel of psychiatric patients and are easily identified on abdominal plain films (Fig. 3-27). Ingested packets of heroin, cocaine, and other illegal drugs may appear on abdominal plain films as round or oval-shaped opacities, sometimes surrounded by a thin crescent of air (double condom sign). These drug packets may cause mechanical bowel obstruction or drug intoxication when leakage or rupture of a packet occurs.

Various iatrogenically-placed feeding or drainage catheters may become dislodged and pass into the small bowel where they appear as tubular filling defects. These include surgical or endoscopic gastrostomy and jejunostomy tubes. Balloon-tip catheters may demonstrate the inflated balloon as well as the tubular portion of the catheter (Fig. 3-28). The Garren-Ed-

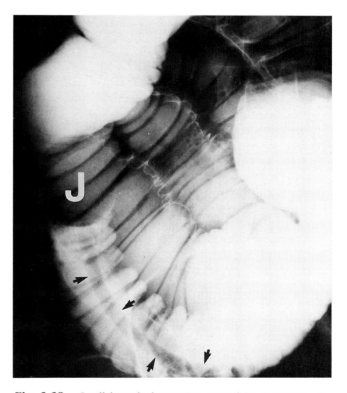

Fig. 3-28   Small bowel obstruction caused by migration of a jejunostomy tube *(arrows)* and impaction of the balloon tip *(J).*

wards gastric bubble, an intragastric balloon once used to treat morbid obesity, has also been reported to spontaneously deflate and migrate into the small bowel where it can cause obstruction.

Erosion of a gallstone into the duodenum can lead to gallstone ileus, a mechanical obstruction caused by impaction of the gallstone in the small bowel, usually at the ileocecal valve. The ectopic gallstone is visible on plain films in approximately 25% of cases. On contrast studies, it may appear as a round or oval-shaped filling defect in the distal small bowel. Associated findings include distal small bowel obstruction and air in the biliary tree (caused by reflux of air through the biliary-enteric fistula). A similar case has been reported in which a renal staghorn calculus eroded into the duodenum and subsequently became impacted at the ileocecal valve.

Air bubbles anywhere in the small bowel and fecal debris refluxed across the ileocecal valve into the distal ileum also appear as intraluminal filling defects.

A lipoma of the small bowel may become extremely pedunculated because of its soft consistency and the repeated mechanical force of peristalsis. An inverted Meckel's diverticulum may also appear almost entirely intraluminal.

EXTRINSIC PROCESSES

Adhesions
Hernias
Organomegaly
Adenopathy
Aortic aneurysm
Other masses
  Mesentery
  Peritoneum

Extrinsic compression of small bowel loops may result from adhesive bands and internal or external hernias.

Focal or diffuse enlargement of abdominal or pelvic organs and distention of other hollow viscera may compress or displace adjacent small bowel. These extrinsic masses cause a spectrum of radiographic appearances depending on their size, location, and relationship to the peritoneal cavity (Fig. 3-29). Although the mass effect typically is smooth, an extrinsic inflammatory or neoplastic mass may evoke serosal tethering or fold thickening. Marked adenopathy caused by inflammatory, infectious, or neoplastic disease can cause similar findings.

An abdominal aortic aneurysm causing extrinsic compression of small bowel may be recognized by cur-

vilinear calcifications outlining the aneurysm or by a pulsatile appearance on fluoroscopy.

Mesenteric masses (cysts, tumors, and abscesses) typically cause focal displacement of bowel loops. Mesenteric extension of leiomyosarcomas or other exoenteric masses arising from the bowel wall can also compress or displace adjacent bowel. Diffuse inflammation or infiltration of the mesentery (retractile mesenteritis, lymphoma, and metastatic disease) may produce separation of bowel loops throughout the abdomen and pelvis.

In the presence of diffuse ascites, supine films demonstrate small bowel loops floating together in the central portion of the abdomen. Focal peritoneal abscesses can produce localized mass effect and inflammation of nearby small bowel.

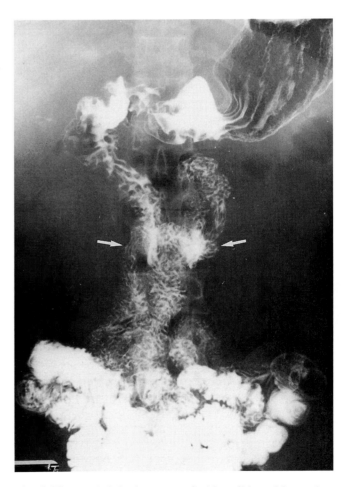

Fig. 3-29   Medial displacement of mid-small bowel loops *(arrows)* resulting from bilateral huge polycystic kidneys.

ULCERATIONS

Nonneoplastic
    Zollinger-Ellison syndrome
    Crohn's disease
    Infections
    Behçet's disease
    Sprue
    Drug-induced
Neoplastic
    Mesenchymal tumors (benign)
    Carcinoid
    Metastases
    Kaposi's sarcoma
    Mesenchymal tumors (malignant)
    Lymphoma
    Adenocarcinoma

Nonneoplastic

Marked gastric hyperacidity as seen in Zollinger-Ellison syndrome can produce an ulcer diathesis affecting the proximal duodenum and less commonly the distal duodenum and proximal jejunum. Marginal ulcerations may complicate subtotal gastrectomy with gastrojejunal anastomosis. These ulcers occur most often in patients with underlying severe peptic ulcer disease and are usually located in the efferent loop just distal to the anastomotic site.

Ulcerations as a result of Crohn's disease can affect any portion of the small bowel and demonstrate a variety of radiographic appearances. Aphthoid ulcers are small, round, and uniform and consist of a central ulceration surrounded by a radiolucent rim of edema. Deeper transverse and longitudinal ulcerations may combine to form a cobblestone pattern in which residual islands of preserved mucosa are separated by the crisscrossing transmural ulcers (Fig. 3-30).

Small bowel infections may also cause ulceration. GI tuberculosis most often involves the ileocecal area where it can cause ulcers and appear radiographically similar to Crohn's disease. CMV enteritis in AIDS may result in ileal ulceration and subsequent perforation. Ileal ulcerations are also seen in enteritis caused by *Salmonella* (typhoid fever), *Yersinia,* and *Campylobacter* organisms. Parasitic infection by the *Strongyloides* and *Anisakis* roundworms may also cause ulcers in the small bowel.

Behçet's disease is a rare systemic vasculitis in which ulcerations occur in the mouth, genitalia, eyes, and GI tract. Ileal ulcerations in this disease may appear either aphthoid or linear.

Ulcerative enteritis is an uncommon condition, ei-

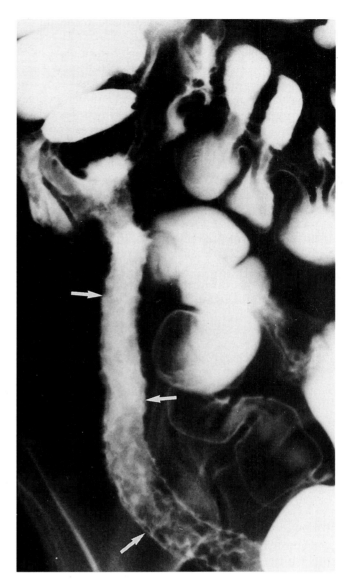

Fig. 3-30 Diffuse ulceration of the neoterminal ileum *(arrows)* represents recurrent Crohn's disease.

ther idiopathic or secondary to sprue, in which ulcerations in the small bowel may lead to fibrosis and focal stricture formation. Small bowel ulcerations can also result from mucosal irritation by ingested enteric-coated potassium chloride tablets.

Neoplastic

In addition to the many inflammatory causes of small bowel ulceration, various neoplastic masses in the small bowel can ulcerate. Benign mesenchymal tumors including leiomyomas and lipomas sometimes bleed because of ulceration of the overlying mucosa. Carcinoid tumors, which demonstrate variable malignant potential, may cause similar findings.

Ulcerating metastases to the small bowel most often result from hematogenous spread of malignant melanoma and less commonly breast carcinoma or lung carcinoma. These masses vary in size and number and may radiographically resemble bull's-eye targets because of the central location of the ulcers. Kaposi's sarcoma can produce similar ulcerated masses in the duodenum and less commonly in the mesenteric small bowel.

Leiomyosarcomas and other less common primary malignant mesenchymal tumors of the small bowel may undergo extensive necrosis and subsequent ulceration. Contrast studies and CT in these lesions demonstrate contrast material filling the large, irregular excavated portion of the mass. Lymphoma, adenocarcinoma, and hematogenous metastases may cause a similar appearance because of infiltration of the bowel wall and resultant ulceration.

FISTULAS

Crohn's disease
Tuberculosis
Radiation
Adjacent inflammatory masses
Postoperative
Malignancy

Small bowel sinus tracts and fistulas may result from extension of preexisting small bowel ulcerations. Sinus tracts and fistulas are common features of severe Crohn's disease and may form between small bowel and adjacent colon, urinary bladder, abdominal wall, or other loops of small bowel (Fig. 3-31). Similar findings can be seen in intestinal tuberculosis. Small bowel fistulas sometimes occur as a late complication of radiation therapy to the abdomen or pelvis.

Involvement of the small bowel by extrinsic processes can lead to the formation of sinus tracts or fistulas. Inflammatory masses of the gallbladder, pancreas, kidney, colon, or pelvic organs may become adherent to an adjacent loop of small bowel and erode into it.

Postoperative sinus tracts and fistulas (enterocutaneous and enteroenteric) may result from interruption or breakdown of enteric anastomoses.

Various neoplastic masses can form fistulous connections involving the small bowel. Primary tumors of the small bowel may invade adjacent bowel loops or other viscera. Likewise, tumors arising from other sites may spread contiguously to involve the small bowel.

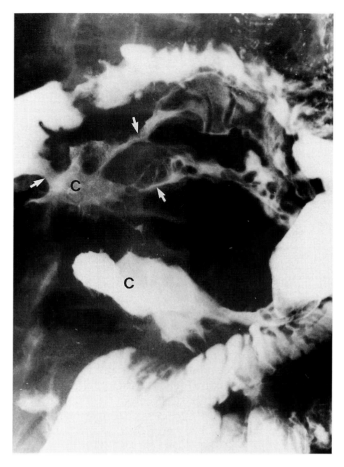

Fig. 3-31 Multiple enteric fistulae *(arrows)* and irregular barium collections *(C)* in a patient with Crohn's disease.

DIVERTICULA

Jejunal
Ileal
Meckel's
Pseudodiverticula

Jejunal and ileal diverticula are less common than duodenal diverticula. These occur along the mesenteric aspect of the bowel wall where penetrating blood vessels have produced focal defects in the muscular layer. Jejunal diverticula may be multiple and large, resulting in bacterial overgrowth (Fig. 3-32). Ileal diverticula, though often multiple, are usually small and located in the terminal portion of the ileum (Fig. 3-33). Diverticulitis, enterolith formation, hemorrhage, and

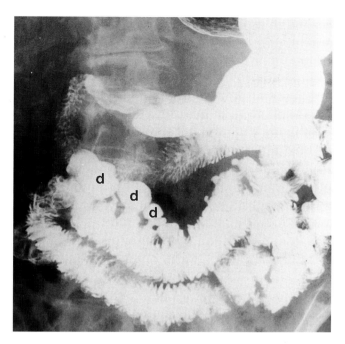

Fig. 3-32   Multiple jejunal diverticula *(d)*.

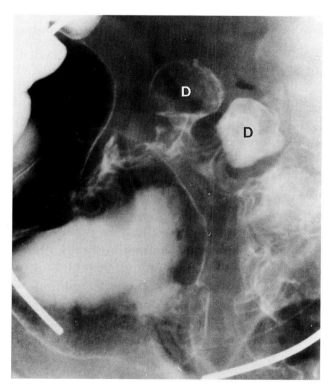

Fig. 3-33   Diverticula *(D)* of the terminal ileum.

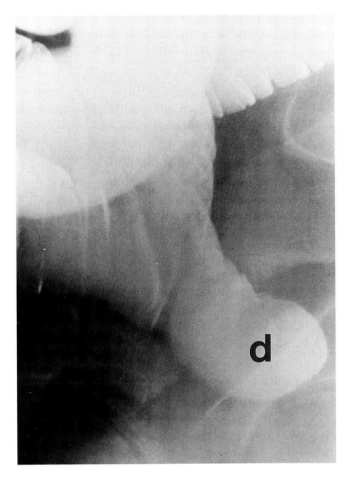

Fig. 3-34   A Meckel's diverticulum *(d)* extends from the distal ileum.

perforation are rare complications of jejunal and ileal diverticula.

Meckel's diverticulum is a congenital abnormality seen in up to 3% of people. Partial persistence of the omphalomesenteric duct results in a diverticulum along the antimesenteric aspect of the ileum, usually within 150 cm of the ileocecal valve. Meckel's diverticulum contains all layers of the bowel wall. Occasionally it first presents during adulthood with hemorrhage and abdominal pain caused by peptic ulceration of sensitive mucosa adjacent to ectopic gastric mucosa within the diverticulum. Diverticulitis, enterolith formation, perforation, and small bowel obstruction are less commonly seen manifestations of Meckel's diverticulum.

Careful fluoroscopy using graded compression is often necessary to demonstrate a Meckel's diverticulum on small bowel follow-through examination because it may otherwise be obscured by overlapping bowel loops (Fig. 3-34). Enteroclysis has proven useful for revealing Meckel's diverticula and demonstrating the characteristic triradiate fold pattern at the junction of the diverticulum and the adjacent segment of ileum. A Meckel's scan using radioactive technetium-99m pertechnetate is sensitive for detecting diverticula that contain ectopic gastric mucosa.

Various abnormalities in the mesenteric small bowel may mimic diverticula. Scleroderma and Crohn's disease may produce asymmetric fibrosis of the bowel wall with subsequent pseudosacculations (Figs. 3-35 and 3-36). Surgically created blind loops and communicating congenital duplications of the small bowel can also resemble diverticula.

In lymphoma, focal aneurysmal dilatation of the lumen, either fusiform or asymmetric, may result from destruction of the autonomic neural plexus by tumor infiltration. Focal saccular dilatation of the ileum may also be seen in ileal dysgenesis, a rare condition of uncertain etiology.

PNEUMATOSIS INTESTINALIS

Idiopathic
Ischemia/infarction
Infection
Inflammation (noninfectious)
Obstruction
Perforation
Trauma (iatrogenic)
Collagen vascular disease
Malabsorption
Pulmonary disease
Steroid therapy

Pneumatosis intestinalis indicates air in the bowel wall. This is idiopathic in approximately 15% of cases and secondary to various underlying diseases in the remaining 85%. Patients with idiopathic pneumatosis are asymptomatic, and the air collections are cystic in appearance. In secondary pneumatosis, the air collections are linear, and the patients usually have signs or symptoms of GI or pulmonary disease (Fig. 3-37).

Small bowel ischemia or infarction can cause mucosal necrosis and extension of luminal air into the bowel wall (Fig. 3-38). Air in the mesenteric and portal veins or pneumoperitoneum may follow with a high incidence of morbidity and mortality.

Infectious and noninfectious enteritis may also cause pneumatosis because of luminal air passing into the bowel wall through mucosal ulcerations. Other factors including luminal distention proximal to strictures and infection of the bowel wall by gas-forming organisms may also play a role in the development of pneumatosis in these cases.

Pneumatosis has been reported following focal perforation of a small bowel diverticulum and iatrogenic

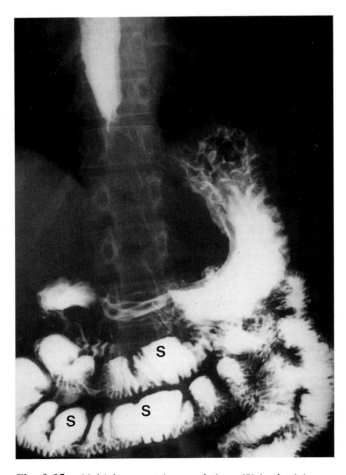

Fig. 3-35 Multiple eccentric sacculations *(S)* in the jejunum in a patient with scleroderma. Note the retained barium in the distal esophagus.

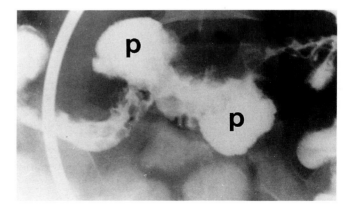

Fig. 3-36 Pseudosacculations *(p)* in the small bowel in a patient with Crohn's disease.

---

trauma caused by indwelling catheters or previous enteric anastomoses. Scleroderma, celiac disease, and other related conditions are rarely complicated by pneumatosis of the small bowel.

Obstructive pulmonary disease can produce pneumatosis secondary to alveolar rupture and subsequent passage of air along interstitial pathways to the mediastinum and, through defects in the diaphragm, to the retroperitoneum, mesentery, and bowel wall.

Pneumatosis has also been reported in patients receiving steroids but may actually be related to the patients' underlying disease rather than to the steroids themselves.

POSTOPERATIVE SMALL BOWEL

Resection
Anastomoses
Intestinal bypass
Stomas and reservoirs

Segmental resection of small bowel with end-to-end anastomosis is a commonly performed procedure in cases of small bowel infarction, perforation, or stenosis. The most frequent complication of this procedure is development of adhesions. In Crohn's disease, segmental small bowel resection is usually avoided whenever possible because of the high incidence of recurrent disease or fistulas at the margins of resection.

Various enteric anastomoses to the stomach, colon, biliary tree, and pancreas have been described. In Bill-

roth II subtotal gastrectomy, afferent and efferent loops of small bowel are anastomosed to the greater curvature of the gastric remnant. The afferent loop has a closed end and consists of the duodenum and a variable length of proximal jejunum. Current surgical construction of the anastomosis favors emptying of the stomach into the efferent loop, thereby avoiding distention of the afferent loop (afferent loop syndrome). A Roux-en-Y anastomosis can be performed simultaneously, connecting the afferent loop to the efferent loop beyond the gastrojejunostomy site. This prevents bile in the duodenum from refluxing into the gastric remnant where it may cause severe bile reflux gastritis.

Following the Billroth II procedure, several complications involving the small bowel may occur. Marginal ulcerations representing peptic ulceration of the jejunal mucosa typically involve the efferent loop just distal to the gastrojejunal anastomosis. In afferent loop syndrome, continued distention of the afferent loop may lead to bacterial overgrowth. Gastrojejunal and jejunogastric intussusception are unusual complications resulting from antegrade or retrograde intussusception at the anastomotic site.

In cases of gastric outlet obstruction, gastrojejunostomy can be used to bypass narrowing of the distal stomach, pylorus, or duodenum. Gastrojejunostomy is also performed in gastric bypass procedures for morbid obesity. Staples form a small gastric pouch that is then anastomosed side-to-side with a loop of proximal jejunum. Important complications of this procedure in-

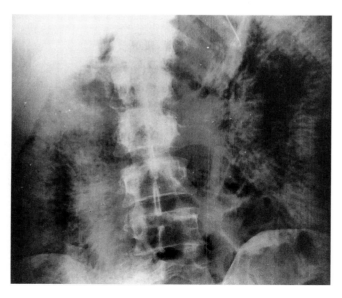

Fig. 3-37 Diffuse linear collections of air in the small bowel wall represent pneumatosis intestinalis.

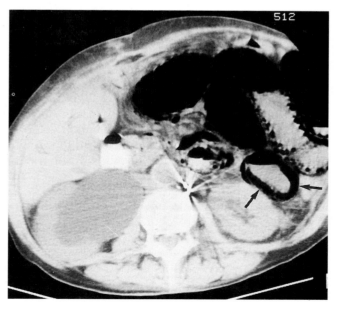

Fig. 3-38 CT shows extensive intramural air *(arrows)* surrounding intraluminal fluid in a patient with small bowel infarction.

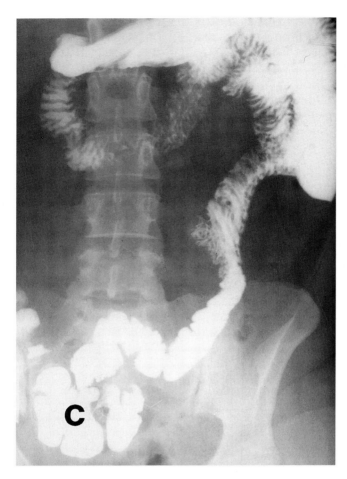

Fig. 3-39 Shortened small bowel secondary to intestinal bypass surgery for obesity. The cecum *(C)* is filled early in the examination.

clude anastomotic leakage and obstruction.

Intestinal bypass procedures were once used for treating morbid obesity but have now been abandoned because of the high incidence of complications (Fig. 3-39). Because of the decreased length of functioning small bowel, malabsorption occurred with subsequent development of gallstones, renal oxalate stones, and liver disease. Bacterial overgrowth also occurred in the lengthy bypassed segment (blind loop syndrome).

Various ileostomy procedures have been developed for patients with total colectomy. The conventional ileostomy consists of a loop of ileum that is brought to the skin surface and empties into a bag. Kock's continent ileostomy represents a surgically created internal ileal pouch just beneath the abdominal wall. In the Kock's continent ileostomy, a segment of ileum acts as a valve, and the patient empties the pouch by intubating it at regular intervals.

Ileoanal reservoir represents anastomosis of the ileum to the distal rectum following resection of rectal mucosa. After the ileum is folded upon itself in the shape of a J or S, the ileal pouch is created and ileoanal anastomosis is performed.

SUGGESTED READINGS
Small Bowel

Balthazar EJ, Gordon R, Hulnick D: Ileocecal tuberculosis: CT and radiologic evaluation, *AJR* 154:499-503, 1990.

Berk RN, Lee FA: The late manifestations of cystic fibrosis of the pancreas, *Radiology* 106:377-381, 1973.

Berk RN, Wall SD, McArdle CB, et al: Cryptosporidiosis of the stomach and small intestine in patients with AIDS, *AJR* 143:549-554, 1984.

Buck JL, Sobin LH: Carcinoids of the gastrointestinal tract, *Radiographics* 10:1081-1095, 1990.

Carlson HC, Breen JF: Amyloidosis and plasma cell dyscrasias: gastrointestinal involvement, *Semin Roentgenol* 21:128-138, 1986.

Dodds WJ, Geenen JE, Stewart ET: Eosinophilic enteritis, *Am J Gastroenterol* 61:308-312, 1974.

Dudiak KM, Johnson CD, Stephens DH: Primary tumors of the small intestine: CT evaluation, *AJR* 152:995-998, 1989.

Gardiner R, Smith C: Infective enterocolitides, *Radiol Clin North Am* 25:67-78, 1987.

Glick SN: Crohn's disease of the small intestine, *Radiol Clin North Am* 25:25-45, 1987.

Goldberg HI, Sheft DJ: Abnormalities in small intestine contour and caliber, *Radiol Clin North Am* 14:461-475, 1976.

Gramm HF, Vincent ME, Braver JM: Differential diagnosis of tubular small bowel, *Curr Imaging* 2:62-68, 1990.

Herlinger H: The small bowel enema and the diagnosis of Crohn's disease, *Radiol Clin North Am* 20:721-742, 1982.

Herlinger H: Why not enteroclysis? *J Clin Gastroenterol* 4:277-283, 1982.

Herlinger H, Maglinte DDT: Jejunal fold separation in adult celiac disease: relevance of enteroclysis, *Radiology* 158:605-611, 1986.

Herlinger H, O'Riordan D, Saul S, et al: Nonspecific involvement of bowel adjoining Crohn disease, *Radiology* 159:47-51, 1986.

James S, Balfe DM, Lee JKT, et al: Small-bowel disease: categorization by CT examination, *AJR* 148:863-868, 1987.

Jones B, Kramer SS, Saral R, et al: Gastrointestinal inflammation after bone marrow transplantation: graft-versus-host disease or opportunistic infection? *AJR* 150:277-281, 1988.

Kelvin FM, Gedgaudas RK, Thompson WM, et al: The peroral pneumocolon: its role in evaluating the terminal ileum, *AJR* 139:115-121, 1982.

Levin B: Mechanical small bowel obstruction, *Semin Roentgenol* 8:281-297, 1973.

Libshitz H, Lindell MM, Dodd GD: Metastases to the hollow viscera, *Radiol Clin North Am* 20:487-499, 1982.

Lund EC, Han SY, Holley HC, et al: Intestinal ischemia: comparison of plain radiographic and computed tomographic findings, *Radiographics* 8:1083-1108, 1988.

Maglinte DDT, Chernish SM, DeWeese R, et al: Acquired jejunoileal diverticular disease: subject review, *Radiology* 158:577-580, 1986.

Maglinte DDT, Herlinger H, Nolan DJ: Radiologic features of closed loop obstruction: analysis of 25 confirmed cases, *Radiology* 179:383-387, 1991.

Maglinte DDT, Lappas JC, Kelvin FM, et al: Small bowel radi-

ography: how, when, and why? *Radiology* 163:297-305, 1987.

Marshak RH, Lindner AE: Malabsorption syndrome, *Semin Roentgenol* 1:138-177, 1966.

Megibow AJ, Balthazar EJ, Hulnick DH: Radiology of nonneoplastic gastrointestinal disorders in acquired immune deficiency syndrome, *Semin Roentgenol* 22:31-41, 1987.

Merine D, Fishman EK, Jones B, et al: Enteroenteric intussusception: CT findings in nine patients, *AJR* 148:1129-1132, 1987.

Merine D, Fishman EK, Jones B: CT of the small bowel and mesentery, *Radiol Clin North Am* 27:707-715, 1989.

Meyers MA: Metastatic seeding along the small bowel mesentery. Roentgen features, *AJR* 123:67-73, 1975.

Orel SG, Rubesin SE, Jones B, et al: Computed tomography vs barium studies in the acutely symptomatic patient with Crohn disease, *J Comput Assist Tomogr* 11:1009-1016, 1987.

Ott DJ, Chen YM, Gelfand DW, et al: Detailed per-oral small bowel examination vs. enteroclysis, *Radiology* 155:29-34, 1985.

Perez C, Llaugher J, Puig J, et al: Computed tomographic findings in bowel ischemia, *Gastrointest Radiol* 14:241-245, 1989.

Pozniak MA, Scanlan K, Yandow D: Ultrasound in the evaluation of bowel disorders, *Semin Ultrasound CT MR* 8:366-384, 1987.

Rubesin SE, Gilchrist AM, Bronner M, et al: Non-Hodgkin lymphoma of the small intestine, *Radiographics* 10:985-998, 1990.

Rubesin SE, Herlinger H, Saul SH, et al: Adult celiac disease and its complications, *Radiographics* 9:1045-1066, 1989.

Scatarige JC, Allen III HA, Fishman EK: Computed tomography of the small bowel, *Semin Ultrasound CT MR* 8:403-423, 1987.

Schatzki R: Small intestinal enema, *AJR* 50:743-751, 1943.

Schwartz S, Boley S, Schultz L, et al: A survey of vascular diseases of the small intestine, *Semin Roentgenol* 1:178-218, 1966.

Seaman WB, Fleming RJ, Baker DH: Pneumatosis intestinalis of the small bowel, *Semin Roentgenol* 1:234-242, 1966.

Teixidor HS, Honig CL, Norsoph E, et al: Cytomegalovirus infection of the alimentary canal: radiologic findings with pathologic correlation, *Radiology* 163:317-323, 1987.

Wiot JF: Intramural small intestinal hemorrhage—a differential diagnosis, *Semin Roentgenol* 1:219-233, 1966.

Yeh H-C, Rabinowitz JG: Ultrasonography of gastrointestinal tract, *Semin Ultrasound CT MR* 3:331-347, 1982.

CHAPTER 4

Pancreas

EXAMINATION TECHNIQUES

The pancreas is a midline retroperitoneal structure located diagonally in the upper abdomen. It consists of the head and uncinate process, body, and tail, and lies in close proximity to the stomach, duodenum, left kidney, spleen, aorta, inferior vena cava, portal and splenic veins, and superior mesenteric vessels.

The pancreas performs important exocrine and endocrine functions. Alkaline fluid secreted into the duodenum through the pancreatic duct neutralizes gastric acid, and the enzymes amylase and lipase aid in the digestion of carbohydrates and fats, respectively. Various hormones, most importantly insulin, glucagon, and gastrin, are formed in the pancreatic islets of Langerhans and are secreted directly into the bloodstream to regulate glucose metabolism (insulin and glucagon) and gastric acid secretion (gastrin).

Abdominal plain films are useful for demonstrating pancreatic calcifications. Upper gastrointestinal (UGI) series shows deformity of the stomach and duodenum secondary to adjacent pancreatic inflammatory or neoplastic disease. Duodenal and proximal jejunal ulcers may also result from hypersecretion of gastric acid in response to a pancreatic gastrinoma (Zollinger-Ellison syndrome). Various methods of hypotonic duodenography have been developed for improved distention of the duodenum and visualization of ampullary and pancreatic head masses.

Cross sectional imaging technique revolutionized pancreatic imaging by allowing direct visualization of the pancreas. Percutaneous drainage of pancreatic or peripancreatic fluid collections and aspiration or biopsy of pancreatic masses are also widely performed using ultrasound guidance or computed tomography (CT) guidance.

Ultrasound of the normal pancreas usually shows homogeneous echogenicity that equals or slightly ex-

ceeds that of the normal liver. Reported measurements of the normal pancreas vary but currently accepted values are 2.6 cm for anteroposterior (AP) diameter of the head, 2.2 cm for that of the body, and 1.5 cm for that of the tail. Advantages of ultrasound compared with CT include lower cost, absence of ionizing radiation, and multiplanar imaging capabilities. The main disadvantage of ultrasound is poor visualization of the pancreas secondary to obesity or overlying bowel gas. Interference by bowel gas may be overcome by having the patient ingest water, thereby distending the stomach and duodenum and forming an acoustic window. Intravenous injection of glucagon may aid sonographic visualization of the pancreas by decreasing intestinal motility. Supplemental examination in prone, decubitus, upright, or oblique positions may be necessary to evaluate the pancreas completely.

Optimal CT demonstration of the pancreas requires a sufficient amount of oral contrast material to opacify the adjacent stomach, duodenum, and proximal jejunum. Rapid infusion of intravenous contrast material provides opacification of adjacent blood vessels and enhancement of the pancreatic parenchyma (Fig. 4-1). Although 10-mm thick axial images are routinely used for evaluating the pancreas, dynamic scanning allows rapid acquisition of contiguous 5-mm or 3-mm thick axial images during peak vascular enhancement. CT is not limited by obesity or overlying bowel gas, and it provides excellent evaluation of associated peripancreatic and extrapancreatic extension of disease.

Magnetic resonance imaging (MRI) of the pancreas offers the advantages of multiplanar imaging capabilities, absence of ionizing radiation, and differentiation between tissue and flowing blood. However, disadvantages include high cost and inability to visualize calcifications. Intravenous injection of glucagon decreases motion artifacts caused by intestinal motility, and various negative and positive contrast agents are available for bowel opacification. Nevertheless, CT is still consid-

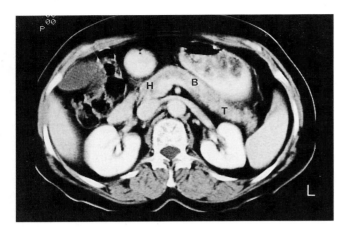

Fig. 4-1   CT demonstrates the normal pancreatic head *(H)*, body *(B)*, and tail *(T)*.

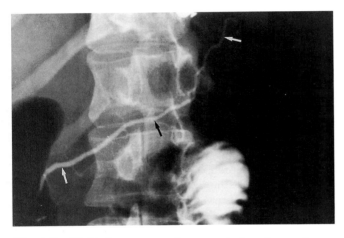

Fig. 4-2   ERCP shows a normal pancreatic duct *(arrows)*.

ered superior to MRI for evaluating the pancreas.

Endoscopic retrograde cholangiopancreatography (ERCP) remains the best method for evaluating the pancreatic duct (Fig. 4-2). Coexistent disease of the biliary tree (e.g. common bile duct narrowing secondary to pancreatic carcinoma, or choledocholithiasis causing pancreatitis) can also be evaluated by ERCP. ERCP is contraindicated in acute pancreatitis because overinjection of the pancreatic duct may cause parenchymal opacification (acinarization) and worsening of pancreatitis. Other disadvantages of ERCP relate to complications of endoscopy in general and potential trauma to the ampulla of Vater during duct cannulation.

Pancreatic angiography for evaluation of pancreatic carcinoma has been largely supplanted by ultrasound and CT. However, both superselective subtraction arteriography and venous sampling are still used for localizing small insulinomas and other functioning islet cell tumors.

Endoscopic ultrasound is a relatively new method that has shown promising results in the detection of pancreatic lesions. The instrument consists of an ultrasound transducer attached to the tip of an endoscope. After positioning the transducer against the gastric or duodenal wall, images of the adjacent pancreas are obtained.

PANCREATIC SIZE

Enlarged
   Pancreatitis
      Acute
      Chronic
   Malignancy
   Fatty infiltration
Atrophic
   Normal aging
   Chronic pancreatitis
   Pancreatic duct obstruction
   Cystic fibrosis
   Other abnormalities

Enlarged

Acute pancreatitis often causes diffuse or focal enlargement of the pancreas secondary to inflammation and edema. Clinically, acute pancreatitis is characterized by abdominal pain radiating to the back. Serum amylase and lipase levels are elevated, and the serum calcium level is often reduced. Acute pancreatitis, although most often occurring secondary to alcohol ingestion or gallstone disease, may also result from various infections, medications, surgical or nonsurgical trauma, and metabolic or systemic disorders.

Abdominal plain films may demonstrate generalized or focal ileus (sentinel loop and colon cut-off sign) or abdominal fat necrosis in which hydrolyzed fat produces a mottled appearance. Chest film findings include basilar subsegmental atelectasis, pleural fluid, and elevation of the left hemidiaphragm. On UGI series, acute pancreatitis may cause widening of the duodenal sweep, thickening of duodenal folds, effacement of folds or a reverse-figure 3 configuration along the inner aspect of the duodenal sweep, enlargement of the major papilla, or anterior displacement of the stomach. These findings are not specific for acute pancreatitis and may also be seen in chronic pancreatitis and in pancreatic carcinoma.

Ultrasound of acute pancreatitis typically demonstrates diffuse or focal pancreatic enlargement, hypoechoic parenchyma, and poorly defined contour. However, ultrasound in these patients is frequently limited by overlying bowel gas caused by intestinal ileus. CT of acute pancreatitis, in addition to showing enlargement and poorly defined contour of the pancreas, may also reveal inflammatory infiltration of peripancreatic and extrapancreatic fat and fascial planes. The pancreatic parenchyma usually shows decreased attenuation secondary to edema or necrosis but on contrast-enhanced scans may appear diffusely hyperdense because of hyperemia. In acute hemorrhagic pancreatitis, a severe form of pancreatitis characterized by parenchymal hemorrhage, inflammation, and destruction, focal areas of increased attenuation are often seen on CT. Both ultrasound and CT are useful for detecting various pancreatic and extrapancreatic fluid collections associated with acute pancreatitis.

ERCP is usually contraindicated in the evaluation of acute pancreatitis because overinjection and manipulation of the pancreatic duct may worsen the pancreatitis.

Chronic pancreatitis is characterized by irreversible destruction of the pancreatic parenchyma. Like acute pancreatitis, chronic pancreatitis may cause focal or diffuse pancreatic enlargement. Common clinical manifestations include abdominal pain radiating to the back and severe diabetes mellitus. Amylase and lipase levels may be elevated, normal, or decreased. Chronic pancreatitis most often results from long-term alcohol ingestion but also occurs secondary to hereditary pancreatitis, trauma, hyperparathyroidism, and malnutrition.

Abdominal films commonly show focal or diffuse pancreatic ductal calculi. Most of the plain film and UGI findings seen in acute pancreatitis may also occur in chronic pancreatitis.

Ultrasound and CT may demonstrate focal or diffuse pancreatic enlargement during acute relapses of chronic pancreatitis. With progression of the disease, diffuse parenchymal atrophy and ductal dilatation result. Ultrasound may demonstrate irregular echogenicity with hyperechoic and hypoechoic areas secondary to fibrosis and edema, respectively. These alterations in parenchymal echo-texture are a sensitive but nonspecific sign of chronic pancreatitis. Other findings of chronic pancreatitis seen on ultrasound and CT include ductal calculi, pseudocysts and other fluid collections, and biliary ductal dilatation.

ERCP is useful in assessing severity and complications of chronic pancreatitis. Typical findings involving

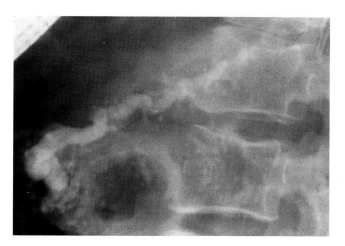

Fig. 4-3   Dilated, tortuous main pancreatic duct and dilated side branches in a patient with chronic pancreatitis.

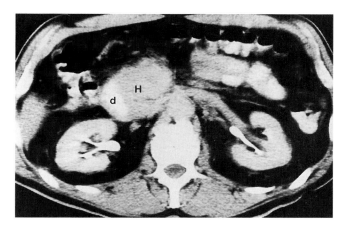

Fig. 4-4   Enlargement of the pancreatic head *(H)* represents pancreatic adenocarcinoma. The adjacent duodenum *(d)* is opacified.

the pancreatic duct include dilatation, irregularity, or beading of the main duct; dilatation of side branches; periampullary ductal stenosis; and filling defects or obstruction caused by ductal calculi (Fig. 4-3). Opacification of the biliary tree during ERCP or percutaneous transhepatic cholangiography (PTC) may reveal smooth stenosis or extrinsic displacement of the common bile duct.

Pancreatic carcinoma, islet cell tumors, and various other neoplasms may cause focal enlargement of the pancreas (Fig. 4-4). Involvement of peripancreatic nodes secondary to lymphoma or metastatic disease may mimic focal or diffuse enlargement of the pancreas itself.

Pancreatic lipomatosis is a disorder in which the parenchyma of the exocrine pancreas is partially or completely replaced by fat. Rarely, massive pancreatic enlargement results from lipomatosis in the form of either diffuse fatty infiltration or multiple nodular fatty masses. This condition, known as lipomatous pseudohypertrophy of the pancreas, is of uncertain etiology but may result from various factors including obesity, cystic fibrosis, diabetes mellitus, alcoholic cirrhosis, and chronic pancreatitis.

Atrophic

The pancreas normally decreases in size with aging and may appear atrophic in elderly patients (without a history of pancreatic disease). Associated findings include pancreatic ductal dilatation and fatty infiltration of the parenchyma.

Chronic pancreatitis often leads to diffuse atrophy of the pancreatic parenchyma. This is associated with parenchymal fibrosis, ductal dilatation, and ductal calculi.

Long-standing obstruction of the pancreatic duct may result in parenchymal atrophy adjacent to the dilated segment of the duct. The obstruction may be the result of an impacted calculus or a benign or malignant tumor and may be located at the ampulla of Vater or anywhere along the course of the pancreatic duct.

Cystic fibrosis (mucoviscidosis) is a common genetic (autosomal recessive) disorder in which abnormally thick mucous secretions lead to pulmonary, pancreatic, and GI dysfunction. The disease may first become evident in the neonate as meconium ileus or in childhood or early adulthood as recurrent pneumonia and progressive pulmonary or pancreatic insufficiency.

In the pancreas, mucus precipitates in the ducts and obstructs the secretion of pancreatic enzymes into the duodenum. This leads to intestinal malabsorption and steatorrhea as well as eventual fibrotic or fatty replacement of the exocrine pancreatic parenchyma. The pancreas may become diffusely atrophic with or without fatty replacement.

Congenital pancreatic hypoplasia (Schwachman syndrome) is a rare genetic disorder characterized by abnormalities of the exocrine pancreas similar to those seen in cystic fibrosis. In pancreatic hypoplasia, atrophy and fatty replacement of the pancreas are associated with various skeletal and hematological abnormalities.

Viral infection, hemochromatosis, and malnutrition may also cause atrophy and fatty replacement of the pancreas.

PANCREATIC MASSES

Solid
   Focal pancreatitis
   Phlegmon
   Ductal adenocarcinoma
   Acinar cell carcinoma
   Other epithelial tumors
   Islet cell tumors
   Lymphoma
   Other nonepithelial tumors
   Metastases
Cystic
   Focal pancreatitis
   Acute fluid collection
   Pseudocysts
   Retention cysts
   Necrosis/abscess
   Congenital cysts
   Microcystic adenoma
   Mucinous cystic neoplasms
   Mucinous pancreatic duct ectasia
   Solid and papillary epithelial neoplasms
   Other cystic tumors

Solid

Acute pancreatitis, though usually a diffuse process, may cause focal enlargement of any portion of the pancreas. The localized inflammatory mass may appear solid, cystic, or inhomogeneous on CT and hyperechoic, normal, or hypoechoic on ultrasound. Focal pancreatic enlargement may also be seen in chronic pancreatitis.

Pancreatic phlegmon represents diffuse pancreatic enlargement and peripancreatic inflammation secondary to acute pancreatitis. It appears inhomogeneous on CT and ultrasound and may resolve completely or worsen, leading to fluid collections, necrosis, or abscess formation.

Pancreatic ductal adenocarcinoma (pancreatic carcinoma) is the most common neoplasm of the pancreas (Table 4-1). It represents 80% of all tumors originating from the ductal epithelium of the exocrine pancreas. Approximately two thirds of pancreatic carcinomas arise in the head of the pancreas, and only 10% to 15% of cases are surgically resectable when first diagnosed. Even when surgical resection is performed, median postoperative survival is less than 20 months.

Clinical signs and symptoms of pancreatic carcinoma are nonspecific and may include abdominal pain, weight loss, jaundice, UGI bleeding, thrombophlebitis (Trousseau's syndrome), and new onset of diabetes mellitus or pancreatitis. Barium studies may demonstrate extrinsic compression or mural invasion of the adjacent stomach, duodenum or transverse colon. However, ultrasound and CT have proven more useful for evaluating the pancreas, pancreatic and biliary ducts, liver parenchyma, and peripancreatic nodes, thereby improving detection of pancreatic carcinoma and allowing determination of resectability. They also provide accurate guidance for percutaneous aspiration and biopsy of primary or metastatic pancreatic carcinoma.

Pancreatic carcinoma typically appears as a focal hypoechoic mass on ultrasound and a hypodense mass on CT (Fig. 4-5). Obstruction of the pancreatic duct by the mass often causes ductal dilatation and atrophy of the adjacent pancreatic parenchyma. Coexistent obstruction of the intrapancreatic segment of the biliary duct may also be seen in cases of carcinoma involving the head of the pancreas. Dilatation of both the pancreatic and biliary ducts is known as the double-duct sign. Although this may also result from intrapancreatic extension of cholangiocarcinoma, it is most commonly caused by carcinoma of the pancreatic head (Fig. 4-6).

Table 4-1 Epithelial neoplasms		
Tumor type	**Texture**	**Histology**
Ductal adenocarcinoma	Solid	Malignant
Acinar cell carcinoma	Solid (partially necrotic)	Malignant
Microcystic adenoma	Cystic (numerous small cysts)	Benign
Mucinous cystic neoplasm	Cystic (fewer and larger cysts)	Premalignant or malignant
Solid and papillary epithelial neoplasm	Solid and cystic	Malignant (low-grade)

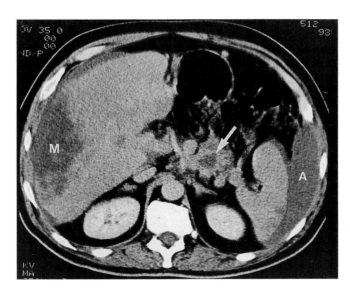

Fig. 4-5   Irregular hypodense mass in the pancreatic tail *(arrow)* represents pancreatic adenocarcinoma. Hepatic metastasis *(M)* and ascites *(A)* indicate disseminated disease.

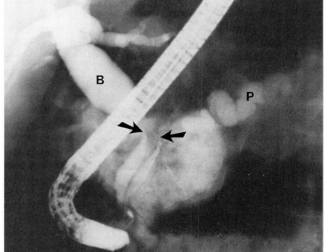

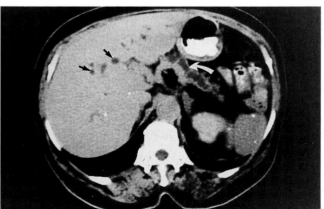

Fig. 4-6   **A,** ERCP shows adjacent narrowing *(arrows)* and proximal dilatation of the biliary *(B)* and pancreatic *(P)* ducts in a patient with pancreatic adenocarcinoma. **B,** CT demonstrates dilatation of the biliary ducts *(arrows)* and pancreatic duct *(curved arrow)*.

Various CT criteria have been established for determining unresectability of pancreatic carcinoma. These include local extrapancreatic extension of tumor, invasion of contiguous organs, hepatic or regional nodal metastases, malignant ascites, and encasement or obstruction of major peripancreatic vessels. Obliteration of fat surrounding the celiac and superior mesenteric arteries, though usually secondary to vascular encasement by pancreatic carcinoma, has been reported in chronic pancreatitis and various nonpancreatic tumors including metastatic disease and lymphoma.

ERCP findings in pancreatic carcinoma include obstruction or encasement of the pancreatic duct (Fig. 4-7). Although involvement is usually irregular and abrupt, it occasionally appears smooth and tapering, mimicking inflammatory disease. Obstruction or encasement of the biliary duct typically affects the intrapancreatic portion of the duct. Less commonly, the proximal common duct or intrahepatic ducts appear narrowed secondary to metastatic disease involving portal nodes or liver parenchyma, respectively. Opacification of an irregular cavity within the pancreas may result from tumor necrosis and subsequent communication between the tumor and the pancreatic duct. In cases of biliary duct obstruction, an internal biliary stent can be placed endoscopically during ERCP in order to achieve decompression.

Similarly, PTC may be performed in cases of biliary duct obstruction secondary to pancreatic carcinoma to detect the level and degree of obstruction. Pancreatic carcinoma may cause irregular or smooth narrowing of the biliary duct. Internal or external biliary drainage can be achieved by percutaneous stent placement immediately following PTC.

The most common angiographic finding in pancreatic carcinoma is encasement of peripancreatic arteries or veins. Less common findings include vascular occlusion, angulation, and displacement. Neovascularity is not a typical feature of pancreatic carcinoma.

Acinar cell carcinoma is a rare tumor arising from acinar cells of the exocrine pancreas (see Table 4-1). This tumor may be associated with elevated serum lipase levels and disseminated intraosseous and subcutaneous fat necrosis. Acinar cell carcinomas usually appear large, lobulated, and partially necrotic when first detected, and liver metastases are often present. Angiography shows moderate vascularity as well as vascular encasement and neovascularity.

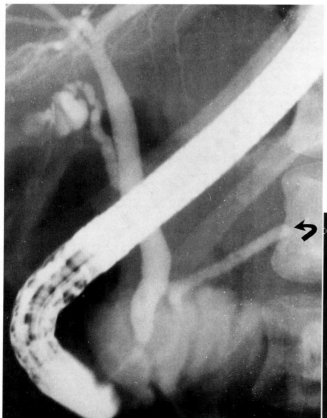

Fig. 4-7   **A,** ERCP shows abrupt occlusion of the midportion of the pancreatic duct *(arrow)* caused by pancreatic adenocarcinoma. **B,** CT reveals the dilated, obstructed duct in the pancreatic body and tail *(arrows)*.

Other rare pancreatic tumors of epithelial cell origin include pleomorphic carcinoma, adenosquamous carcinoma, and pancreatoblastoma. Radiographic findings are similar to those of pancreatic ductal adenocarcinoma.

Tumors arising from the islet cells of the pancreas produce a variety of clinical and radiographic findings. Islet cells, classified as APUD cells because of their chemical properties of **a**mine **p**recursor **u**ptake and **d**ecarboxylation, elaborate various hormones including insulin, glucagon, gastrin, and somatostatin (Table 4-2). APUD cells migrate from neural crest tissue during embryological development and are found not only in the pancreas but throughout the GI tract and in endocrine organs including thyroid, parathyroid, and adrenal medulla.

Pancreatic islet cell tumors are divided into functioning and nonfunctioning types. The functioning types are hormonally active and are further divided according to the hormone that they produce and the subset of islet cells from which they arise. Functioning islet cell tumors may be associated with multiple endocrine neoplasia type I (MEN I or Wermer's syndrome), an autosomal dominant disease characterized by hyperplasia or neoplasia of the pituitary and parathyroid glands. Islet cell tumors occur in 45% to 80% of cases of MEN I. These tumors are usually multiple and may involve any subset of islet cells. Islet cell tumors are also found in approximately 20% of patients with von Hippel-Lindau disease, an autosomal dominant syndrome that includes central nervous system hemangioblastomas, retinal angiomas, renal cell carcinoma, and pheochromocytoma.

Insulinoma, the most common type of functioning islet cell tumor, originates from the beta islet cell and produces insulin. Approximately 90% of these tumors are benign, solitary, and measure less than 2 cm in diameter at the time of diagnosis. They produce a symptom complex known as Whipple's triad, which consists of hypoglycemia central nervous system abnormalities related to hypoglycemia (including confusion, loss of consciousness, and seizures), and rapid response to oral or intravenous administration of glucose.

Clinical symptoms and laboratory evaluation usually lead to early diagnosis of insulinoma, and radiological studies are primarily indicated for localizing the tumor before surgical resection. Angiography using superselective injections can detect up to 80% to 90% of insulinomas and typically demonstrates a well-defined hypervascular mass. CT typically shows a small enhancing mass that may deform the pancreatic contour. Ultrasound reveals a hypoechoic, solid mass. Because of the small size of most insulinomas, careful technique is essential for radiographic detection (CT with dynamic bolus and thin axial slices; real-time or high frequency intraoperative ultrasound).

Gastrinoma, the second most common type of functioning islet cell tumor, arises from the alpha-1 islet cell and produces gastrin. Approximately 60% of these tumors are malignant, and 50% to 66% have metastasized when first diagnosed. Elevated serum gastrin levels produce the Zollinger-Ellison syndrome, in which increased output of gastric acid in the stomach leads to an ulcer diathesis in the duodenum and proximal jejunum. In 10% to 40% of patients with Zollinger-Ellison syndrome, pancreatic gastrinomas are associated with MEN I.

As a result of the small size and sometimes ectopic location of primary gastrinomas, imaging studies have not proven reliable in their detection. However, because gastrinomas frequently metastasize, CT and ultrasound are useful for demonstrating extrapancreatic disease and determining an appropriate course of treatment. In the absence of metastases, surgical resection of the primary tumor is curative. If metastases are present, however, gastric acid hypersecretion can be controlled by either total gastrectomy or medical treatment with histamine H_2 receptor antagonists or omeprazole.

Tumor type	Cell of origin	Hormone produced	Malignancy (% cases)	Clinical findings
Table 4-2 Functioning islet cell tumors				
Insulinoma	Beta	Insulin	10	Hypoglycemia
Gastrinoma	Alpha-1	Gastrin	60	Zollinger-Ellison syndrome
Glucagonoma	Alpha-2	Glucagon	80	Diabetes mellitus, necrolytic migratory erythema
Vipoma	Delta-1	VIP	50	WDHA syndrome
Somatostatinoma	Delta	Somatostatin	67 (4/6 reported cases)	Diarrhea, weight loss

VIP, Vasoactive intestinal polypeptide; *WDHA*, watery diarrhea, hypokalemia, and achlorhydria.

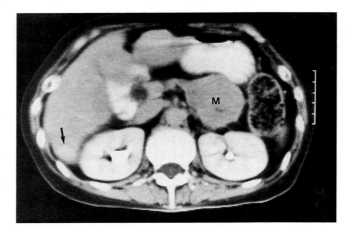

Fig. 4-8 Contrast-enhanced CT shows a large soft tissue mass *(M)* in the pancreatic tail and an enhancing mass in the right lobe of the liver *(arrow)* in a patient with metastatic pancreatic glucagonoma. (From Goodman P, Kumar R: Diagnostic radiology case number 11, *Intern Med* 12(2):46, 88, 1991.)

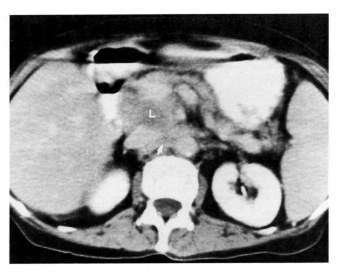

Fig. 4-9 Hypodense masses occupying the peripancreatic *(L)* and interaortocaval regions *(arrow)* represent non-Hodgkin's lymphoma.

Glucagonoma arises from the alpha-2 islet cell and produces glucagon. This slow-growing tumor is malignant in approximately 80% of cases and is often large and metastatic when first diagnosed. It usually occurs in the body or tail of the pancreas and metastasizes to the regional lymph nodes or liver (Fig. 4-8). Pancreatic glucagonomas and their liver metastases are typically hypervascular. Clinical findings include diabetes mellitus, anemia, weight loss, hypoaminoacidemia, and necrolytic migratory erythema (a recurrent skin rash that may blister and crust).

Vipoma (VIPoma) originates in the delta-1 islet cell and secretes VIP (vasoactive intestinal polypeptide). This tumor is malignant in 50% of cases and occurs most often in the pancreatic body and tail. Originally described by Verner and Morrison in 1958, vipoma produces a syndrome characterized by watery diarrhea, hypokalemia, achlorhydria, and hypovolemia (WDHA or WDHH syndrome). The primary tumor typically appears large and hypervascular on angiography.

Somatostatinoma, a rare tumor arising in the delta islet cell, produces somatostatin. Of the few reported cases of somatostatinoma, most were hypervascular, malignant, and associated with diarrhea and weight loss.

Nonfunctioning (or nonhyperfunctioning) islet cell tumors do not produce the clinical symptoms typical of their functioning counterparts. Although nonfunctioning tumors may actually secrete hormones, the type or amount of hormone produced cannot be detected or measured.

Nonfunctioning islet cell tumors are usually large

and metastatic at the time of diagnosis. They cause nonspecific clinical symptoms related to focal mass effect, including abdominal pain, jaundice, and GI bleeding or obstruction. Although typically hypervascular, nonfunctioning tumors may undergo focal necrosis because of their large size. Imaging studies are useful for demonstrating both the large primary tumor and local or distant metastases.

Lymphoma rarely occurs as a primary tumor of the pancreas. More commonly, pancreatic involvement results from secondary spread of non-Hodgkin's lymphoma. Lymphoma may affect the pancreas, peripancreatic lymph nodes, or both (Fig. 4-9). Though typically large with solid, uniform texture, pancreatic lymphoma may appear cystic or inhomogeneous on cross sectional imaging studies. Other radiographic findings of lymphoma include displacement of the pancreatic duct and vessels by the mass and displacement of the pancreas itself by adjacent peripancreatic adenopathy. Lymphoma may mimic pancreatic carcinoma but is less likely to cause vascular or ductal encasement.

Other rare pancreatic tumors of nonepithelial cell origin include hemangiomas, lymphangiomas, and sarcomas.

Metastasis to the pancreas usually occurs through contiguous spread from adjacent organs including the colon and stomach. Hematogenous metastases that may involve the pancreas include renal cell carcinoma, hepatoma, melanoma, leiomyosarcoma, and carcinoma of the breast, lung, ovary, or prostate. Pancreatic metastases are usually asymptomatic but may cause recurrent acute pancreatitis. Radiographically, pancreatic metas-

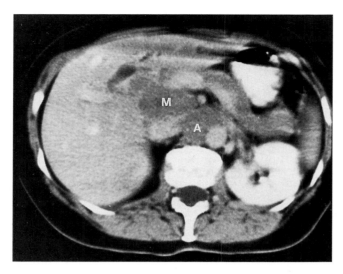

Fig. 4-10 Hypodense masses in the peripancreatic *(M)* and interaortocaval regions *(A)* represent metastatic oat cell carcinoma of the lung.

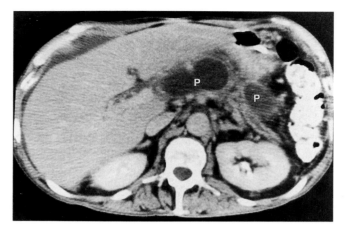

Fig. 4-11 Cystic masses *(P)* represent pancreatic pseudocysts.

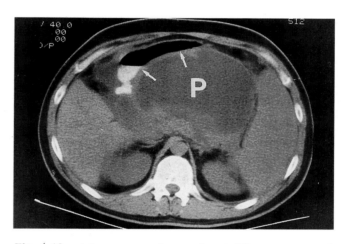

Fig. 4-12 A large pancreatic pseudocyst *(P)* compresses and displaces the adjacent stomach *(arrows).*

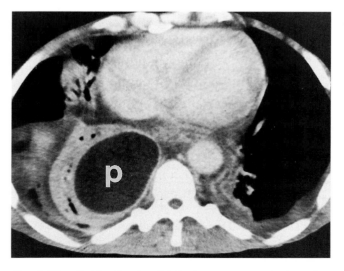

Fig. 4-13 Fluid collection *(p)* in the posterior right hemithorax represents a pseudocyst surrounded by pulmonary consolidation.

tases may appear solid or cystic and demonstrate variable degrees of vascularity. Metastatic disease involving peripancreatic lymph nodes surrounding the head of the pancreas may mimic a primary pancreatic tumor (Fig. 4-10).

Cystic

Inflammatory pancreatic cystic lesions include focal acute pancreatitis, acute fluid collections, pseudocysts, retention cysts, necrosis, and abscesses.

Focal acute pancreatitis may produce a cystic-appearing pancreatic mass resulting from localized edema. This appears hypoechoic on ultrasound and shows low attenuation on CT.

Acute fluid collections occur secondary to release of pancreatic secretions from ruptured pancreatic ductules in acute pancreatitis. These collections may be confined to the pancreas or extend into the surrounding tissues. Acute fluid collections lack a fibrous capsule.

Unlike acute fluid collections, pseudocysts are surrounded by a fibrous capsule. However, they lack an epithelial lining and therefore are not considered true cysts. Pseudocysts occur in approximately 10% of patients with acute pancreatitis but are more commonly associated with chronic pancreatitis (Figs. 4-11 and 4-12). Although usually located in the pancreas or peripancreatic region, pseudocysts may occur in areas distant from the pancreas (Fig. 4-13). Other causes of pseudocysts include trauma and surgery. Although uncomplicated pseudocysts appear cystic on CT and ultrasound, superimposed hemorrhage or infection may cause the fluid contents to appear complex or inhomogeneous.

Retention cysts result from focal obstruction of pancreatic ductules. The cysts are usually small and lined by epithelium. Although most often seen in chronic pancreatitis, retention cysts may also occur in pancreatic carcinoma, gallbladder disease, ampullary stenosis, acute pancreatitis, and various parasitic diseases associated with acute pancreatitis including ascariasis and clonorchiasis. Hydatid disease of the pancreas may demonstrate multiseptated cysts that represent the Echinococcal daughter cysts.

Pancreatic necrosis represents devitalized pancreatic tissue secondary to acute pancreatitis and resultant ischemia (Fig. 4-14). This produces diffuse or localized decrease in density of the pancreatic parenchyma on CT. Pancreatic abscess formation or fistulization to an adjacent hollow viscus may complicate pancreatic necrosis, forming gas collections within the pancreatic parenchyma in 25% of cases. Pancreatic abscess develops in approximately 4% of patients with pancreatitis and may require prompt surgical debridement and drainage.

Congenital pancreatic cysts have an epithelial lining and are therefore classified as true cysts. Solitary congenital cysts vary in size and may appear unilocular or multilocular. They are seen mostly in neonates and result from abnormal segmentation of rudimentary pancreatic ducts. CT and ultrasound demonstrate their fluid content and thin wall.

Multiple congenital cysts are usually associated with adult polycystic kidney disease, von Hippel-Lindau disease, or cystic fibrosis. Multiple pancreatic cysts occur in 10% of patients with adult polycystic kidney disease and in 25% to 72% of patients with von Hippel-Lindau disease. The pancreatic cysts occurring in cystic fibrosis represent the sequelae of chronically dilated pancreatic ductal structures.

Intrapancreatic choledochal cysts and duodenal duplication cysts are other congenital lesions that can mimic true pancreatic cysts. Duplication or enterogenous cysts of the pancreas itself are extremely rare.

Cystic tumors of the pancreas represent 5% to 15% of pancreatic cystic masses (see Table 4-1). Approximately half of these tumors are classified as microcystic adenoma (serous cystadenoma or glycogen-rich cystadenoma) and the other half as macrocystic or mucinous cystic neoplasms (mucinous cystadenoma and cystadenocarcinoma). These tumors arise from ductal epithelium of the exocrine pancreas, and together account for approximately 6% of nonfunctioning pancreatic neoplasms.

Microcystic adenomas can occur in any portion of the pancreas and are composed of numerous small

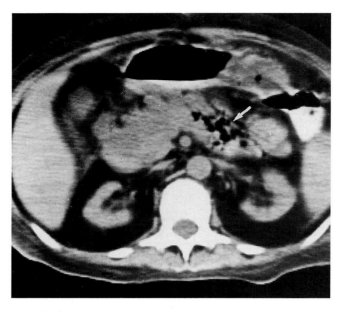

Fig. 4-14   Numerous air bubbles *(arrow)* in the pancreatic tail of a patient with pancreatitis and pancreatic necrosis.

cysts, each measuring 0.1 to 2.0 cm in diameter. The cysts are lined by low cuboidal epithelium containing glycogen. These slow-growing tumors, though often discovered incidentally, may become quite large and produce symptoms of bowel or biliary duct obstruction. About 80% of cases are first detected after age 60, and the female to male ratio is 1.5:1. Microcystic adenoma occurs with increased incidence in patients with von Hippel-Lindau disease. Though generally considered a benign lesion, a single case of malignancy in microcystic adenoma was recently reported.

CT of microcystic adenoma typically demonstrates a low attenuation mass on noncontrast scans and a honeycombed or spongy appearance on contrast-enhanced scans as a result of hypervascularity of the septa (Fig. 4-15). Overall attenuation of the mass on contrast-enhanced scans varies from solid to cystic. A central scar with or without calcification is often present.

On ultrasound, microcystic adenoma appears primarily hyperechoic or hypoechoic, depending on the size of cysts and the number of fibrous septa. Angiography typically reveals hypervascularity and neovascularity, but hypovascular lesions have also been described.

Mucinous cystic neoplasms occur most often in the tail of the pancreas and are rarely seen in the pancreatic head. They are typically composed of no more than six cysts with each cyst measuring more than 2 cm in diameter. The cysts are lined by tall columnar epithelium that produces mucin. The tumors are usually large and bulky when first detected. The mean age

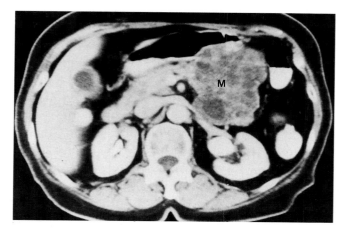

Fig. 4-15 Large mass *(M)* composed of numerous small cysts represents a microcystic adenoma of the pancreatic tail.

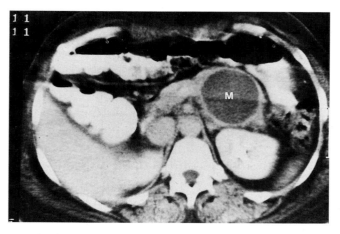

Fig. 4-16 Large unilocular cystic mass *(M)* in the pancreatic tail represents a mucinous cystic neoplasm.

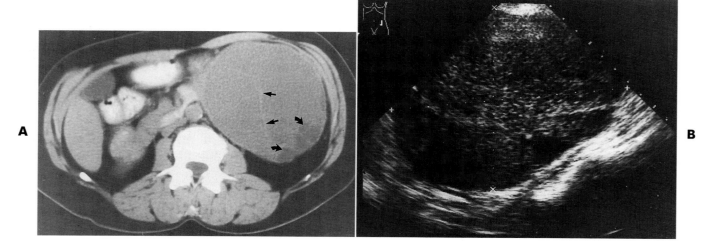

Fig. 4-17 **A,** CT shows a large cystic mass containing septations *(arrows)* and mural nodules *(curved arrows)* in a patient with mucinous cystic neoplasm of the pancreas. **B,** Ultrasound demonstrates numerous internal echoes throughout the mass.

of patients with mucinous cystic neoplasms is 50 years old, and females are affected 6 to 8 times more often than males. Mucinous cystadenoma, the benign form of mucinous cystic neoplasm, is generally considered premalignant.

CT and ultrasound of mucinous cystic neoplasms show a multilocular or, less often, unilocular cystic lesion that may contain septations, papillary projections, or mural nodules (Figs. 4-16 and 4-17). Although contrast-enhanced CT may show enhancement of the septa and cyst wall, these areas are better visualized using ultrasound. Angiography reveals a hypovascular mass, and peripheral curvilinear calcifications are found in approximately 15% of cases. In the absence of meta-

static disease, benign and malignant lesions are difficult to distinguish radiographically.

Mucinous pancreatic duct ectasia (ductectatic mucinous cystadenoma and cystadenocarcinoma) is a rare tumor of the pancreatic duct that demonstrates histological features similar to those of mucinous cystic neoplasms. This tumor consists of clusters of small thin-walled cysts that cause dilatation of the side branches of the main pancreatic duct. This tumor occurs most often in the uncinate process of the pancreas and may undergo malignant transformation.

Solid and papillary epithelial neoplasms of the pancreas (papillary cystic tumor) are rare tumors arising from acinar cells (see Table 4-1). They most often af-

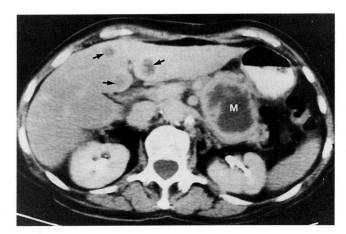

Fig. 4-18 Irregular cystic mass *(M)* represents necrotic adenocarcinoma of the pancreatic tail. Hypodense hepatic lesions *(arrows)* indicate metastases.

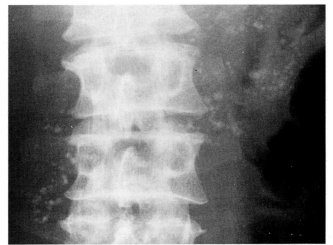

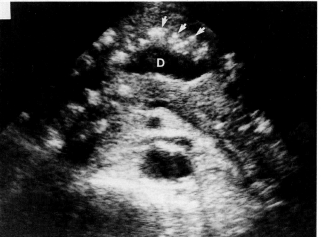

Fig. 4-19 **A,** Speckled calcifications in the midabdomen represent pancreatic calculi secondary to chronic pancreatitis. **B,** Ultrasound demonstrates a markedly dilated pancreatic duct *(D)* and multiple pancreatic calcifications *(arrows).*

fect young women and can arise in any portion of the pancreas. These large, well-circumscribed masses usually contain both solid and cystic areas resulting from focal necrosis and hemorrhage. Calcifications and septations rarely occur. These tumors are considered low-grade malignancies with good prognosis following resection.

Cystic islet cell tumors of the pancreas result from central necrosis of nonfunctioning or functioning islet cell tumors. These lesions are locally invasive and potentially or frankly malignant. A similar cystic appearance may be seen in necrotic pancreatic ductal adenocarcinoma and in metastatic lesions involving the pancreas (Fig. 4-18). Other rare pancreatic tumors that may appear cystic on radiographic studies include acinar cell carcinoma, cystic teratoma, lymphoma, hemangioma, lymphangioma, sarcoma, and various types of anaplastic carcinoma.

CALCIFICATIONS

Pancreatitis
Pseudocysts
Neoplasms
Hyperparathyroidism
Cystic fibrosis
Malnutrition
Other causes

Radiographically visible pancreatic calcifications occur in approximately 50% of patients with chronic pancreatitis secondary to alcohol ingestion. The calcifications lie within the pancreatic ducts and vary in size,

shape, and distribution (Fig. 4-19).

Hereditary pancreatitis is an unusual form of chronic pancreatitis that demonstrates autosomal dominant genetic transmission. The disease begins in childhood and recurs throughout adult life. It is characterized by a high incidence of pancreatic calculi, which typically appear larger than those occurring in other forms of chronic pancreatitis. Patients with hereditary pancreatitis have a 20% chance of developing pancreatic carcinoma.

Pancreatic pseudocysts sometimes demonstrate curvilinear calcification in the cyst wall (Fig. 4-20). These calcifications appear similar to those seen in mucinous cystic neoplasms of the pancreas.

Mucinous cystic neoplasms contain peripheral curvi-

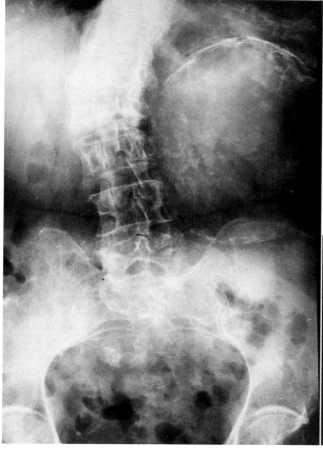

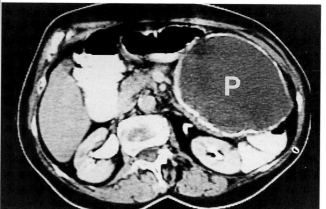

Fig. 4-20   A, Large, peripherally calcified mass in the left upper quadrant represents a pancreatic pseudocyst. **B,** CT demonstrates homogeneous cystic contents *(P).*

A

B

linear calcifications in approximately 15% of cases (Fig. 4-21). Microcystic adenomas occasionally demonstrate stellate calcification within a central fibrous scar on plain films or CT.

Dystrophic calcification may occur in solid and papillary epithelial neoplasms. Calcifications have also been reported in nonfunctioning islet cell tumors and rarely in gastrinomas associated with MEN I syndrome. Cavernous lymphangiomas of the pancreas are rare tumors that may contain calcifications in dilated lymphatic channels.

Hyperparathyroidism may cause pancreatitis and pancreatic calcifications, most likely as a result of hypercalcemia.

Pancreatic calcifications in cystic fibrosis typically appear granular and may be either focal or diffuse. Calcium precipitates within dilated pancreatic ductules secondary to obstruction by mucous plugs or within the pancreatic parenchyma secondary to extravasation of pancreatic enzymes from ruptured ductules and acini. Pancreatic calcifications in cystic fibrosis are often associated with marked pancreatic fibrosis and diabetes mellitus.

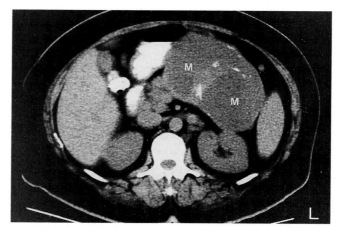

Fig. 4-21   Large cystic mass *(M)* containing partially calcified septations represents mucinous cystic neoplasm of the pancreas.

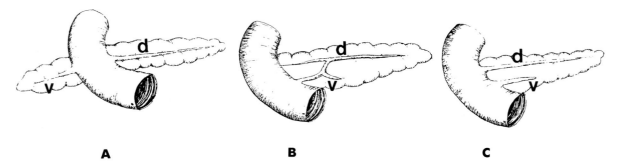

Fig. 4-22   Diagrams illustrate the relationship of the ventral *(v)* and dorsal *(d)* pancreatic ducts **A,** before fusion, **B,** following fusion, and **C,** in pancreas divisum.

In tropical countries, an idiopathic form of pancreatitis associated with pancreatic ductal calculi may result from malnutrition caused by a diet low in protein and high in carbohydrates.

Peripheral calcifications have been reported in congenital pancreatic cysts associated with von Hippel-Lindau disease. Hydatid cysts, though rarely occurring in the pancreas, may also calcify peripherally.

Other unusual causes of intraparenchymal pancreatic calcifications include previous trauma, hematoma, abscess, and infarction. A calcified aneurysm of the adjacent celiac or splenic artery may similate an intrapancreatic mass.

CONGENITAL ANOMALIES

Annular pancreas
Pancreas divisum
Ductal duplications
Ectopic pancreas
Short pancreas
High fusion of pancreatic and common bile ducts

The pancreas develops from the embryological fusion of dorsal and ventral buds of the foregut. The dorsal duct drains the body, tail, and superior portion of the head of the pancreas into the minor papilla, and the ventral duct drains the uncinate process and inferior portion of the pancreatic head into the major papilla. Following fusion of the two ducts, the main duct of Wirsung, consisting of the ventral duct and the proximal segment of the dorsal duct, continues to drain into the major papilla. The distal segment of the dorsal duct, which drains into the minor papilla, partially regresses to form the accessory duct of Santorini (Fig. 4-22).

Annular pancreas is a rare congenital abnormality in which a ring of pancreatic tissue encircles the duodenum at or above the papilla of Vater. Normally, the left ventral bud atrophies and the right ventral bud moves dorsally during growth and rotation of the duodenum. However, in annular pancreas, evidence indicates that the embryological left ventral bud persists, causing the ventral pancreas to form a ring around the duodenum. Depending on the degree of obstruction, this may present as an acute surgical condition in the newborn or be asymptomatic throughout life. Annular pancreas may also first become symptomatic in adulthood, producing epigastric pain, early satiety, and vomiting secondary to duodenal obstruction. Gastric and duodenal peptic ulcer disease and pancreatitis also occur with increased incidence in long-standing annular pancreas.

Typical findings of annular pancreas on UGI series include eccentric or concentric narrowing of the descending duodenum with associated mucosal effacement but without ulceration or mucosal destruction. The proximal duodenum may become dilated, and reversed peristalsis and dilatation of the duodenum distal to the annular narrowing have also been described. CT scan may demonstrate the annulus surrounding and constricting the descending duodenum. On ERCP, opacification of the ventral duct encircling the descending duodenum is diagnostic of annular pancreas.

Recommended treatment of annular pancreas presenting in adulthood is surgical bypass of the narrowed segment of duodenum. Simple division of the pancreatic annulus is often insufficient for relief of symptoms, because of the frequent association of duodenal stenosis and fibrosis at the site of long-standing narrowing. Division of the annulus with transection of the annular duct may also lead to pancreatitis and pancreatic fistula.

Pancreas divisum represents a common congenital abnormality of the pancreas, with an incidence of up to 11% recorded in an autopsy series. This anomaly re-

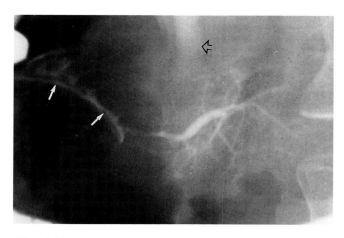

Fig. 4-23 ERCP shows a short, tapering ventral pancreatic duct, indicating pancreas divisum. The cannula of the endoscope extends into the major papilla *(arrows)*. Contrast material partially opacifies the common bile duct *(open arrow)*.

sults from failure of fusion of the embryological dorsal and ventral buds. Consequently, the dorsal and ventral ducts remain separate, with the dorsal duct draining the body, tail, and superior portion of the head of the pancreas into the minor papilla, and the ventral duct draining the uncinate process and inferior portion of the pancreatic head into the major papilla (Fig. 4-22).

On ERCP of pancreas divisum, injection of contrast material into the major papilla opacifies the short, tapering ventral duct (Fig. 4-23). Visualization and cannulation of the minor papilla is often difficult because of its small size but when accomplished demonstrates opacification of the long dorsal duct extending along the pancreatic body and tail. Thin-section CT may reveal lobulation of the pancreatic head, separation of the ventral and dorsal portions of the pancreas by a fat cleft, or failure of fusion of the ventral and dorsal ducts. Pancreatitis may occur with increased incidence in patients with pancreas divisum, possibly caused by impeded drainage of the bulk of the pancreatic parenchyma through the small minor papilla. However, the association of pancreatitis and pancreas divisum remains controversial.

Duplications of the ventral or dorsal pancreatic ducts represent rare embryological abnormalities that have been documented on ERCP.

Ectopic or aberrant pancreas (pancreatic rest) represents pancreatic tissue occurring in extrapancreatic sites, most commonly along the greater curvature of the distal gastric antrum or in the periampullary portion of the descending duodenum. The ectopic tissue is

typically small and submucosal in location. A tiny central umbilication that may represent a primitive pancreatic duct is sometimes noted. Ectopic pancreas, though usually asymptomatic, may cause GI hemorrhage or obstruction, biliary obstruction, or small bowel intussusception. Rarely, inflammatory or neoplastic pancreatic lesions may arise within ectopic pancreatic tissue.

Short pancreas is characterized by congenital absence of the pancreatic body and tail and a rounded appearance of the pancreatic head. This most likely results from agenesis of the dorsal pancreas and may occur as an isolated finding or in association with the polysplenia syndrome.

The pancreatic duct and the common bile duct normally enter the major papilla either separately or through a short common channel. Abnormally high fusion of the ducts forms a long common channel which, by allowing pancreatic secretions to reflux into the common bile duct, may predispose to the development of a choledochal cyst.

TRAUMA

Pancreatic injury occurs in 3% to 12% of patients with blunt abdominal trauma. Clinical symptoms suggesting pancreatic injury are nonspecific. However, elevated serum amylase levels are found in 90% of patients with blunt trauma to the pancreas.

Pancreatic injuries include contusion, laceration, and transection (fracture) and most often result from compression of the pancreatic body against the spine. Thin-section contrast-enhanced CT scan of the pancreas may demonstrate focal or diffuse pancreatic enlargement and extension of blood into the peripancreatic and retroperitoneal tissues. An area of decreased density perpendicular to the long axis of the pancreas may be seen immediately following trauma, suggesting a contusion or hematoma. Within hours to days, a clear zone of disruption through the pancreatic parenchyma may become evident, indicating a laceration or transection. Ultrasound is sometimes able to demonstrate these findings but frequently is limited by overlying bandages or by bowel gas secondary to intestinal ileus. Laceration of the pancreatic duct resulting from pancreatic transection is best evaluated by ERCP.

Pancreatic injury is accompanied by trauma to other visceral structures in 75% of cases and is fatal in 10% to 20% of cases. Surgical treatment of pancreatic transection usually consists of partial resection (when the body or tail is injured) or repair (when the head is injured). Complications of pancreatic trauma occur frequently and include chronic pancreatitis, pseudocysts, pancreatoenteric fistulas, and abscesses.

POSTOPERATIVE PANCREAS

Resection
Cystogastrostomy
Puestow's procedure
Pancreatic transplantation

Surgical resection of the pancreas may be partial or complete. After resection of the tail or of the body and tail, the residual pancreas appears shortened.

The standard Whipple's procedure consists of resection of the pancreatic head and neck, subtotal gastrectomy, duodenectomy, gastrojejunostomy, pancreaticojejunostomy, and choledochojejunostomy. A total rather than a partial pancreatectomy is sometimes performed, leading to severe diabetes mellitus.

Cystogastrostomy or marsupialization represents a surgical anastomosis of a pancreatic pseudocyst to the adjacent gastric wall. This procedure allows the pseudocyst to drain internally and eventually resolve. A UGI series or CT scan using oral contrast material typically demonstrates opacification of the pseudocyst through the patent anastomosis.

Puestow's procedure represents a side-to-side pancreaticojejunostomy. It is performed to allow drainage of the dilated but nonobstructed pancreatic duct in chronic pancreatitis.

Pancreatic transplantation is an increasingly performed procedure for managing patients with severe diabetes mellitus. A cadaver-donor pancreas and adjacent periampullary segment of duodenum are placed in the recipient's pelvis with vascular anastomoses to iliac vessels and duodenal anastomosis to the dome of the urinary bladder. Complications include acute and chronic transplant rejection, intraperitoneal or extraperitoneal leakage, fluid collections (hematomas, abscesses, and pseudocysts), fistulas, and various vascular abnormalities.

Cystography has proven useful for detecting anastomotic leaks and fistulas by allowing opacification of the adjacent duodenal segment (Fig. 4-24). CT is useful for evaluating intraabdominal fluid collections and providing guidance for percutaneous drainage procedures and pancreatic biopsies. MRI has shown some promising results in detecting pancreatic transplant rejection.

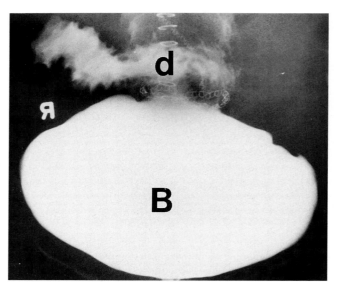

Fig. 4-24   Cystogram following pancreatic and renal transplantation shows opacification of the urinary bladder *(B)* and transplanted duodenum *(d)*.

SUGGESTED READINGS
Pancreas

Axon ATR: Endoscopic retrograde cholangiopancreatography in chronic pancreatitis: Cambridge classification, *Radiol Clin North Am* 27:39-50, 1989.

Balthazar E: CT diagnosis and staging of acute pancreatitis, *Radiol Clin North Am* 27:19-37, 1989.

Balthazar EJ, Robinson DL, Megibow AJ, et al: Acute pancreatitis: value of CT in establishing prognosis, *Radiology* 174:331-336, 1990.

Bolondi L, LiBassi S, Gaiani S, et al: Sonography of chronic pancreatitis, *Radiol Clin North Am* 27:815-833, 1989.

Buck JL, Hayes WS: Microcystic adenoma of the pancreas, *Radiographics* 10:313-322, 1990.

Burdeny DA, Kroeker MA: CT appearance of the ventral pancreas, *J Can Assoc Radiol* 39:190-194, 1988.

Clark LR, Jaffe MH, Choyke PL, et al: Pancreatic imaging, *Radiol Clin North Am* 23:489-501, 1985.

Dodds WJ, Wilson SD, Thorsen MK, et al: MEN I syndrome and islet cell tumors of the pancreas, *Semin Roentgenol* 20:17-63, 1985.

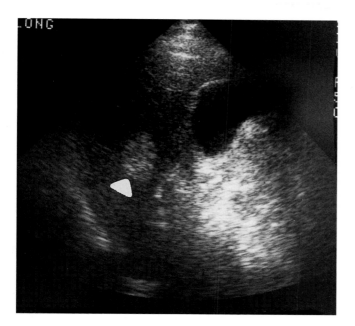

Fig. 5-11   Ultrasound of the liver shows a well-defined echogenic lesion within the liver *(arrowhead)*, representing the most common ultrasonic finding in small- to moderate-sized hemangiomas.

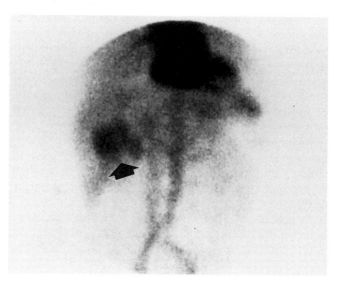

Fig. 5-13   Radionuclide tagged red blood cells demonstrate a focal area of increased uptake in the right lobe of the liver typical of hemangioma *(arrow)*.

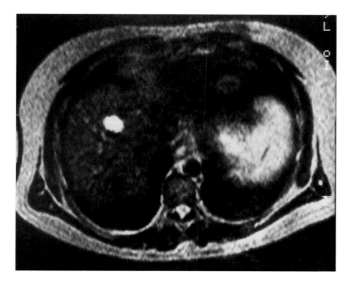

Fig. 5-12   Image obtained through the liver on T2-weighted MRI scan demonstrates a high signal intensity in a rounded hepatic hemangioma.

in small lesions. Larger cavernous hemangiomas with fibrosis and thrombus formation may also give an atypical appearance on MRI and can be confused with other liver lesions.

Radionuclide imaging utilizing tagged red blood cells has also been occasionally used in an attempt to clarify a questionable hepatic lesion that may be a hemangioma (Fig. 5-13). In similar fashion, uptake is seen at the edge of the lesion and delayed imaging shows gradual fill-in. The nuclear scan suffers from exactly the same weaknesses as that described for CT.

Although there has been a general hesitancy about doing direct aspiration biopsy of these questionable lesions, there is a slowly developing consensus that a thin needle aspiration biopsy is the method of definitive clarification and diagnosis. Relative contraindications in this diagnostic approach are patients with coagulopathies and patients in whom the lesion is immediately subcapsular in position.

Metastatic Disease

Secondary metastatic lesions to the liver are quite common. Generally, the detection of such lesions is a grave prognostic indicator. In the past, it has been observed that only about 5% of patients with untreated liver metastatic disease will survive 1 year beyond detection.

CT imaging of liver metastatic lesions has demonstrated that they come in all sizes, shapes, and numbers. The lesions can be focal or they can be diffuse. By far the most common appearance of hepatic metastatic disease on CT is a low attenuation lesion with respect to the surrounding liver, although isodense and hyperdense lesions are encountered (Figs. 5-14 and 5-15). There may be degrees of peripheral ring enhancement similar to that observed in hemangioma, although the centripetal opacification is uncommon. The central portion of the lesion may be near fluid density in lesions large enough to undergo central necrosis. Calcifications are not common and tend to be seen in younger patients with aggressive primary lesions, such as mucinous adenocarcinomas of the colon, stomach, or ovary.

In general, focal metastatic disease is not difficult to detect if the lesion is greater than 1 cm. However, metastatic disease superimposed on a fatty liver can present a diagnostic dilemma.

The diffuse form of metastatic involvement of the liver does occasionally occur and can be especially difficult if IV-contrast enhancement is not utilized. Moreover, certain types of diffuse metastatic disease that are hypervascular in nature, such as islet cell tumors and carcinoids, may become isodense during the contrast enhancement of the liver. For this reason, both preenhancement and postenhancement images of the liver are recommended for the evaluation of the liver for possible metastatic disease.

In the late 1970s, an interest in the possible resection of solitary liver metastatic lesions was revived. Indeed, this approach has resulted in increased survival times in a select subgroup of patients.

Of course, imaging techniques are not sufficiently sensitive to ensure that the liver is truly free from all disease. At best, we can attest to the fact that no metastatic disease is seen or that there is disease apparently limited to one lobe. The presence of extrahepatic nodal disease will, of course, negate the possibility of hepatic resection regardless of the state of the liver.

The increasing interest in the possibility of selective hepatic resection for metastatic disease has resulted in several attempts to refine the CT evaluation of the liver in an attempt to improve its sensitivity for metastatic disease detection.

At the moment the best approach appears to be CTAP. Most lesions are believed to be largely supplied by blood drawn from the hepatic arterial system while normal liver tissue derives most of its blood supply from the portal venous system. In CTAP, the portal system is flooded with contrast while dynamically scanning the liver. This results in increased contrast at the lesion/parenchymal interface and makes subtle, smaller, or otherwise invisible lesions more discernible. Indeed, CTAP has resulted in improved sensitivity in the detection of liver metastatic disease.

CTAP requires arterial puncture and the advance-

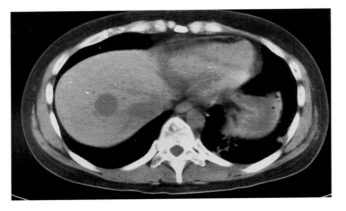

Fig. 5-14 CT through the dome of the liver demonstrates an isolated metastatic lesion.

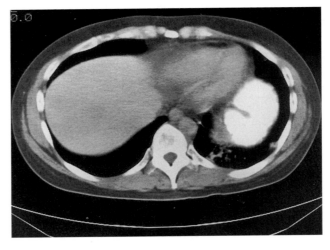

Fig. 5-15 In the same patient in Fig. 5-14 after IV administration of contrast material, the well-defined lesion seen on the preenhancement scan has become isodense.

ment of a catheter tip to the celiac axis and subsequent selective catheterization of the splenic artery or superior mesenteric artery. The splenic artery may be preferred because of dilution factors and streaming artifacts associated with superior mesenteric artery injection portography. Following placement of the catheter tip in the splenic artery, an injection bolus of 60 to 80 ml is given, followed by dynamic imaging of the liver (Fig. 5-16).

Sonography has not proven to be the diagnostic imaging method of choice for hepatic metastatic disease when CT or MRI capabilities are available. The false negative rate is generally higher than CT, and apart from distinguishing fluid from solid tissue, lesion characterization is often limited and nonspecific.

At the moment, CT continues to be the imaging modality bearing the burden for the detection of hepatic

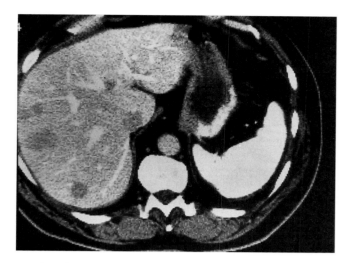

Fig. 5-16 Demonstration of CTAP with injection of the splenic artery. Note the hyperdense appearance of the spleen and a portion of the gastric wall. Several defects are now clearly demonstrated predominantly in the right lobe of the liver.

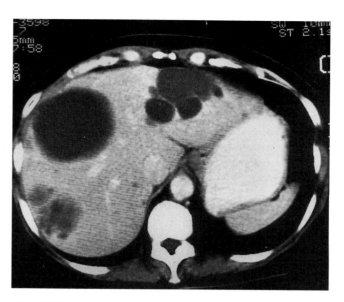

Fig. 5-17 CT scan through the liver of female patient demonstrates multiple, benign hepatic cysts of varying size.

metastatic disease. Recent studies comparing CTAP and MRI sensitivity in the detection of hepatic metastatic lesions have been conflicting. MRI sensitivities have been reported ranging between 57% to 95%. The sensitivity using CTAP has been reported around 85%.

Cysts

The simple congenital hepatic cyst is extremely common. These probably arise from developmental defects in bile duct development in utero. It is rare for these lesions to be symptomatic, and liver function is usually unaffected. They tend to be more common in females and more commonly localized to the right lobe of the liver. The size of the cyst can be quite variable from 5 mm to 10 to 12 cm. Most of these congenital cysts have an epithelial lining and are filled with clear or cloudy fluid.

Cysts can occur as an isolated hepatic lesion or as multiple lesions involving both lobes of the liver. When the cysts are multiple, concomitant cystic disease of the kidneys, pancreas, and ovaries may be present. In 20% to 50% of patients with polycystic disease of the kidneys, hepatic cysts can be identified.

CT imaging of hepatic cysts will disclose a sharp, well-circumscribed, low attenuation lesion with extremely thin or no discernible walls (Fig. 5-17). Cysts are usually round. The internal content is homogeneous and low-density with Hounsfield numbers approaching those of water. Generally, no change will occur in the internal density of the cysts with intravenous enhancement, although the cyst itself will give the ap-

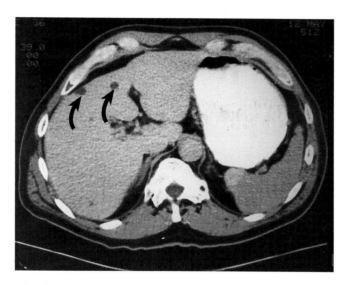

Fig. 5-18 Two small cysts *(curved arrows)* seen near the margin of the liver and measuring approximately 1 cm, confirmed by ultrasound.

pearance of being more lucent because of the increased density in the surrounding liver tissue. Very small cysts are very difficult to evaluate and are difficult to get a cursor on to obtain accurate density numbers (Fig. 5-18).

Ultrasound can often be extremely helpful in distinguishing a simple cyst from a low-density solid lesion, such as an abscess, necrotic tumor, echinococcal cyst, or a cystic neoplasm. The ultrasound characteristics are a typical focal well-defined anechoic defect within the liver, through-transmission, and acoustic enhancement of the far wall.

MRI characteristics of hepatic cysts are also characteristic with a low signal on T1-weighted images and a very high signal on T2-weighted images (Fig. 5-19). The relatively long T1 and T2 values are helpful in differentiating simple cysts from most hepatic neoplasms. It should be recalled, however, that a hemangioma can give a similar signal pattern. In addition, difficulties may also be encountered when imaging infected or bloody cysts.

Hepatocellular Carcinoma

Hepatocellular carcinoma or hepatoma is a slow growing but, nevertheless, malignant lesion originating in liver parenchymal cells. Distant metastatic involvement is unusual but has been reported. However, 75% of patients have contiguous or lymphatic extrahepatic spread of tumor at the time of diagnosis and are unresectable. In addition, portal vein thrombosis is seen in up to 50% of patients. Invasion of the hepatic venous system can result in a Budd-Chiari–type picture.

The tumor appears to be more common in females and is relatively common in the Far East with its etiology attributed to the presence of various parasites, especially liver flukes, diet, and a high incidence of hepatitis B.

In the West, the tumor is much less common. However, a very definite relationship between hepatic cirrhosis and hepatocellular carcinoma does exist with almost 75% of patients with hepatocellular carcinoma having either cirrhosis or a history of cirrhosis. There may also be an increased risk of hepatocellular carcinoma in patients with hemochromatosis of the liver.

In addition, certain other risk factors have been described. The use of oral contraception is thought to relate to an increased incidence over the last 3 decades. Moreover, in recent years, the use of anabolic steroids has thought to place individuals at an increased risk for this disease.

Patients often present with cachexia, weakness, right upper quadrant pain, and weight loss. Clinically, an enlarged liver is commonly detected.

The CT pattern may demonstrate a solitary mass or multiple masses with a dominant lesion and multiple satellite lesions. The mass is usually of low attenuation (Fig. 5-20). A small number of patients (less than 10%) may have some calcification within the lesion. In addition, the size of the lesion may be exaggerated on CT evaluation by the presence of regional portal vein thrombosis in up to 50% of patients. This may be seen on CT imaging as regional wedgelike shapes of low-density projecting peripherally.

In patients with a background of cirrhosis, involvement of the liver with hepatocellular carcinoma tends to be more diffuse and thus presents more of a diagnostic difficulty in attempting to differentiate between regenerating nodules, metastatic disease, or primary hepatic carcinoma.

Multiple patterns have been described for the ultrasonographic presentations of this lesion. These can

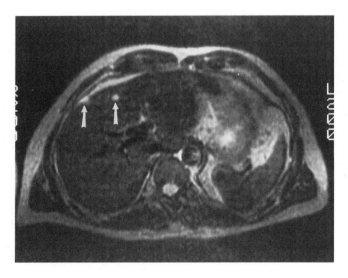

Fig. 5-19   T2 weighted MRI image of liver demonstrates two small hepatic cysts near the liver margin *(arrows)*.

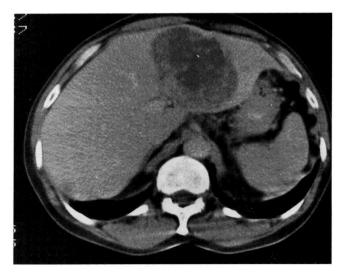

Fig. 5-20   Large inhomogeneous lesion occupying and expanding most of the left lobe of the liver, representing a hepatocellular carcinoma.

range from discrete echogenic to relatively echo-free lesions. They can have a mixed echo pattern, or there may be diffuse disease. MRI of hepatocellular carcinoma approaches CT in its accuracy. In large lesions, findings can be nonspecific and to some extent will be dependent upon the amount of fibrosis and necrosis within the lesion (Fig. 5-21). Generally, this lesion displays low-signal intensity on the T1-weighted images with an increase in signal intensity on T2-weighted images. MRI has proven to be, however, quite superior in demonstrating vascular involvement by this tumor.

Fibrolamellar hepatocellular carcinoma is a rare variety of hepatocellular carcinoma more commonly seen in younger patients. There is a tendency for intralesion calcification, and a better prognosis.

Adenomas

Hepatic adenomas are focal, well-differentiated benign lesions of the liver. They are usually solitary. Ninety percent or more of these lesions are found in females. The lesions are generally well-encapsulated. There has been an increasing incidence of hepatic adenomas over the last 3 decades, possibly relating to the increased use of oral contraception. There is also said to be an increased incidence of hepatic adenomas in some glycogen storage diseases.

Generally, the malignant potential of hepatic adenomas is considered quite low. Yet, the suspected increased incidence of hepatocellular carcinoma in the female population on birth control pills does raise the question of some degree of malignant potential.

These lesions tend to be hypervascular, and internal hemorrhage can lead to blood-filled cysts within the adenoma (Fig. 5-22). They are usually asymptomatic. When symptoms do occur, they usually occur acutely and are a result of bleeding in 50% of the cases. The adenomas can be subcapsular or pedunculated on the edge of the liver, and bleeding can occur into the peritoneal cavity, resulting in a surgical emergency. The incidence of bleeding in hepatic adenomas is increased among women taking birth control pills.

Hepatic adenomas present as discrete masses, usually solitary on dynamic CT scanning. They are commonly hyperdense. If hemorrhage or internal necrosis has occurred, the tumor can be heterogeneous in its appearance with focal areas of low attenuation (Figs. 5-23 and 5-24). Ultrasound will demonstrate variable patterns, depending on the presence of intralesional bleeding. This will result in a decreased echogenicity within the lesion. Otherwise, the adenoma will be seen as a hyperechoic solid lesion (Fig. 5-25).

Like hepatocellular carcinoma, hepatic adenomas are best demonstrated on T2-weighted MRI images.

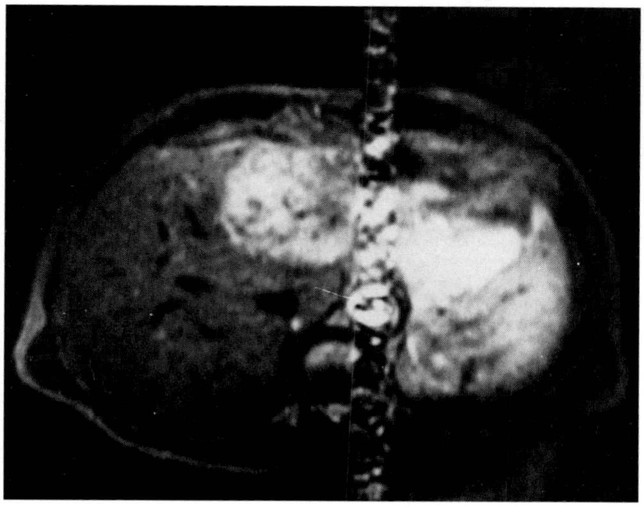

Fig. 5-21 MRI scan in the same patient as Fig. 5-20 demonstrates high signal within the lesion on T2-weighted image.

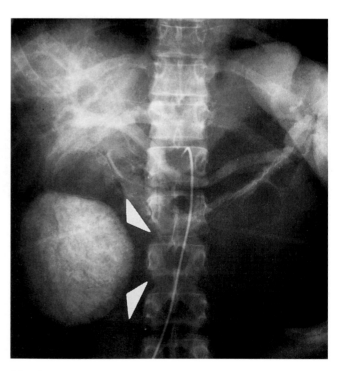

Fig. 5-22 Vascular study during venous phase on patient with pedunculated hepatic adenoma demonstrates well-defined hypervascular lesion *(arrowheads).*

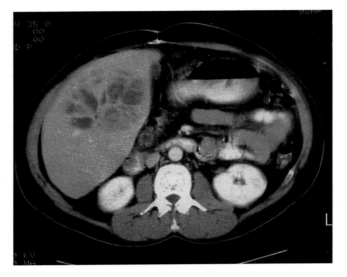

Fig. 5-23   Large heterogeneous lesion involving the lower portion of the right lobe of the liver that proved to be a hepatic adenoma in a 30-year-old female.

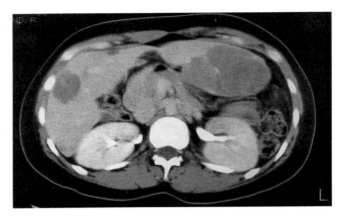

Fig. 5-24   CT scan of the abdomen obtained on a young female after abdominal trauma demonstrates multiple inhomogeneous low-density lesions of the liver that proved to be multiple adenomas.

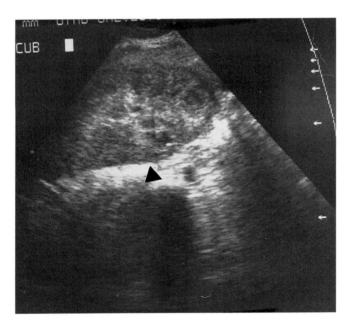

Fig. 5-25   Ultrasound in young female with hepatic adenoma demonstrates a large hyperechoic lesion *(arrowhead)*.

Focal Nodular Hyperplasia

This relatively uncommon lesion is very similar in its histological appearance to hepatic adenoma. The etiological origins are unclear. Unlike hepatic adenomas, there is much less of a tendency for the lesion to bleed or rupture. Generally, focal nodular hyperplasia (FNH) is asymptomatic. A small proportion of the patients may have vague right upper quadrant pain.

Most patients are female (70% to 80%), in the 30 to 40 years of age range. Again a relationship between FNH and the use of birth control pills has been postulated. This, however, is still somewhat controversial.

The lesions can be single, or more commonly multiple. The mass is composed of normal liver parenchymal elements often partitioned into bundles by fibrous bands radiating from a large central scar. This configuration is seen in approximately 60% of patients with

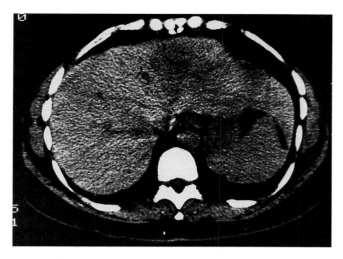

Fig. 5-26   FNH of the liver seen in a female as ill-defined area of low attenuation in the left lobe of the liver.

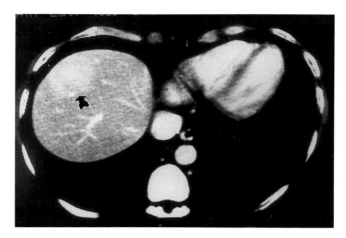

Fig. 5-27   Postenhancement CT image through the dome of the liver demonstrates increased enhancement *(arrow)* within solitary FNH lesion in a female patient.

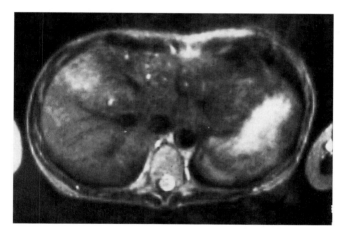

Fig. 5-28   In the same patient in Fig. 5-27, a MRI scan through the same region shows relative increase in signal intensity at the lesion site.

FNH. The size of the lesions can vary from 1 to 20 cm. They are most commonly seen in the right lobe of the liver.

CT imaging may demonstrate an isodense or hypodense lesion on the unenhanced scans (Fig. 5-26). Like hepatic adenomas, there is an increase in homogeneous enhancement in the lesion following IV-contrast enhancement (Fig. 5-27). There may be an area of low attenuation in the center of the lesion if a central stellate area of scarring is present. It is difficult to differentiate between hepatic adenoma and FNH on CT scanning.

The ultrasound appearance is that of a mass which may appear somewhat less echogenic than the surrounding normal liver. Unfortunately, it can also appear isoechoic with the surrounding liver. Identification of the central scar may be helpful and is manifested by dense internal echos.

MRI may be helpful. There is a tendency for the lesion to be isodense on all pulse sequences. If the central scarring complex is present, this tends to have a low signal on T1-weighted images and somewhat higher signal on T2-weighted images (Fig. 5-28). On technetium sulphur colloid scans, FNH can show normal or near normal uptake and may be indistinguishable from surrounding liver tissue, whereas a hepatic adenoma is almost always a cold defect.

Abscesses

Hepatic abscesses can be bacterial, parasitic, or mycotic. The bacterial or pyogenic abscesses are focal collections of pus within the liver. They are relatively uncommon today. Most pyogenic abscesses occur as an extension of infection ascending through the biliary tree, ascending cholangitis. Hematogenous spread through the portal vein or the hepatic artery or direct contiguous spread from an adjacent site of infection can also be a cause for hepatic abscess formation. It can be also seen in posttraumatic events involving the liver.

Most commonly a gram-negative organism is involved. The clinical course without therapeutic intervention is almost uniformly a rapid downhill decline and death.

The patient can present with a variety of symptoms including fever, chills, sweating, right upper quadrant pain, pleuritic pain, nausea, and vomiting. Many patients will have abnormal liver function tests, and up to one third of the patients will present with some degree of jaundice. The size of the lesions can be quite variable from 1 cm to 18 to 20 cm. The smaller the abscess, the higher the probability of multiple sites within the liver. In fact, approximately two thirds of cases have multiple lesions. Eighty percent of the lesions occur in the right lobe of the liver. The CT evaluation of the liver will generally disclose a low attenuation lesion with a peripheral rim that usually enhances following IV contrast. Internally, there may be septations or papillary projections (Fig. 5-29). In about one fifth of the cases there may also be gas bubbles detected. Air-fluid levels are identified on occasion. Lesions may be solitary or multiple, or there may be a grouping of lesions, generally in the right lobe with one large and several small adjacent lesions (Fig. 5-30). The CT appearance can be simulated by metastatic disease, although the clinical presentations are quite dif-

ferent. Needle aspiration is the most helpful method of differentiation. MRI of hepatic abscesses provides no additional specificity above CT imaging. Ultrasound generally demonstrates a focal area of decreased echogenicity. If there is gas within the abscess, or internal septations, internal echoes are generated.

Hepatic amoebic abscesses, although common in many parts of the world, are only rarely seen in the United States and Canada. It is thought that they are secondary to colonic amoebiasis. It is estimated that approximately 5% of these patients will have hepatic abscesses. Amoebic abscesses can also be seen within the lungs and brain. The organism, *Entamoeba histolytica,* is thought to access the liver through the portal venous system. For that reason, the lesions tend to be peripheral in location. The classical "anchovy sauce" appearance of the contents of hepatic amoebic abscess results from a combination of internal liquefaction, hepatonecrosis, and bleeding. The cysts are mostly solitary with thick, shaggy walls. Complications of these amoebic abscesses include rupture upward through the diaphragm into the pleural or pericardial spaces or downward into the peritoneal cavity.

The patient will almost always present with abdominal pain. Fever, weight loss, and symptoms relative to colonic involvement may also be present. Diagnosis is usually made by history, clinical presentation, and positive hemagglutination titers. Although considerable reluctance to do a needle aspiration of these lesions existed in the past, this procedure is being done today, with little or no occurrence of the catastrophic complications once anticipated. The CT appearance of amoebic abscesses in the liver is similar to pyogenic ab-

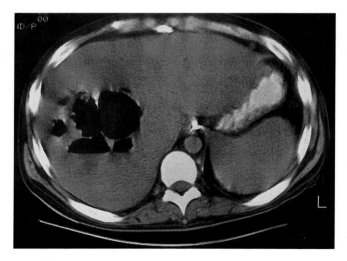

Fig. 5-29   Large hepatic abscess occupying most of the right lobe of the liver. Note the internal septations, air-fluid levels, and wall irregularity of the lesion.

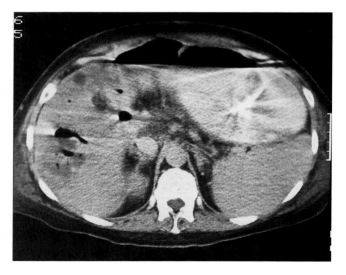

Fig. 5-30   CT images obtained through liver of patient with multiple, small hepatic abscesses in the right lobe of the liver.

scesses. However, there is a tendency for amoebic abscesses to be unilocular (Fig. 5-31). Ultrasound often demonstrates a lesion with ill-defined walls around a generally solitary or ovoid lesion located near the liver capsule. Decreased echogenicity within the lesion is encountered.

Echinococcal infection of the liver (hydatid cyst disease) can occur in two forms, *Echinococcus granulosus* or *Echinococcus multilocularis*. The former is more likely to involve the liver with large encapsulated cysts.

Although the parasite primarily involves the colon, at least half of the cases with extracolonic disease have hepatic involvement. Animals, particularly dogs, are the chief mediators of hydatid disease. The ingested eggs hatch in the patient's stomach and upper small bowel and reach the liver through the portal system. In the liver, the larvae will encyst and for a long period of time the patient may be asymptomatic. Symptoms develop as the size of the cyst increases. Occasionally, the parasite will die, the fluid be absorbed, and an encapsulated, calcified lesion is all that remains. However, in cases of viable, long-standing cysts, calcifications may also occur in the wall. The major clinical problems arise as a result of complications associated with the cysts. These can be a result of the pressure on the biliary system raising the possibility of obstructive jaundice. The most significant complication is rupture into the peritoneal cavity, alimentary canal, or the biliary tree. Indeed, cephalad development of the cysts could result in rupture into the pleural cavity. Rupture, especially into the peritoneum, is accompanied by pro-

found shock, peritonitis, and possibly anaphylaxis. Prognosis following intraperitoneal rupture is poor.

As would be expected, the disease is relatively common in sheep raising, and to a lesser extent, cattle raising areas in the world. However, with increased mobility and worldwide travel common today, the dissemination of this along with other diseases that were relatively confined to endemic regions of the world is now seen with more frequency in North America.

Hydatid cyst involvement of the liver is manifested by low attenuation lesions on CT. Focal areas of additional attenuation within the cysts are usually indicative of daughter cysts. Calcification may be identified in the rims. Infection or bleeding can result in alteration of the CT appearance. Occasionally, the detached cyst membrane may be seen on CT. This is analogous to the well-known water lily sign seen in the lungs of patients with pulmonary involvement. This finding has been described after cyst aspiration, and is highly specific for hydatid disease. The sonographic findings can be variable. Cyst wall calcification may be present. Otherwise, a well-defined mass with good through-transmission may be identified. Daughter cysts within the lesion are particularly helpful in making the diagnosis.

Mycotic abscesses of the liver are almost always multiple in nature and small. These are commonly seen in immunocompromised patients and frequently are accompanied by multiple small abscesses within the spleen as well. The most common organism is *Candida albicans* (Fig. 5-32).

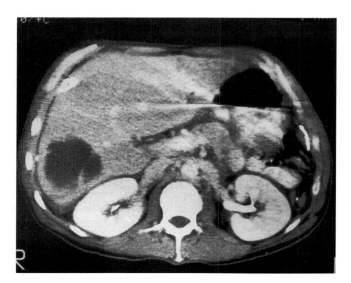

Fig. 5-31 CT scan through the liver of a patient with known amoebic abscess of the posterior right lobe. Note the well-defined margins of the abscess on this enhanced scan as well as the internal septation.

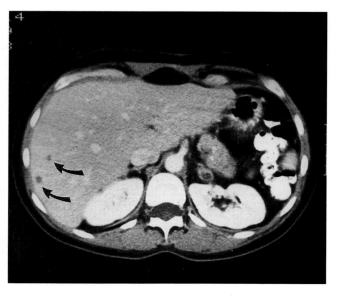

Fig. 5-32 CT scan through the liver of patient who has recently undergone bone marrow transplant. At least two small abscesses are seen in the periphery of the right lobe of the liver *(curved arrows)*, representing hepatic candidiasis.

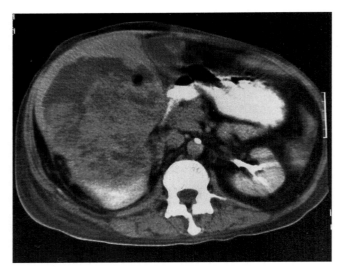

Fig. 5-33 CT scan through the lower portions of the right lobe of the liver demonstrates a huge inhomogeneous mass occupying and expanding most of the inferior portion of right lobe of the liver, representing an angiosarcoma of the liver.

Angiosarcoma

This is a rare tumor of particular interest because of its association with Thorotrast and the industrial carcinogen, vinyl chloride. During the 1940s and 1950s a radioactive colloid suspension of thorium dioxide, called Thorotrast, was injected intravenously for hepatosplenic imaging. Unfortunately, the radioactivity put the individual at high risk for malignant induction. Patients chronically exposed to arsenic or to vinyl chloride in the manufacture of plastics have also been found to have a significant risk for this tumor. Generally, CT evaluation of these patients discloses a large, irregular low-attenuation lesion within the liver that may manifest peripheral enhancement during the dynamic phase (Fig. 5-33).

Other causes of solitary low-attenuation lesions of the liver include lipomas. These are unusual but do occur in about 10% of patients with renal angiomyolipomatosis. The CT appearance of this lesion is characteristic.

Biliary Cystadenoma and Cystadenocarcinoma

This rare tumor arises from the bile ducts but will most commonly appear as a liver lesion on CT. Eighty percent of the cases are seen in middle-aged women. They are usually large, solitary lesions with low-attenuation characteristics on CT. They will often demonstrate multiple loculations, which are lined with biliary epithelium.

The patients present with abdominal pain, upper abdominal mass, and occasionally jaundice as well as constitutional symptoms. The tumor tends to be slow growing. CT evaluation will also demonstrate enhancement along the margin and the septum of the lesion. This unusual septal enhancement occurs as a result of papillary growth along the septum, which is seen in the cystadenocarcinoma. Lesser degrees of papillary growth can be seen in the cystadenoma. The cystadenoma, however, usually demonstrates a thin septum and little or no enhancement. However, absolute differentiation between the cystadenoma and the cystadenocarcinoma will ultimately require surgical removal of the lesion and subsequent pathological evaluation. Surgical resection of these lesions often yields excellent results.

MULTIPLE DEFECTS

Metastatic Disease
Focal Nodular Hyperplasia
Hepatic Cysts
Abscesses
Hemangioma
Caroli's Disease
Epithelioid Hemangioendothelioma
Regenerating Nodules
Peliosis Hepatis

Many of the lesions that have been previously discussed and can present as a solitary lesion within the liver may also present as multiple lesions. To avoid redundancy, they will be mentioned and only briefly discussed in the following section.

Metastatic Disease

Multiple bilobar metastatic involvement is a common presentation and results in the typical low-attenuation lesions previously described. Hypervascular metastatic lesions are much less common but include such malignancies as carcinoid, islet cell carcinomas, renal cell carcinomas, and some pancreatic cancers.

Lymphoma involves the liver in 20% to 50% of the cases of Hodgkin's disease. This may be higher in non-Hodgkin's lymphomas. The hepatic involvement can be multiple and nodular, giving multiple, low-attenuation lesions on CT examination. Alternatively, the involvement may be diffuse, resulting in an inhomogeneous enlarged liver (Fig. 5-34). Primary hepatic lymphoma has been described in the literature, although the existence of such a lesion is disputed. Other lesions that can rarely involve the liver with focal nodular lesions include Burkitt's lymphoma and leukemia.

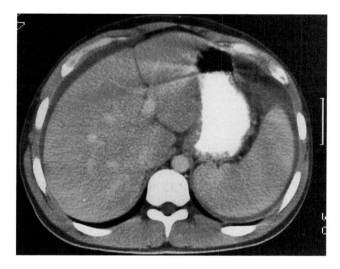

Fig. 5-34 CT through the liver in a 27-year-old patient with lymphoma. The liver is diffusely and homogeneously infiltrated with lymphoma. Note the perihepatic fluid.

Focal Nodular Hyperplasia

Although usually solitary, FNH can present as multiple hepatic lesions.

Hepatic Cysts

Hepatic cysts are commonly multiple. Along with hemangiomas, they represent the most common CT and ultrasound lesions incidentally encountered in the liver.

Abscesses

In about 50% of the cases, abscesses are multiple in the liver. Most abscesses that result from bacteremia and the entrance of microorganisms through the hepatic artery tend to be multiple and bilobar. In adults, as previously mentioned, most pyogenic hepatic abscesses are associated with bile duct infections.

Hemangiomas

In about 10% of patients, hemangiomas are multiple.

Caroli's Disease

Cavernous ectasia of the biliary tract (Caroli's disease) is actually a disease of bile ducts, in which cystic dilatation of the ducts occurs. In its severe form, it can look like multiple cystic lesions of the liver on CT.

Recently, a central dot sign within the apparent cystic lesions in the liver on CT, following IV contrast, has been described. This central dot is felt to represent portal vein surrounded by the dilated biliary ducts. This finding when present may result in an increased degree of specificity for the diagnosis on CT examination.

Epithelioid Hemangioendothelioma

Epithelioid hemangioendothelioma is a rare vascular tumor most commonly seen in adults. It often starts as a multinodular lesion of the liver and may progress to a more diffuse pattern. The usual CT findings include multiple, low-attenuation lesions with a low-attenuation halo around all the lesions. These are slow-growing, indolent, but progressive lesions.

Regenerating Nodules

Regenerating nodules, seen in cirrhotic livers, are also referred to as adenomatous hyperplasia or nodular hyperplasia of the liver. There is no definite capsule around the lesion. They are generally considered precancerous lesions in cirrhotic livers. Often these nodules can contain malignant foci. It is extremely difficult to distinguish between a small, well-differentiated hepatocellular carcinoma and a regenerating nodule. CT portography probably provides the best imaging method to distinguish between the two at this time. Because regenerating nodules tend to have an abundance of portal blood supply as opposed to diminished portal blood supply for hepatocellular carcinomas, portography provides a helpful method in distinguishing them. MRI of regenerating nodules tends to show a low signal on T2-weighted images, as opposed to hepatocellular carcinoma, which tends to have a high signal on T2-weighted images.

Peliosis Hepatis

Peliosis hepatis is considered a rare lesion but is being seen with increasing frequency over the last decade. This is thought to relate to the increasing use of androgenic anabolic steroids. The condition is manifested by multiple, blood-filled cysts throughout the liver. The earliest cases were thought to be a result of advanced tuberculosis or cancer. However, recently, peliosis hepatis in human immunodeficiency virus (HIV)-infected patients with associated cutaneous bacillary angiomatosis, a pseudoneoplastic vascular proliferation containing bacteria, has been reported. Peliosis has also been reported involving the spleen. Multiple small intrahepatic cystic lesions may be seen on CT and ultrasound of the liver.

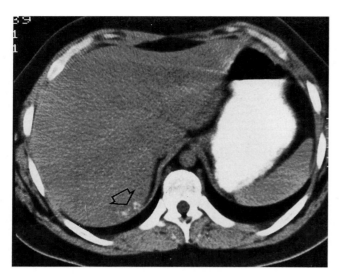

Fig. 5-35 Calcifications seen in a small metastatic lesion in the posterior aspect of the right lobe of the liver *(arrow)*. The primary tumor was a mucinous carcinoma of the colon.

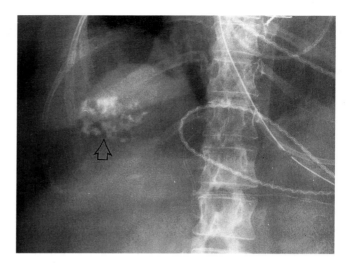

Fig. 5-36 Plain film of the abdomen demonstrates flocculent calcification *(arrow)* in an old intrahepatic abscess.

CALCIFICATION

Granulomatous Diseases
   Histoplasmosis
   Tuberculosis
   Sarcoidosis
Metastatic Disease
Hepatocellular Carcinoma
Abscesses
Cysts
Hemangiomas
Hematomas
Tertiary Syphilis
Parasites

Granulomatous Diseases

Granulomatous diseases excite the immune system in a specific manner that results in a characteristic inflammatory response. The particular response results in the formation of a granuloma that commonly calcifies after a period of time. Granulomatous inflammatory responses, especially without caseation, are nonspecific and frequently the offending organism cannot be identified unless associated with other systemic or laboratory findings.

The most common granulomatous disease seen in North America is histoplasmosis, which is endemic in certain regions of the United States. In its postinfectious state, it is seen as tiny punctate calcifications scattered throughout the liver and possibly the spleen. However, tuberculosis, rickettsial infection, bacterial,

viral, fungal, or even parasitic involvement of the liver can give a similar pattern. In addition, patients with sarcoid may have liver involvement in a similar pattern.

Primary hepatic granulomatous disease tends to have little or no calcifications associated with it. This would include primary biliary cirrhosis and so-called granulomatous hepatitis as well as granulomatous hepatic lesions resulting from drug toxicities.

Metastatic Disease

Calcifications within hepatic metastatic lesions are unusual. They have been described in association with mucinous (colloid) lesions of the colon or stomach. These are typically tiny stippling calcifications seen focally within the liver (Fig. 5-35).

Hepatocellular Carcinoma

Calcification within hepatocellular carcinoma is unusual, and it is said that less than 10% of these lesions calcify. If the calcification is present in the right clinical circumstances, the possibility of a fibrolamellar hepatocellular carcinoma may be considered because these lesions more frequently (30%) demonstrate calcification.

Abscesses

Calcification may be seen in the wall of old pyogenic or amoebic abscesses. Often this is a result of chronic, organized inflammation, secondary infection, or even bleeding into the wall of the lesion (Fig. 5-36).

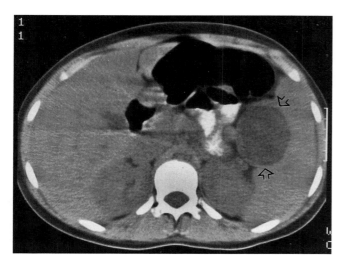

Fig. 5-43 A large splenic epithelial cyst *(arrows)* is seen during a CT examination for patient with diagnosis of appendicitis.

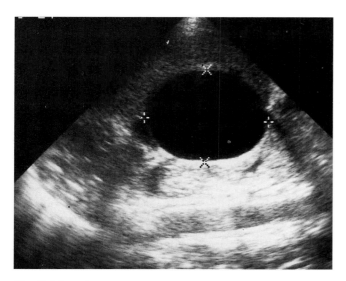

Fig. 5-44 The same patient in Fig. 5-43 also underwent ultrasound examination of the spleen that demonstrated typical appearance of a large, well-defined splenic cyst.

They are most commonly found in adults and are presumed to be of the traumatic origin. The cyst wall may be calcified and no epithelial lining is present. These account for approximately 80% of splenic cysts. True epidermoid cysts, on the other hand, are less common (approximately 20%) and are lined by stratified squamous epithelium. These cysts are felt to be congenital in origin (Figs. 5-43 and 5-44). Calcification can be seen in the wall of both acquired and congenital types of splenic cysts. The cysts can be quite variable in their size and generally contain clear fluid, although turbid or bloody contents may also be present. There is no sexual predilection for the congenital type of cyst. Congenital splenic cysts are not felt to represent part of the spectrum of more widespread cystic disease involving the pancreas, kidney, and liver. These usually occur as incidental findings within the spleen of asymptomatic patients. On rare occasions, the splenic cyst may be complicated by hemorrhage, rupture, or even infection.

Pancreatic pseudocysts involving the tail of the pancreas can occasionally give the appearance of splenic cysts on CT. The cyst may be adherent to and indenting the splenic capsule or can actually invade the substance of the spleen.

Echinococcal cysts involving the spleen are not common. Less than one third of cases of hydatid disease have splenic involvement.

Primary Neoplastic Lesions

Hemangiomas are the most common benign neoplasms of the spleen. These are almost always asymptomatic and are incidental findings. It is possible that a large splenic hemangioma or diffuse splenic hemangiomas could lead to splenomegaly, although this is rare. The lesions are usually solitary. Lymphangiomas occur in the spleen and are less common than hemangiomas. Distinguishing between the two can be impossible. It has been suggested that lymphangiomas occur more commonly in the subcapsular region than hemangiomas.

Splenic hamartomas are uncommon and are almost always asymptomatic. The majority are solitary. CT demonstration of these lesions may show a well-defined, solitary splenic lesion with homogeneous or mixed cystic components.

Primary malignant lesions of the spleen are rare. These are generally angiosarcomas, and unlike in the liver, there appears to be no direct relationship between Thorotrast and development of splenic angiosarcomas. Patients with these tumors carry a poor prognosis, often having widespread metastatic disease at the time of diagnosis. Primary malignant fibrous histiocytomas of the spleen have been reported but are extremely rare.

Metastatic Disease

Surprisingly, apart from lymphomatous involvement, secondary hematogenous metastatic lesions to the

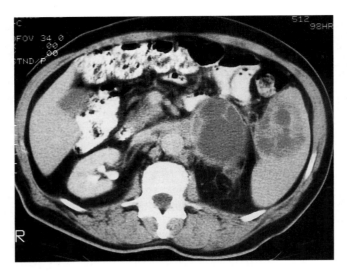

Fig. 5-45 CT scan through the midabdomen demonstrates a cystic neoplastic lesion of the tail of the pancreas. There has also been metastatic spread of the lesion to the spleen.

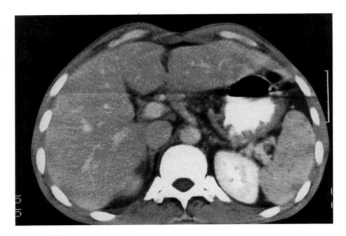

Fig. 5-46 Multiple, tiny splenic abscesses are seen in this immunoimpaired patient. These were found to be tuberculosis.

spleen are quite unusual (Fig. 5-45). A number of different explanations have been put forward to explain this scarcity of splenic metastatic disease, although none is fully satisfying. Metastatic lesions to the spleen do tend to occur when there is a widespread dissemination of tumor throughout the body. In such patients, splenic involvement is found in less than 4% at autopsy.

Lymphoma

As previously discussed, both Hodgkin's and non-Hodgkin's lymphoma, can involve the spleen. The involvement can be diffuse or it can be focal. The focal lesions can be solitary or more commonly multiple. These are usually demonstrated on CT as low-density lesions or on MRI as high signal lesions on T2-weighted images.

Abscesses

Large solitary focal abscesses of the spleen are fortunately an uncommon condition as they generally are associated with high mortality. These lesions tend to be poorly encapsulated and have intermediate densities on CT. There is often enhancement of the rim during the contrast phase of CT examination.

More recently, widespread disseminated microabscesses occurring in both liver and spleen have been seen predominantly in immunosuppressed patients (Fig. 5-46). They are commonly due to *Candida albicans* and on occasion tuberculosis. CT appearance demonstrates multiple areas of low attenuation within the spleen and commonly in the liver as well.

Focal Infarctions

In any condition where the potential of systemic emboli is possible, such as in cardiac valvular disease, emboli can become lodged within the vasculature of the spleen and result in splenic infarctions. These, in the early stage, are hemorrhagic in their appearance but eventually become smaller, fibrotic, and more dense. Quite often, they are associated with left upper quadrant pain and initially there may be some mild splenomegaly. Vascular thrombosis within the spleen and resultant infarctions may also be seen in disease processes such as leukemia, particularly of the chronic myelogenous variety, and are also quite commonly encountered in patients with sickle cell disease, eventually leading to splenic atrophy. Splenic infarcts secondary to septic emboli may also be encountered as a result of bacterial endocarditis.

INCREASED DENSITY

Thorotrast
Hemochromatosis
Autoamputation
Trauma

On routine CT of the abdomen (particularly unenhanced), the tissue density of the spleen is slightly less than that of the liver. There are relatively few conditions that result in true increased splenic density. The use of contrast agent Thorotrast in earlier decades has been previously discussed. It is possible for the spleen

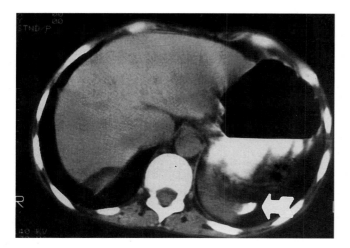

Fig. 5-47 CT scan demonstrates a tiny, calcified shrunken spleen posterior to the stomach *(arrow)* in this patient with sickle cell anemia. The spleen has undergone autoamputation.

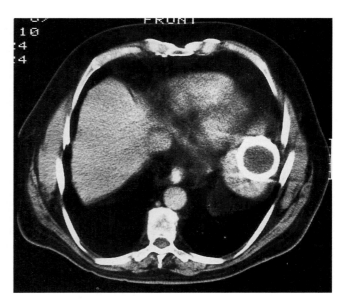

Fig. 5-48   CT scan demonstrates an old splenic abscess that is densely calcified in the wall.

to demonstrate increased density in cases of hemochromatosis. In a small, shrunken nonfunctioning spleen having undergone autoamputation, the spleen may appear increased in density (Fig. 5-47). This most commonly occurs as chronic sequela of sickle cell disease. Splenic trauma with diffuse bleeding throughout the spleen in the acute stage will result in increased density in the subcapsular region or possibly diffusely throughout the spleen.

CALCIFICATIONS

Histoplasmosis
Tuberculosis
Brucellosis
Phleboliths
Old infarction
Old healed abscesses
Cyst wall calcifications
Pneumocystis carinii infection

The most common cause of calcification in the spleen is previous histoplasmosis in which small punctate calcifications are identified within a normal-sized spleen. Tuberculosis and brucellosis may also result in calcifications. Phlebolith formation within the spleen with calcification is rare but can potentially occur. The possibility that old focal areas of infarction will calcify must also be a consideration. Old healed abscesses within the spleen, particularly microabscesses, may also lead to residual calcification (Fig. 5-48). Old hematomas can readily calcify. Calcification can be seen in

the walls of both acquired and congenital cysts. In addition, focal calcifications in abdominal organs, including the spleen, have been described in AIDS patients with disseminated *Pneumocystis carinii* infections.

SELECTED READING
Liver

Acunas B, Rozanes I, Acunas G, et al: Hydatid cyst of the liver: identification of detached cyst lining on CT scans obtained after cyst puncture, *AJR* 156:751-752, 1991.

Baker ME, Silverman PM: Nodular focal fatty infiltration of the liver: CT appearance, *AJR* 145:79-80, 1985.

Beggs I: The radiology of hydatid disease, *AJR* 145:639-648, 1985.

Bradley DW, Maynard JE: Etiological and natural history of post-transfusion and enterically transmitted non-A, non-B hepatitis, *Semin Liver Dis* 6:56-63, 1986.

Brunt PW: Alcohol and the liver, *Gut* 12:222-229, 1971.

Casarella WJ, Knowles DM, Wolff M, et al: Focal nodular hyperplasia and liver cell adenoma: radiologic and pathologic differentiation, *AJR* 131:393-402, 1978.

Choi BI, Han MC, Kim CW: Small hepatocellular carcinoma versus small cavernous hemangioma: differentiation with MR imaging at 2.0T, *Radiology* 176:103-106, 1990.

Choi BI, Yeon KM, Kim SH, et al: Caroli disease: central dot sign in CT, *Radiology* 174:161-163, 1990.

Dachman AH, Ros PR, Goodman ZD, et al: Nodular regenerative hyperplasia of the liver: clinical and radiologic observations, *AJR* 148:717-722, 1987.

Dodds WJ, Erickson SJ, Taylor AJ, et al: Caudate lobe of the liver: anatomy, embryology, and pathology, *AJR* 154:87-93, 1990.

Egglin TK, Rummeny E, Stark DD, et al: Hepatic tumors: quantitative tissue characterization with MR imaging, *Radiology* 176:107-110, 1990.

Ferrucci JT: Liver tumor imaging: current concepts, *AJR* 155:473-484, 1990.

Furui S, Itai Y, Ohtomo K, et al: Hepatic epithelioid hemangioendothelioma: report of five cases, *Radiology* 171:63-68, 1989.

Grace ND, Powell LW: Iron storage disorders of the liver, *Gastroenterology* 67:1257-1283, 1974.

Heiken JP, Weyman PJ, Lee JK, et al: Detection of focal hepatic masses: prospective evaluation with CT, delayed CT, CT during arterial portography, and MR imaging, *Radiology* 171:47-51, 1989.

Holley HC, Koslin DB, Berland LL, et al: Inhomogeneous enhancement of liver parenchyma secondary to passive congestion: contrast-enhanced CT, *Radiology* 170:795-800, 1989.

Khuroo MS, Zarger SA, Mahajan R: Echinococcus granulosus cysts in the liver: management with percutaneous drainage, *Radiology* 180:141-145, 1991.

LaBerge JM, Laing FC, Federle MP, et al: Hepatocellular carcinoma: assessment of resectability by computed tomography and ultrasound, *Radiology* 152:485-490, 1984.

Landay MJ, Setaiwan H, Hirsh G, et al: Hepatic and thoracic amoebiasis, *AJR* 135:449-454, 1980.

Langer JC, Rose DB, Keystone JS, et al: Diagnosis and management of hydatid disease of the liver, *Ann Surg* 199:412-417, 1984.

Lee MJ, Saini S, Hamm B, et al: Focal nodular hyperplasia of the liver: MR findings in 35 proved cases, *AJR* 156:317-320, 1991.

Lewis E, Bernardino ME, Barnes PA, et al: The fatty liver: pitfalls of the CT and angiographic evaluation of metastatic disease, *J Comput Assist Tomogr* 7:235-241, 1983.

Lewis JW Jr, Koss N, Kerstein MD: A review of echinococcal disease, *Ann Surg* 181:390-396, 1975.

Ludwig J: Drug effects on the liver, *Dig Dis Sci* 24:785-796, 1979.

Markos J, Veronese ME, Nicholson MR, et al: Value of hepatic computerized tomographic scanning during amiodarone therapy, *Am J Cardiol* 56:89-92, 1985.

Matsui O, Kadoya M, Kameyama T, et al: Adenomatous hyperplastic nodules in the cirrhotic liver: differentiation from hepatocellular carcinoma with MR imaging, *Radiology* 173:123-126, 1989.

Matsui O, Kadoya M, Kameyama T, et al: Benign and malignant nodules in cirrhotic livers: distinction based on blood supply, *Radiology* 178:493-497, 1991.

Matsui O, Takashima T, Kadoya M, et al: Liver metastases from colorectal cancers: detection with CT during arterial portography, *Radiology* 165:65-69, 1987.

Mitchell MC, Biotnott JK, Kaufman S, et al: Budd-Chiari syndrome: etiology, diagnosis and management, *Medicine* 61:199-218, 1982.

Murphy BJ, Casillas J, Ros PR, et al: The CT appearance of cystic masses of the liver, *Radiographics* 9:307-322, 1989.

Nadell J, Kosek J: Peliosis hepatis: twelve cases associated with oral androgen therapy, *Arch Pathol Lab Med* 101:405-410, 1977.

Nelson RC, Chezmar JL: Diagnostic approach to hepatic hamangiomas, *Radiology* 176:11-13, 1990.

Nelson RC, Chezmar JL, Sugarbaker PH, et al: Preoperative localization of focal liver lesions to specific liver segments: utility of CT during arterial portography, *Radiology* 176:89-94, 1990.

Partin JS, Partin JC, Schubert WK, et al: Serum salicylate concentrations in Reye's disease, *Lancet* 1:191-194, 1982.

Perkocha LA, Geaghan SM, Yen TSB, et al: Clinical and pathological features of bacillary peliosis hepatis in association with human immunodeficiency virus infection, *N Engl J Med* 323:1581-1586, 1990.

Rao BK, Brodell GK, Haaga JR, et al: Visceral CT findings associated with Thoratrast, *J Comput Assist Tomogr* 10:57-61, 1986.

Rummeny E, Weissleder R, Stark DD, et al: Primary liver tumors: diagnosis by MR imaging, *AJR* 152:63-72, 1989.

Terrier F, Becker CD, Triller JK: Morphologic aspects of hepatic abscesses at computed tomography and ultrasound, *Acta Radiol Diagn* 24:129-137, 1983.

Torres WE, Whitmire LF, Gedgaudas-McClees K, et al: Computed tomography of the hepatic morphologic changes in cirrhosis of the liver, *J Comput Assist Tomogr* 10:47-50, 1986.

Vasile N, Lardé D, Zafrani ES, et al: Hepatic angiosarcoma, *J Comput Assist Tomogr* 7:899-901, 1983.

Wall SD, Fisher MR, Amparo EG, et al: Magnetic resonance imaging in the evaluation of abscesses, *AJR* 144:1217-1221, 1985.

Yang PJ, Glazer GM, Bowerman RA: Budd-Chiari syndrome: computed tomographic and ultrasonographic findings, *J Comput Assist Tomogr* 7:148-150, 1983.

Spleen

Amorosi EL: Hypersplenism, *Semin Hematol* 2:249-285, 1965.

Baron JM, Weinshelbaum EI, Block GE: Splenic rupture associated with bacterial endocarditis and sickle cell trait, *JAMA* 205:112-114, 1968.

Bensinger TA, Keller AR, Merrell LF, et al: Thorotrast-induced reticuloendothelial blockage in man, *Am J Med* 51:663-668, 1971.

Berkman WA, Harris SA, Bernardino ME: Nonsurgical drainage of splenic abscesses, *AJR* 141:395-356, 1983.

Brinkley AA, Lee JK: Cystic hamartoma of the spleen: CT and sonographic findings, *J Clin Ultrasound* 9:136-138, 1981.

Burke JS: Surgical pathology of the spleen: an approach to the differential diagnosis of splenic lymphomas and leukemias, part I, diseases of the white pulp, *Am J Surg Pathol* 5:551-563, 1981.

Castellino RA: Hodgkin disease: practical concepts for the diagnostic radiologist, *Radiology* 159:305-310, 1986.

Dachman AH, Ros PR, Murari PJ, et al: Nonparasitic splenic cysts: a report of 52 cases with radiologic-pathologic correlation, *AJR* 147:537-542, 1986.

Dodds WJ, Taylor AJ, Erickson SJ, et al: Radiologic imaging of splenic anomalies, *AJR* 155:805-810, 1990.

Freeman MH, Tonkin AK: Focal splenic defects, *Radiology* 121:689-692, 1976.

Gebbie DAM, Hamilton PJS, Hutt MSR, et al: Malarial antibodies in idiopathic splenomegaly in Uganda, *Lancet* 2:392-393, 1964.

Gill PG, Souter RG, Morris PJ: Splenectomy for hypersplenism in malignant lymphomas, *Br J Surg* 68:29-33, 1981.

Halgrimson CG, Rustad DG, Zeligman BE: Calcified hemangioma of the spleen (letter), *JAMA* 252:2959-2960, 1984.

Louie JS, Pearson CM: Felty's syndrome, *Semin Hematol* 8:216-220, 1971.

Pearson HA, Spencer RP, Cornelius EA: Functional asplenia in sickle cell anemia, *N Engl J Med* 281:923-926, 1969.

Peters SP, Lee RE, Glew RH: Gaucher's disease: a review, *Medicine* 56:425-442, 1977.

Pryor DS: Splenectomy in tropical splenomegaly, *Br Med J* 3:825-828, 1967.

Radin DR, Baker EL, Klatt EC, et al: Visceral and nodal calcification in patients with AIDS-related pneumocystis carinii infection, *AJR* 154:27-31, 1990.

Strijk SP, Wagener DJT, Bogman MJ, et al: The spleen in Hodgkin disease: diagnostic value of CT, *Radiology* 154:753-757, 1985.

Svartholm EG, Haglund U: Splenic resection for benign cyst, *Acta Chir Scand* 151:491-494, 1985.

Weed RI: Hereditary spherocytosis: a review, *Arch Intern Med* 135:1316-1323, 1975.

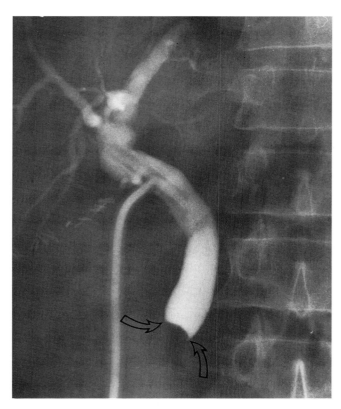

Fig. 6-6   T-tube cholangiogram demonstrates a rounded filling defect in the distal common bile duct *(arrows)* raising the possibility of an impacted stone.

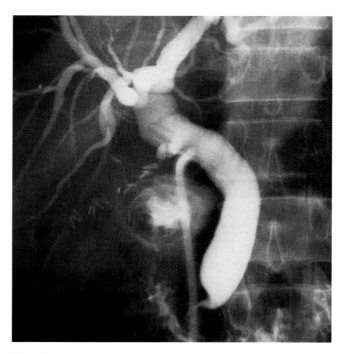

Fig. 6-7   In the same patient as Fig. 6-6 following the administration of IV glucagon, the apparent filling defect in the distal common bile duct has disappeared and represented spasm of the sphincter of Oddi.

be less defined and more ovoid. There may be some changing of configuration as the filling defect moves. Blood clots almost never result in obstruction.

Benign Polypoid Lesions

Benign bile duct tumors are uncommon, but when present, most frequently present as small, rounded filling defects on the margin of the duct. These include such benign lesions as adenomas and papillomas, as well as fibromas, neurofibromas, lipomas, hamartomas, and carcinoids. These lesions are usually solitary, although multiple filling defects are present in biliary papillomatosis, a very rare condition in which multiple papillomas are seen. This condition reputedly carries an increased risk of cholangiocarcinoma.

Parasites

A number of parasitic infestations can affect the biliary system and result in typical filling defects within the common bile duct. The most common is the roundworm, *Ascaris lumbricoides*. The problem is

worldwide, with the greatest prevalence in developing nations and rural areas where overcrowding and unsanitary environments are common. The ingested ova hatch in the small bowel and usually make that site their habitation. The worm is capable of ascending the small bowel and reaching the duodenum. This proximal migration can result in some of the worms passing into the common bile duct, leading to degrees of biliary obstruction and possible secondary infection. Quite often, this is accompanied by pancreatitis, either as a secondary effect or as a result of worm migration into the pancreatic duct. Linear intraluminal filling defects are demonstrated on contrast studies of the common bile duct.

Liver flukes, most commonly seen in the Far East, are being occasionally seen in North America and Western Europe with the increase in worldwide travel. The cysts are ingested, usually with raw fish. The larvae hatch in the duodenum and migrate to the liver and biliary system where they can produce biliary obstruction and recurrent cholangitis. There is an increased incidence of cholangiocarcinoma in chronic infestation.

Hydatid echinococcal cysts of the liver can also occasionally communicate with the biliary tree and discharge daughter cysts into the biliary system, resulting in filling defects.

DUCTAL NARROWING

Postinflammation
Postsurgical
Sclerosing Cholangitis
Ascending Cholangitis
Extrinsic Obstructive Processes
Cholangiocarcinoma
Adjacent Malignant Lesions
Ampullary and Periampullary Processes
Biliary Atresia

Postinflammation

Chronic pancreatitis is one of the most frequent causes of common bile duct narrowing. This narrowing occurs as a result of changes in the pancreatic head, consisting of edema, chronic inflammation, and eventually fibrosis resulting in a mass effect. The combination of mass and cicatrization about the intrapancreatic portion of the common bile duct results in a smooth, tapered narrowing. Approximately 25% of these patients will have sufficient narrowing to induce obstructive jaundice. When the stricture is the result of mass effect secondary to inflammation and edema and less due to cicatrization, the severity of the stricture may not be permanent and some degree of relief may be observed as the pancreatic inflammatory process subsides. Prolonged strictures, resulting mostly from fibrotic changes about the common bile duct in the intrapancreatic portion, can result in permanent liver

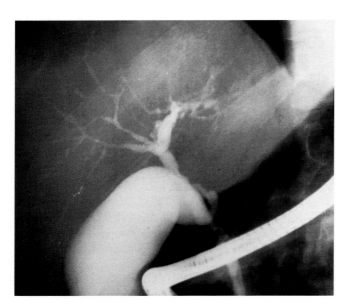

Fig. 6-8 ERCP in a 32-year-old patient with ulcerative colitis and sclerosing cholangitis demonstrates intrahepatic areas of segmental narrowing.

damage if unrelieved. These patients will eventually go on to develop cirrhosis. This type of stricture is not very amenable to dilatation and the definitive treatment is choledochoduodenostomy or a choledochojejunostomy.

The configuration of smooth, narrow tapering over a 2 to 4 cm segment of the distal common bile duct in its intrapancreatic portion is benign in most cases. However, occasionally malignancy may present in such a manner. In a patient with no clinical or radiological evidence of pancreatitis or gallstone disease, one should be suspicious.

Other causes of stricture resulting from inflammation/fibrosis include trauma resulting from difficult stone passage, ischemic and inflammatory damage that can occur as a result of hepatic artery chemotherapy infusion, as well as external penetrating and blunt trauma. Recurrent biliary infections may also result in stricture formation. Sclerosing cholangitis will be discussed separately.

Postsurgical

Another important cause of benign strictures is accidental injury to the bile duct during cholecystectomy. The inadvertent placement of a ligature or a hemostat around the common bile duct or common hepatic duct is the most common injury. Most frequently the trauma involves the common hepatic duct, and depending upon the degree of injury and the severity of the stricture, the patient may present with symptoms within weeks or years of the injury. Acutely, the patient may be jaundiced or experience intermittent attacks of cholangitis. About 25% of these patients develop ductal stones above the stricture. Long-term, unrelieved strictures will eventually lead to obstructive biliary cirrhosis and liver failure.

Careful fundal to ductal dissection by the surgeon to clearly identify the common hepatic and common bile duct, as well as routine use of intraoperative cholangiography, reduces the incidence of these injuries.

Sclerosing Cholangitis

Sclerosing cholangitis is a progressive, inflammatory process involving all or parts of the bile duct system. Frequently, it involves the biliary system diffusely with both extrahepatic and intrahepatic involvement. The inflammation results in diffuse thickening of the bile duct walls. Quite commonly, the degree of severity varies segmentally (Fig. 6-8). The disease appears to be more common in men by a 2:1 ratio.

A number of conditions are associated with sclerosing cholangitis, with ulcerative colitis being the most frequently observed. A third to one half of patients with sclerosing cholangitis have associated inflammatory bowel disease. Conversely, only 1 in 100 patients with ulcerative colitis will develop sclerosing cholangitis. The relationship is not understood. However, some regression in the severity of the disease has been reported in patients with ulcerative colitis who have had total colectomies.

Other conditions associated with sclerosing cholangitis include Crohn's disease, Riedel's thyroiditis, and retroperitoneal and mediastinal fibrosis.

The imaging diagnosis is best obtained either by ERCP or PTC. Although the small sclerosed ducts are difficult to aspirate with the percutaneous transhepatic approach, the use of the Chiba skinny needle in recent years has made the success rate somewhat higher.

Diffuse or localized areas of alternating narrowing and relative dilatation are seen involving both the intrahepatic and extrahepatic biliary system. The differential considerations include a slow-growing scirrhous type of bile duct carcinoma, as well as the possibility of congenital cystic disease when the strictures are segmental. In addition, it should be noted that a secondary bile duct sclerosis can occur above chronic partial obstructions of benign causes. The appearance will be similar to primary sclerosing cholangitis, and a clear limitation of the changes in the extrahepatic system should at least raise the suspicion of this possibility. These changes are thought to most likely be a result of the chronic recurrent cholangitis associated with partial obstruction.

Ascending Cholangitis

As previously discussed, chronic recurrent ascending cholangitis proximal to a long-term partial obstruction of the common hepatic or common bile duct results in proximal bile stasis, dilatation, potential development of primary stone formation, and bacterial cholangitis. Both intrahepatic and extrahepatic ducts can be involved in a secondary sclerosing (ascending) cholangitis. The resultant changes in the biliary system can be indistinguishable from primary sclerosing cholangitis. These are usually seriously ill patients with a biliary system, which, in the worst scenerio, is filled with pus at the height of the infectious process. Numerous small pericholangitic abscesses may form and make the diagnosis somewhat easier. If untreated, the condition is usually fatal. Treatment and multiple recurrences of the infectious process are usually the scenario for the sclerosing ductal changes. Although the treatment of the septic process is primary, the definitive treatment consists of relieving the distal obstructive process.

Occasionally, tiny common bile duct diverticula are encountered that may be indicative of previous ascending cholangitis (Fig. 6-9).

Recently, nonbacterial types of ascending cholangitis have been described in patients with acquired immune deficiency syndrome (AIDS), with a radiological picture very similar to primary sclerosing cholangitis. Biliary *Cryptosporidium,* although uncommon, is being encountered with more frequency with the increasing number of AIDS patients. Biliary cytomegalovirus (CMV) and moniliasis, although extremely uncommon, may produce similar pictures in the immunocompromised patient.

Extrinsic Obstructive Processes

Stricture of the intrapancreatic portion of the common bile duct is a well-known result of both acute and chronic pancreatitis involving the pancreatic head. This has been discussed previously. However, metastatic spread in the porta hepatis or the peripancreatic or periduodenal region can also, on occasion, cause

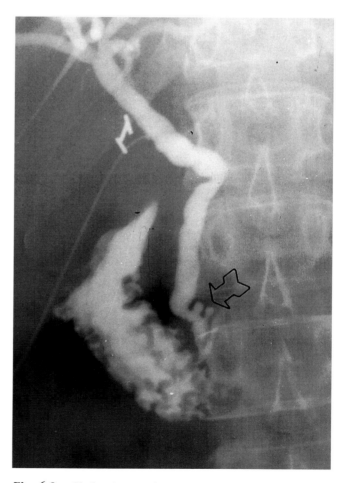

Fig. 6-9   Cholangiogram demonstrates several small diverticula *(arrow)* in the distal common bile duct associated with slight narrowing and irregularity but no obstruction.

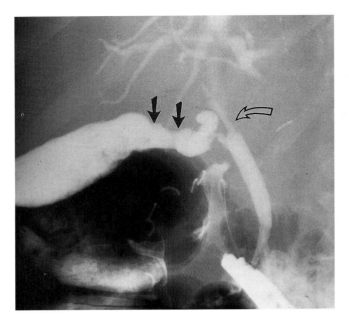

Fig. 6-10 ERCP demonstrates a lesion arising from the neck of the gallbladder *(arrows)* narrowing the gallbladder neck, cystic duct, and the adjacent common hepatic duct *(curved arrow)*.

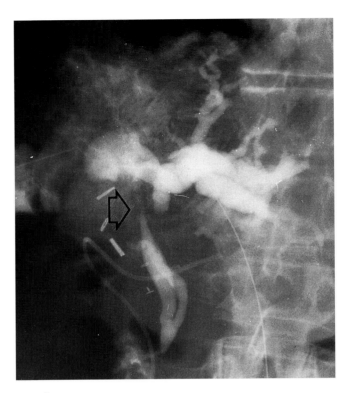

Fig. 6-11 Cholangiography demonstrates marked dilatation of the intrahepatic biliary system with tapered narrowing extending over 3 to 4 cm of the common hepatic duct at the level of the bifurcation, representing a sclerosing cholangiocarcinoma *(arrow)*.

sufficient extrinsic compression to cause bile duct narrowing and obstruction. Tumors from the gastrointestinal tract, lung, or breast are most commonly involved.

Lymphomatous nodes, although large and bulky, seldom result in sufficient extrinsic pressure to seriously narrow the common hepatic or common bile duct except when accompanied by desmoplastic changes.

Mirizzi syndrome and Mirizzi-like syndrome are unusual conditions that result in degrees of biliary obstruction. Mirizzi syndrome classically refers to a stone impacted in the neck of the gallbladder or the cystic duct, with the mass of the stone and accompanying inflammatory changes causing compression and narrowing of the adjacent common bile duct. Malignant masses arising from the neck of the gallbladder or the cystic duct region can result in a Mirizzi-like picture as a result of contiguous spread, involvement of the common bile duct, and biliary narrowing and obstruction (Fig. 6-10).

Cholangiocarcinoma

This lesion is uncommon but associated with high mortality. It occurs most often in adults 50 to 70 years old. Five percent of the patients have associated ulcerative colitis, almost always pancolonic in its distribution. These patients do not always have sclerosing

cholangitis, but the risk of malignancy increases with the presence of sclerosing cholangitis. There is also increased risk in any condition that results in chronic bile stasis, including Caroli's disease, choledochal cysts, and widespread cystic disease of the liver. There is also an increased risk with chronic parasitic infections of the biliary system, biliary papillomatosis as well as in certain environmental circumstances, such as encountered in the chemical industry.

The most common presentation of cholangiocarcinoma is a short area of biliary stenosis. This is occasionally accompanied by marked desmoplastic changes, and on rare occasion, the lesion can resemble sclerosing cholangitis. Approximately half of the tumors are located in the region of the bifurcation of the main biliary ducts (Klatskin tumors) (Fig. 6-11). Morphologically, these lesions can be focally stenotic (most common), as well as polypoid or diffusely scirrhous in nature. CT and ultrasound are often unable to demonstrate the tumor, although the secondary effects of biliary obstruction are readily identified using these modalities. ERCP is very helpful, but in cases with high-grade obstructive lesions, PTC is superior in that it is able to show the proximal extent of the lesion. The

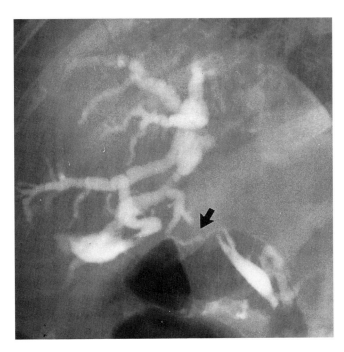

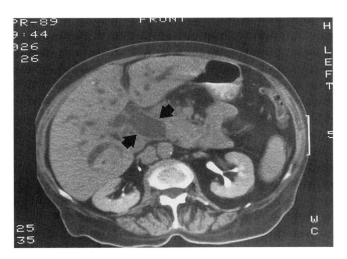

Fig. 6-13   A patient with pancreatic carcinoma presenting with biliary obstruction. A CT section through the region of the common bile duct demonstrates a grossly dilated common bile duct *(arrows)* and intrahepatic system.

Fig. 6-12   Cholangiogram in a patient with known breast cancer and disseminated metastatic disease demonstrates obstruction of the biliary system at the level of the common hepatic duct *(arrow)* as a result of metastatic disease in the porta hepatis.

value of MRI in this lesion is debatable. There is some suggestion that the tumor may be more visible on certain MRI protocols. However, at this point MRI does not occupy a primary or even secondary place in the imaging workup.

The most common lesion pattern is a short, irregular stricture, although smooth margins are not infrequent. The polypoid form has the best prognosis while the scirrhous the worst. Only a small number of patients are candidates for any form of surgical resection. For the remainder, once the diagnosis has been firmly established, biliary drainage is the goal. This can be accomplished by stenting the narrowed segment either from below (ERCP) or above (PTC).

Adjacent Malignant Lesions

Malignant lesions arising in the tissues adjacent to the biliary system, such as the liver, in the case of hepatoma, or occasionally hepatic metastatic lesions, can result in biliary stenosis caused by compression or invasion (Fig. 6-12). A similar pattern can be seen with cancer of the pancreatic head. Moreover, cancer of the ampulla of Vater will commonly constrict the distal common bile duct leading to proximal distention.

Ampullary and Periampullary Processes

Carcinoma of the ampulla of Vater is often a nonspecific entity that includes lesions arising from the distal common bile duct, the pancreatic duct, and the adjacent duodenum. The appellation is more regional than histological, and in many instances it is impossible to histologically differentiate these tumors. True periampullary carcinomas are relatively rare. Carcinomas of the pancreatic head are 3 to 4 times more common (Fig. 6-13). Whereas the survival rate with pancreatic carcinoma is usually not reckoned beyond a year, the survival rate for true periampullary lesions can hold a much better prognosis, with 5-year survival rates as high as 40% in patients with negative nodes. Jaundice resulting from common bile duct obstruction is one of the most common presenting symptoms in this patient group along with weight loss and anorexia. A palpable gallbladder (Courvoisier's gallbladder) is seen in at least 25% of the patients.

Other assorted ampullary and periampullary processes that may result in biliary duct obstruction include polyps arising in the periampullary region. These are uncommon, but adenomas, particularly the villous type, are the most frequently encountered lesion (Fig. 6-14). Carcinoids of the periampullary region have also been described along with most of the other benign tumors of the GI tract.

Periampullary fibrosis or papillary stenosis can occur as a result of chronic inflammatory changes in the region. The difficult passage of a gallstone may account for some of the stenotic changes observed. It may also

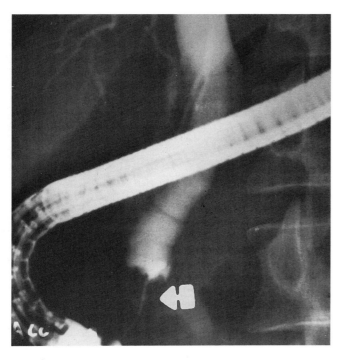

Fig. 6-14 ERCP examination demonstrates some dilatation of the common bile duct with narrowing distally *(arrow)*. The finding was persistent and proved to be a villous adenoma of the duodenum with extension into the distal common bile duct.

be possible that some of the stenosis could be iatrogenic as a result of previous failed sphincterotomies or repeated cannulations.

Duodenal diverticula are a common and mostly innocuous finding on UGI examinations. Most of the diverticula occur in the juxtaampullary region, and the ampulla may actually empty into the diverticulum. In most instances, this provides little or no problem. However, under certain circumstances, the anatomical arrangement becomes important. If the ampulla empties into the diverticulum and there are duodenal inflammatory changes involving the diverticulum, the possibility of inflammatory and edematous changes resulting in some obstruction to the outflow of bile and pancreatic secretions is increased. This is uncommon. Moreover, if the diverticulum is sufficiently large and bulky, it may present a mechanical difficulty by impressing the distal common bile duct.

Finally, when the papilla is located within a diverticulum, the risk of papillary injury during cannulation is increased.

Biliary Atresia

This is defined as luminal obliteration of either the intrahepatic or the extrahepatic bile ducts during the neonatal period. It is the most common cause of jaundice and liver-related death in neonates. It may be congenital, although there is some suspicion that the lesions are the result of intrauterine, biliary or hepatic infections and inflammation resulting in sclerosing changes within the ductal system.

The symptoms usually develop shortly after birth, and without liver transplantation the life expectancy depends on the degree of biliary patency present. Life expectancy, in general, is approximately 2 years.

Of interest is the ongoing problem of trying to sort out the confusion surrounding the two neonatal conditions, biliary atresia and neonatal hepatitis. Even with liver biopsies, a clear differentiation may not be possible. It is this interesting observation that has led some to suggest that biliary cirrhosis and neonatal hepatitis may be manifestations of the same disease process.

DUCTAL DILATATION

Obstruction
Choledochal Cysts
Caroli's Disease
Bacterial Cholangitis
Postcholecystectomy

Obstruction

There is clearly some overlapping of the radiological problems of biliary stenosis and bile duct dilatation, in that one commonly leads to the other. Our classification in this and the following section is at best arbitrary, choosing to emphasize the primary pathophysiological process. It should be noted that the most common cause of biliary duct distention is obstruction, many of the causes of which have been previously discussed. The problem of a dilated biliary ductal system will be viewed in this section from the perception of the dilated ducts as the primary problem instead of as the sequela of some other problem such as stenosis.

Choledochal Cysts

Choledochal cysts are not true cysts but rather cystic dilatations of the biliary tree. The condition is quite uncommon, although the Japanese report a higher incidence than the rest of the world. The changes in the biliary tree are thought to be congenital, although there is some evidence to suggest that some cases may be acquired as a result of an anomalous configuration of the pancreaticobiliary junction and subsequent reflux of pancreatic secretions into the bile duct. Whether the dilatation is congenital or acquired, it appears that it is a progressive process and it is interest-

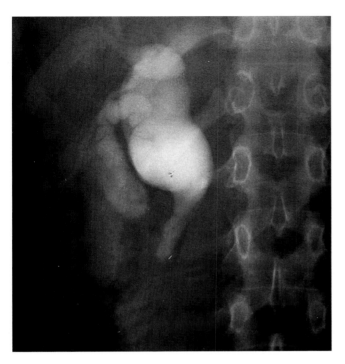

Fig. 6-15 Choledochal cyst: Cholangiogram demonstrates focal dilatation involving part of the common bile duct and common hepatic duct.

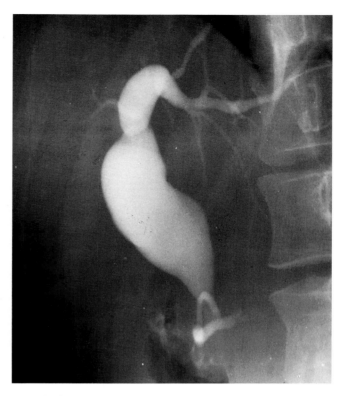

Fig. 6-16 Choledochal cyst: Retrograde cholangiogram demonstrates fusiform dilatation of the entire common bile duct.

ing to note that choledochal cysts are only infrequently encountered in infancy.

The original classification of choledochal cysts divided them into three categories. The first and most common presentation (80% to 90%) is manifested by a cystic dilatation of the entire common bile duct (type 1A). A subtype of this (type 1B) is focal dilatation of the common bile duct (Fig. 6-15). Another subtype (type 1C) is fusiform dilatation of the common bile duct (Fig. 6-16). In the type 1 form of choledochal cysts, the lesion is solitary and limited, and neither the cystic duct nor the intrahepatic system is involved. The cystic dilatation can be fusiform or saccular in configuration.

In type 2 (about 2% of all cases), a well-defined diverticulum with an ostium is seen arising from the common bile duct. The remainder of the biliary tree is usually normal. If the diverticulum becomes sufficiently large, it may begin to extrinsically compress, narrow, and obstruct the common bile duct.

Type 3 choledochal cyst is a choledochocele, in which there is cystic dilatation of the intraduodenal portion of the common bile duct and protrusion into the duodenal lumen (2% to 5% of all cases).

In recent years two categories have been added. These include type 4A, which consists of multiple intrahepatic and extrahepatic segmental cystic dilatations

(Fig. 6-17), and an extremely uncommon type, type 4B, which is limited to extrahepatic segmental cystic dilatations. The condition designated as type 5, which is a pattern of multiple intrahepatic cystic dilatations with sparing of the extrahepatic system (also known as Caroli's disease) will be discussed separately.

Every medical student is familiar with the clinical triad of right upper quadrant pain, mass, and jaundice, which is said to represent the classical findings of choledochal cysts. As is frequently the case, the classical findings are found in only a minority of patients (22% to 40%). Right upper quadrant pain or discomfort is the most common symptom and is frequently attributed to the gallbladder, misdirecting the initial workup. Other clinical presentations include cholangitis and pancreatitis. Gallstones are found in a higher than expected number of patients who present as adults, and acute cholecystitis or gallstone-related pancreatitis can occasionally be the presenting problem. In many instances, the correct diagnosis is not made preoperatively.

Imaging methods of choice include ERCP and PTC, which permit the morphology of the ductal systems to be seen in detail. Ultrasound, CT, and radionuclide scans may also be helpful, but in many cases, it is impossible to rule out an obstructing process as the cause of ductal dilatation.

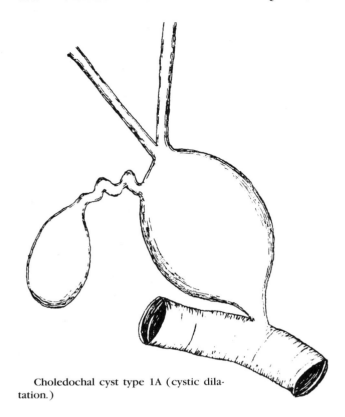

Choledochal cyst type 1A (cystic dilatation.)

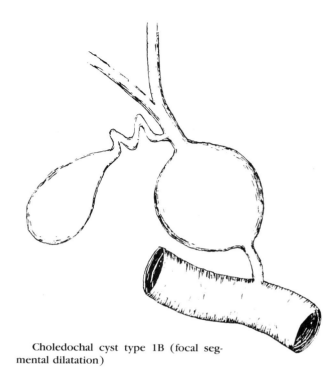

Choledochal cyst type 1B (focal segmental dilatation)

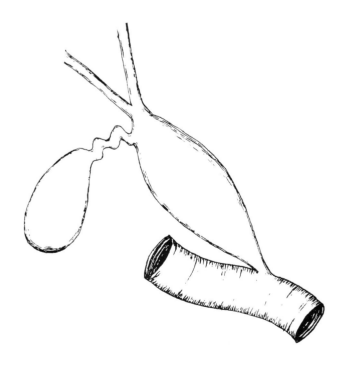

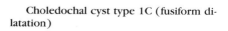

Choledochal cyst type 1C (fusiform dilatation)

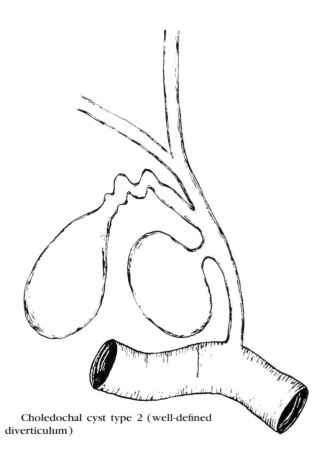

Choledochal cyst type 2 (well-defined diverticulum)

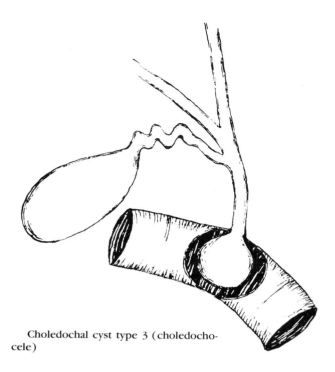

Choledochal cyst type 3 (choledochocele)

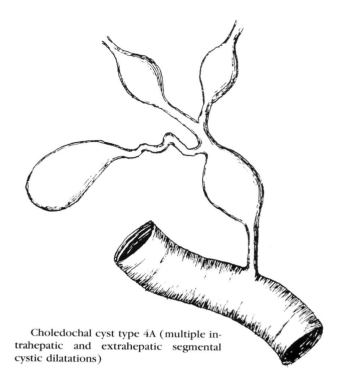

Choledochal cyst type 4A (multiple intrahepatic and extrahepatic segmental cystic dilatations)

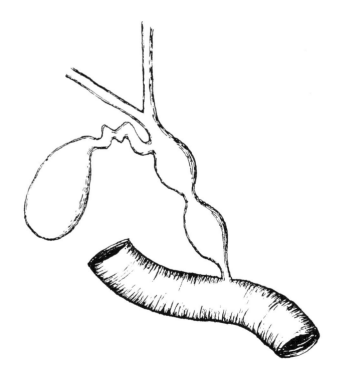

Choledochal cyst type 4B (extrahepatic segmental cystic dilatations)

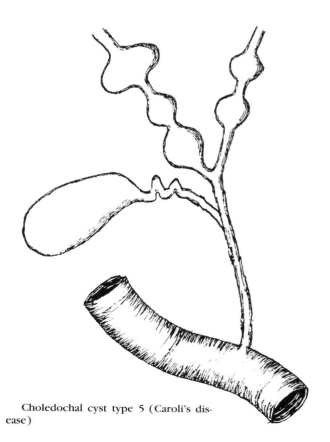

Choledochal cyst type 5 (Caroli's disease)

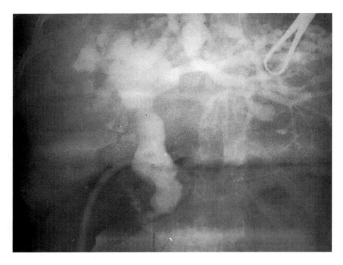

Fig. 6-17   T-tube cholangiogram demonstrates multiple biliary cystic changes throughout the extrahepatic and intrahepatic system.

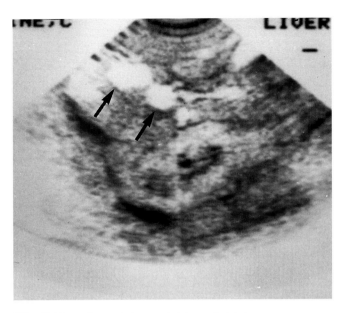

Fig. 6-18   Ultrasound examination of the liver in a patient with Caroli's disease demonstrates multiple cysts *(arrows)*.

Caroli's Disease

Caroli's disease, also designated as type 5 choledochal cystic disease, is a condition usually limited to the intrahepatic ductal system and manifested by segmental saccular dilatations within a nonobstructed system. For some unknown reason, portions of the ductal system are spared in some patients. The process results in stasis and all the attendant complications associated with biliary stasis, including infection and stone formation. It is these complications that usually cause patients to seek medical attention. Liver function and portal blood flow are generally well preserved.

The disease is quite rare and is probably seen with considerably more frequency in written and oral board examinations than in actual practice. The course of the process is linked to the predisposition to develop bacterial cholangitis, as well as a very definite increased risk for cholangiocarcinoma. These patients have approximately 100 times increased risk for the development of this cancer.

It should be noted that some controversy exists as to the etiology of the condition. It is believed by some that it is but one manifestation of a spectrum of a more generalized disease process that includes renal tubular ectasia (medullary sponge kidney), congenital hepatic fibrosis, and intrabiliary sacculations. Renal tubular ectasia, as well as renal cystic disease, is seen in almost 80% of reported cases. There is also an increased incidence of pancreatic cyst formation.

Ultrasound and CT demonstrate multiple intrahepatic cysts (Figs. 6-18 and 6-19), but differentiation from polycystic disease may not be possible without luminal contrast studies, such as ERCP or PTC. These studies clearly demonstrate the ductal origin of the cystic structures and provide a better opportunity to evaluate potential complications.

Bacterial Cholangitis

Recurrent bacterial cholangitis can result in changes in the intrahepatic ductal system that appear very similar to Caroli's disease, although the clinical courses are quite different. Numerous sacculations and strictures are the usual pattern in chronic disease (Fig. 6-20). Chronic recurrent cholangitis is uncommon in North America and Europe. However, in the Far East, it is among the most common causes of abdominal emergencies admitted to the hospital. The extrahepatic ducts can also be involved. The most important etiological factor is the antecedent presence of intrabiliary parasitic disease that results in an increased incidence of stone formation, obstruction, and subsequent infection. Additional complications of infectious cholangitis commonly encountered in the Orient include liver abscesses, secondary pancreatitis, biliary and gallbladder-enteric fistulas, as well as thromboembolic vascular disease.

Postcholecystectomy

It has been asserted that the common bile duct can become mildly dilated following cholecystectomy. The issue is controversial, and postsurgical common bile

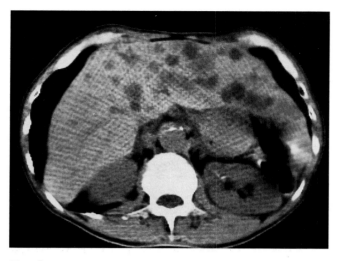

Fig. 6-19   CT of a patient with Caroli's disease demonstrates multiple cystic changes more prominently seen in the left lobe of the liver. Although most of the cysts seem discrete, some give the appearance of being part of the branching biliary system, suggesting this diagnostic possibility.

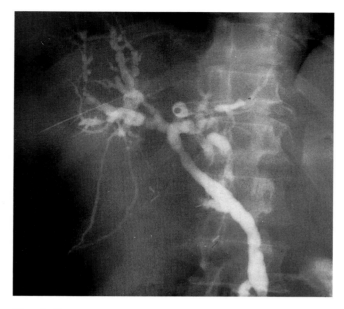

Fig. 6-20   PTC in a patient with infectious cholangitis demonstrates multiple strictures and sacculations of the intrahepatic system.

duct dilatation is not accepted by everyone. The literature reports the results of studies supporting both perspectives. However, episodic right upper quadrant pain is seen in 5% to 40% of postcholecystectomy patients. In such symptomatic patients, there is an increased incidence of mild common bile duct dilatation.

MISCELLANEOUS

Pneumobilia
Bile Peritonitis and Biloma

Pneumobilia

By far the most common cause of pneumobilia is previous diverting surgery for biliary obstruction, such as choledochojejunostomy or choledochoduodenostomy. Patients who have had previous sphincterotomies during ERCP may also reflux air from the duodenum into the biliary system. Any condition that undermines the competence of the sphincter of Oddi, whether it be traumatic, inflammatory, neoplastic, or iatrogenic, can result in air in the biliary system. On plain abdominal films, the air is seen as linear branching lucencies, and during UGI studies, barium may also be seen within the biliary system. The air collections within the biliary system are generally centralized as a result of the centripetal flow of bile. This observation helps distinguish air in the biliary system from air in the portal venous system, which is carried peripherally.

One of the more interesting causes of air in the biliary system is biliary-enteric fistula. This condition is discussed in more depth in the gallbladder section, as the fistulous connection is almost always between the gallbladder and the adjacent bowel. Most cases involve the duodenum, although fistulous connection from the gallbladder to the colon can occur (Fig. 6-21). Even less common is a fistulous connection to the stomach. These conditions most commonly occur as a result of chronic cholecystic inflammation combined with erosion of a stone through the gallbladder wall and communication with the adjacent bowel lumen. In about half the cases, a permanently open fistulous tract remains, and air can be seen within the biliary tree.

In most inflammatory conditions of the duodenum, even the more severe peptic processes, the biliary system will be unaffected. However, reflux of air into the biliary tree has been seen on rare occasion in patients with severe involvement of the duodenum with Crohn's disease. Whether this is due to distortion, deformity, and subsequent incompetence of the sphincter of Oddi or a result of fistulous connections between the duodenum and common bile duct is not clear.

Occasionally, a periampullary neoplastic process can also sufficiently affect the sphincter of Oddi to induce incompetence and reflux of air.

Rarely, biliary air may be seen in asymptomatic patients with no evidence of current disease or history of previous disease or surgery. This finding may relate to anomalous pancreaticobiliary duct relationships.

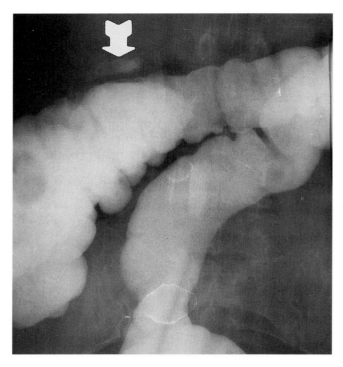

Fig. 6-21 Film from a barium enema demonstrates barium filling of a small, tubular structure adjacent to the colon and just superior to the hepatic flexure *(arrow)* that proved to be a small, contracted gallbladder continuous with the colon as a result of a fistulous connection.

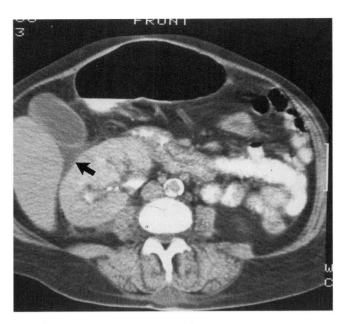

Fig. 6-22 CT section through the lower portion of the gallbladder in a patient with severe inflammation and gangrene of the gallbladder wall and a pericholecystic bile collection *(arrow)*.

Bile Peritonitis and Biloma

Leakage of bile from either the gallbladder or the biliary ductal system can occur as a result of several conditions. Focal bile leakage after biliary surgery, or after PTC is not uncommon, although serious consequences associated with these leaks are much less common. Abdominal trauma, particularly penetrating trauma, is another important cause of bile leakage. Serious free spillage of bile into the peritoneal cavity can result in bile peritonitis with the clinical picture of an acute surgical abdomen. If the bile leakage is sequestered and loculated, usually in the right upper quadrant of the abdomen, a biloma develops. Bilomas that mature for a few weeks usually are round and have a thin capsule. Patients will present with abdominal tenderness and a mass in the right upper quadrant in most cases. However, the biloma can occur in the midabdomen or left upper quadrant in about a third of the cases. If the biloma ruptures, the clinical presentation is more dramatic, similar to that of frank bile peritonitis. Additionally, a biloma can also decompress itself by eroding into an adjacent hollow viscus and possibly setting up a fistulous connection between the bowel and biliary system.

Gallbladder perforation is also a known complication in acute cholecystitis in approximately 10% of cases (Fig. 6-22). The spillage of infected bile (which is almost always the case in this complication of acute cholecystitis) into the peritoneal cavity results in a fulminating peritonitis that requires immediate surgical intervention. Approximately half the patients with acute cholecystitis and perforation of the gallbladder will form a biloma that will usually become infected as well. This may present several days to weeks after the perforation as a pericholecystic abscess.

GALLBLADDER

Examination techniques

Oral cholecystogram (OCG) In February 1924, a method for opacifying the gallbladder was reported by Graham and Cole in the *Journal of the American Medical Association.* The original contrast agent utilized was the sodium salt of tetrabromophenolphthalein. In the ensuing decades, more efficient and safer cholecystographic agents have been developed. Iopanoic acid (Telepaque), a triiodobenzene ring compound, was introduced in the 1950s and along with variations has been the standard oral cholecystographic agent used to date.

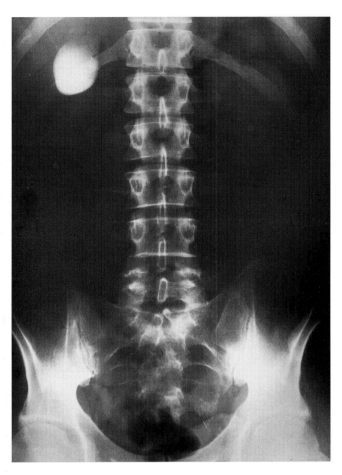

Fig. 6-23 Normal opacification of the gallbladder following the ingestion of oral cholecytographic contrast material.

Being mostly lipid soluble, orally administered iopanoic acid is readily absorbed from the gut into the portal bloodstream where it is bound to serum albumin and transported to the liver. In the hepatocyte, the bound cholecystographic agent undergoes conjugation in a manner similar to bilirubin. It is then excreted into the biliary ductal system where it ultimately collects in the gallbladder. In the fasting, fat-restricted patient, gallbladder contractability is diminished and the contrast agent remains within the gallbladder where concentration can occur as a result of water absorption. In most patients, within 18 to 24 hours following the ingestion of the contrast agent, the gallbladder is sufficiently opacified for imaging (Fig. 6-23).

Not all of the ingested contrast agent is absorbed. Some will pass through the small bowel into the colon and appear as dense flecks of contrast sprinkled throughout the lower bowel. Not all conjugated contrast is retained in the gallbladder. In the bowel, the conjugated excreted contrast agent will be seen as a homogeneous, hazy, luminal opacity. In addition, it has also been estimated that a sizeable amount (up to one third) of conjugated agent is excreted through the kidneys. As a result, renal toxicity is a known but rare complication of oral cholecystography.

For years, the usual dosage regimen has consisted of 3 gm (6 tablets) of the oral contrast. Approximately 30% of patients will have faint or no opacification of the gallbladder following this dose regimen. It has been found that two thirds of these patients will demonstrate gallbladder visualization following the administration of a second 3-gm dose. Unfortunately, this two-dose schedule is incorrectly referred to as a double-dose examination in many radiology departments and occasionally results in a patient receiving 6 gm (12 tablets) oral contrast agent at the same time. This may actually reduce the chances of opacification because of the significant diarrhea this dosage often causes. The correct application of this regimen, which is now routinely used by many institutions, is to administer 6 gm of the contrast agent to the patient divided into 3 gm doses over a 2-day period. This is done while a fat-restrictive diet is observed.

In a diseased or obstructed gallbladder, little or no opacification occurs. In a diseased nonobstructed gallbladder, the reason for nonopacification may relate to the inability of the sick gallbladder to concentrate the bile and hence the contrast agent. On the other hand, inflammatory changes involving the wall of the gallbladder, in particular the mucosal surface, resulting in edema and hyperemia may impair the integrity of the gallbladder mucosa. This increases its permeability to the contrast agent, and some of the contrast may escape the gallbladder via absorption through the mucosal surface with vicarious excretion through the kidneys.

Although the failure to opacify the gallbladder following a repeat-dose examination is presumptive evidence of gallbladder disease, it should be remembered that there may be other causes of nonopacification not directly related to gallbladder pathology, and these causes must be excluded. Some of them include the following:

Problems with patient compliance Most commonly the problem of patient compliance is a result of failure on the part of the patient to understand the instructions with respect to the ingestion of the tablets and dietary restrictions. These problems are best avoided by a careful explanation to the patient accompanied by a simple set of written instructions and the phone number of a person within the department who may be reached if the patient has any questions or concerns.

Failure to reach the absorbing surface Unless the contrast reaches the absorbing surfaces of the small bowel in adequate amounts, insufficient absorption will occur and poor opacification will be the result. This can occur for a number of reasons. Diverticula anywhere in the gut proximal to these absorbing surfaces can sequester contrast, resulting in a much diminished flow distally. These diverticula can be located in the esophagus, the gastric fundus, or in the duodenum or jejunum. Patients with or without diverticula who are sick, immobile, and limited to the supine position may also sequester the contrast material in the fundus of the stomach. Gastric outlet obstruction, of any cause, whether inflammatory or neoplastic, can result in lack of presentation of the contrast to the small bowel. A patient with constant vomiting may lose much of the contrast before it reaches the small bowel. Patients with gastric atony or gastrocolic fistulas can also be expected to present some difficulty in achieving opacification of the gallbladder.

Absorbing surface abnormalities Absorbing surface abnormalities are a relatively uncommon cause of nonopacification, even among patients with known inflammatory bowel disease and malabsorption syndromes that affect the absorbing surface of the small bowel. Occasionally, a patient with Crohn's disease or extensive small bowel resection who has a normal gallbladder can show nonopacification at OCG because of inadequate absorption. Patients with severe acute pancreatitis and accompanying malabsorption may also fall into the same category.

Hepatic abnormalities Because the contrast agent must undergo conjugation within the hepatocyte before being excreted into the biliary system, the presence of normal hepatic function is necessary to undertake OCG examination. Patients with elevated bilirubin levels (above 2 mg%), whether from primary hepatocellar disease or from biliary ductal obstructing processes, are not candidates for OCG examinations. Diminished opacification or nonopacification occurs in these patients not only because of the impairment of the intrahepatic capacity to transport the contrast agent but also because the contrast agent molecule competes with bilirubin for the hepatobiliary-excretion mechanisms.

The use of the OCG fell off dramatically during the 1980s with the widespread use of ultrasound in the evaluation of the gallbladder. In recent years, its use increased modestly for a period concomitant with the use of biliary lithotripsy to evaluate for stone size, number, and calcification.

Despite the decrease in the number of OCGs being performed in the United States, it should be remembered that this is a simple, safe, inexpensive, and very accurate method for examination of the gallbladder. Its sensitivity in detecting gallstones approaches that of ul-

trasound, while the cost of ultrasound ranges from 1½ to 2 times that of an OCG. The sensitivity for detection of gallstones with OCG is said to be around 94%, compared to 98% with ultrasonography.

A significant limitation of the OCG is that diagnostic information is limited to the gallbladder. However, in a patient presenting with a clinical history and symptoms that are most consistent with gallstone disease, an OCG may still be considered a reasonable first step in the evaluation of the patient. Filming procedure for the OCG includes upright, oblique, and compression views of the gallbladder.

Ultrasound Ultrasound has the advantage of being noninvasive and utilizes no ionizing radiation. It is highly accurate in detecting gallstones. It can provide additional valuable information regarding gallbladder wall thickness and pericholecystic abnormalities as well as an evaluation of the liver and pancreas (Fig. 6-24).

With the widespread use of real-time ultrasound, this method of imaging has now become the primary diagnostic modality for gallbladder and biliary pathology. In instances where the OCG is contraindicated, ultrasound is always an effective alternative. This applies in jaundiced patients with abnormal bilirubin levels, as well as in patients with known allergies to iodinated contrast material. Any patient with known structural abnormalities, such as high small bowel obstruction or gastric outlet obstruction, will predictably have an unsuccessful OCG examination. In these instances, ultrasound should always be considered as the first choice.

In any instance where the OCG examination is not

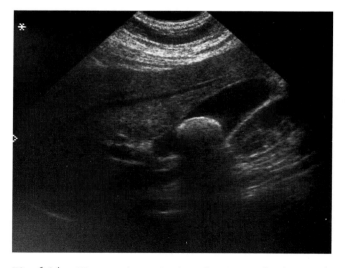

Fig. 6-24 Ultrasound examination of patient with a large, solitary gallstone casting a prominent acoustic shadow.

conclusive or there is nonopacification of the gallbladder, ultrasound is indicated.

Radioisotope studies Direct radionuclide imaging of the biliary system and gallbladder may be obtained using technetium-99m–labeled derivatives of iminodiacetic acid (HIDA, DISIDA, Mebrofenin), which are excreted directly into the biliary tract and can demonstrate patency with a high degree of sensitivity. Its most obvious use is in the evaluation of cystic duct patency in patients presenting with signs and symptoms of acute cholecystitis.

Following the administration of the radionuclide, concentration can be detected within the liver within 5 to 10 minutes. Usually by 40 to 60 minutes the biliary system, including the gallbladder, common bile duct, and possibly the cystic duct, may be seen, with some activity already present within the adjacent small bowel loops. Cholecystokinin (CCK) or an analog may be given before the examination to contract and empty the gallbladder and thus possibly promote filling during the study. This maneuver should be considered in patients in whom normal dietary stimulation of the gallbladder is ineffective.

In some instances, the efficiency of gallbladder contraction and emptying can be determined using the same agent by measuring uptake over the gallbladder before and after intravenous injection of CCK. There is an assumption that some patients who have no evidence of stones or inflammation but who present with symptoms similar to those seen in gallstone disease suffer from biliary dyskinesia, which can give identical symptoms. This diagnosis is somewhat controversial.

Non-visualization of the gallbladder after 1 hour is usually indicative of cystic duct obstruction. Delayed gallbladder visualization beyond 1 hour after the common bile duct and the adjacent bowel have already been identified does not necessarily rule out the possibility of acute cholecystitis, although such a finding would be unusual. More commonly, delayed visualization of the gallbladder is associated with chronic cholecystitis. Generally speaking, the longer the delay, the greater the likelihood of chronic cholecystitis.

Computed tomography and magnetic resonance imaging CT cannot be considered a primary examination technique for gallbladder evaluation at this time. If gallstones are calcified, they may be detected on CT scanning depending upon the location of the stones and the size of the thicknss of the slices. Most stones, however, being composed of cholesterol, tend to blend into the bile environment within the gallbladder and are often not seen. However, pericholecystic fluid or masses can be well-demonstrated on CT. MRI has not played any significant role to date in the evaluation of gallbladder disease.

DILATED GALLBLADDER

Physiological
Courvoisier's Gallbladder
Hydrops of the Gallbladder
Neuromuscular Abnormalities

Physiological

Patients undergoing prolonged fasting or starvation will accumulate increased amounts of bile within the gallbladder, with resultant distention of the organ. These people also experience an increased risk of stone formation. A similar picture is encountered in patients on prolonged hyperalimentation. Following bone marrow transplant, patients will commonly show some distention of the gallbladder on ultrasound and CT of the abdomen. Often this is accompanied by sludge or stone formation. The exact cause of these findings are not clear at this time.

Courvoisier's Gallbladder

Progressive, painless enlargement of the gallbladder with late development of jaundice has long been recognized as a high probability sign for pancreatic cancer with secondary involvement and narrowing of the distal common bile duct (Fig. 6-25). Other lesions, such as carcinoma of the ampulla of Vater or the peripapillary duodenum, can also result in a similar clinical presentation. Additionally, benign processes, such as villous adenomas or carcinoids involving the region of

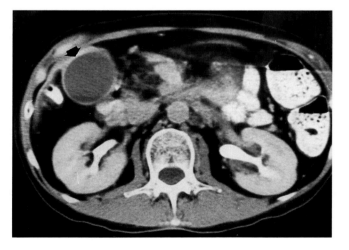

Fig. 6-25 CT of a patient with known carcinoma of the pancreas and marked passive dilatation of the biliary system and gallbladder *(arrows)*.

the papilla, have been noted to result in Courvoisier's sign. The general clinical significance of the Courvoisier's gallbladder is that a palpable nontender gallbladder in a jaundiced patient is more likely to be related to a neoplastic process than to an inflammatory process or a stone. Progressive, slow obstruction of a normal gallbladder will result in a considerable amount of painless distention. Conversely, distention in chronic disease is less likely, even with significant obstruction, because of gallbladder wall thickening and fibrosis. Distention secondary to stones is commonly intermittent, incomplete, and very painful. Inexplicably, some patients with complete cystic duct obstruction who do not present in the acute stage can go on to manifest one of several conditions associated with chronic aseptic cystic duct obstruction. These include porcelain gallbladder, milk of calcium bile, cholesterol impregnation of the gallbladder wall and mucosal surface (strawberry gallbladder), and hydrops of the gallbladder.

Hydrops of the Gallbladder

In most instances, patients with gallstone obstruction of the gallbladder neck or cystic duct will present with acute cholecystitis. These patients will frequently have a distended, painful gallbladder. The treatment of acute cholecystitis may be variable, depending on the condition of the patient and operative risks. Most commonly, early surgery is favored. However, in a small number of individuals who have chronic obstruction of the cystic duct, the gallbladder can distend and become surprisingly large. It contains a clear or mucoid, milky aseptic bile. This is the condition known as hydrops of the gallbladder. Some of these patients will have little or no history of gallbladder disease and the finding can be incidental. However, most patients will have degrees of right upper quadrant discomfort and possibly biliary colic. These patients are almost never jaundiced, unless some intervening process results in common bile duct obstruction. Complications of hydrops of the gallbladder include gallbladder empyema (when the gallbladder content becomes infected), perforation, or, rarely, infarction. While radionuclide imaging is the examination of choice in suspected acute cholecystitis, ultrasound has been found to be a superior method of evaluation in the chronic situation, with remarkably easy and quick identification of the dilated, distended gallbladder. If the obstructing stone can be demonstrated in the gallbladder neck or cystic duct, the diagnosis is complete.

Neuromuscular Abnormalities

Gallbladder atony and enlargement are common among patients with diabetes mellitus, occurring in up to half of the patients with insulin-dependent diabetes. The incidence may be higher in patients with peripheral vascular disease or diabetic neuropathy. Additionally, patients with diabetes have a decreased ability to empty the gallbladder, with resultant increased bile stasis and increased risk of stone formation. The increased size of the gallbladder relates to contractile abnormalities of the muscular wall of the gallbladder secondary to neuromuscular changes associated with the disease.

Postvagotomy patients may demonstrate increased gallbladder size. An increased incidence of gallstone formation in this group has also been observed. Truncal vagotomies are more frequently associated with increased gallbladder volume and selective vagotomies less so.

SMALL, SHRUNKEN GALLBLADDER

Chronic Cholecystitis
Cystic Fibrosis

Chronic Cholecystitis

The term chronic cholecystitis has meant different things to different people in various specialties. In a few patients, obstruction of the cystic duct results in hydrops of the gallbladder with intermittent or persistent symptoms. These patients may be said to have developed chronic cholecystitis. However, more frequently chronic cholecystitis refers to the condition seen in patients who have chronic inflammatory changes in the gallbladder wall with associated thickening of the wall. The gallbladder is small and often contracted, and in 95% of the cases contains numerous stones. This pattern is probably the most commonly encountered form of gallbladder inflammation seen at surgery. These patients frequently suffer from intermittent biliary colic resulting from intermittent cystic duct obstruction. Typically the pain is severe, in the right upper abdomen, possibly radiating to the back or shoulder. The pain has a tendency to escalate shortly after the onset of symptoms and diminish slowly over the next few hours, as opposed to acute cholecystitis where the pain continues to increase and is prolonged beyond 5 or 6 hours.

The diagnosis of chronic cholecystitis may be suggested on CT or ultrasound studies where a small, contracted gallbladder is demonstrated with a thickened wall and gallstones (Fig. 6-26). Small amounts of pericholecystic fluid may be seen, although this is more common in acute cholecystitis. The diagnosis can also be suggested by biliary scintigraphy when the gallbladder is seen to fill in a delayed fashion either spontane-

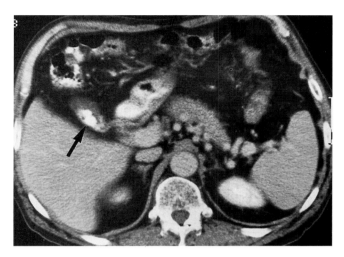

Fig. 6-26   CT examination through the inferior aspect of the liver demonstrates a small, contracted gallbladder containing several calcified stones *(arrow)*.

ously or with pharmacological assistance, such as the administration of 2 mg of IV morphine to induce spasm of the sphincter of Oddi.

Cystic Fibrosis

Gallbladder changes are seen in approximately one third of patients with cystic fibrosis. A small, hypoplastic gallbladder is not uncommon among this group. In addition, the bile is somewhat thicker than normal and it is assumed that some impairment of bile flow is present, accounting for the increased incidence of gallstones. These changes are unusual in infancy and are usually seen during the teen years.

FILLING DEFECTS

Artifacts and Spurious Filling Defects
Gallstones
Nonadenomatous Polyps
Adenomatous Polyps
Carcinoma of the Gallbladder
Metastatic Disease

Artifacts and Spurious Filling Defects

One of the more common problems encountered with the OCG examination is that of spurious lucencies projected over the gallbladder and mimicking gallstones. These are usually air bubbles in the adjacent hepatic flexure of the colon or the duodenal bulb. If multiple positional views are routinely obtained, this is

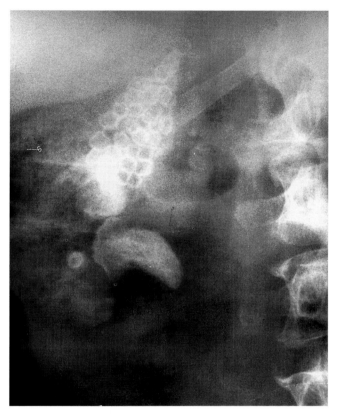

Fig. 6-27   Right upper quadrant coned-down view of supine abdomen of a patient with numerous faceted gallstones filling the entire gallbladder. Adjacent to this can be seen prominent renal calcifications.

usually not a serious problem. Routine compression views will also diminish the potential of mistaking overlying air bubbles for gallstones.

Occasionally, a tiny, persistent filling defect in the neck of the gallbladder can be seen, representing a slight invagination of the cystic duct into the neck of the gallbladder lumen.

Calcification in the anterior ribs, liver, right kidney, lymph nodes in the right upper quadrant, pancreatic head, and abdominal wall projecting over the gallbladder can be occasionally mistaken for calcified stones (Fig. 6-27). Supine, upright, and compression views as a routine part of the examination should deal with the problem. In some instances, fluoroscopy may be required to sort out some of these calcifications.

Gallstones

It is estimated that approximately 20 million people in the United States have gallstones. Of these an estimated 500,000 will annually undergo cholecystectomy. Unfortunately, the estimates of the prevalence of gallbladder disease depend to a large extent on the method by which information is gathered and the type of imaging techniques utilized. Many of the epidemiological studies have produced incidences based upon interviews or questionnaires regarding a history of gallbladder surgery or reported findings of gallstones on previous imaging studies. The figures thus arrived at are, at best, loose estimates of the prevalence of the disease. Realistically, we probably do not know with certainty what the incidence is and have probably underestimated it. We do know, however, that most removed gallstones (80%) are composed of cholesterol, while the remainder contain a variety of calcium salts. Approximately 15% of all gallstones are sufficiently calcified to be seen on plain films of the abdomen. Stones that are predominantly pigmented tend to occur in patients with hemolytic types of anemias, such as sickle cell disease. Cholesterol stone formation is more common in females than males, slightly more common in whites, and much more common in native American Indians. Moreover, there is a relationship between obesity and the incidence of gallstone formation, particularly in young women. Other etiological factors include chronic liver disease, the use of certain types of antilipidemic agents, as well as hyperalimentation.

Most gallbladder stones are never diagnosed. Many patients with stones are asymptomatic, while others have vague nonspecific symptoms. Only a fraction of patients come to cholecystectomy. Interestingly, the heightened attention to alternative therapies for the treatment of cholelithiasis has brought about a renewed interest in the composition as well as the pathophysiological processes that lead to the formation of gallstones. Gallstone pharmacological dissolution, as well as biliary lithotripsy or combinations of both therapies, have been used in the contemporary treatment of gallstones.

As previously mentioned, 15% of gallstones can be diagnosed on plain films of the abdomen. Plain film diagnosis of cholesterol stones with fissured interiors containing gas is a rare occurrence and a curious phenomenon of gallstone formation (Fig. 6-28). When present, this is usually manifested by cross-shaped or stellate thin lucencies in the right upper quadrant. This has been referred to as the Mercedes-Benz sign and is pathognomonic of gallstones (Fig. 6-29).

However, the principal method of imaging gallstones is ultrasonography or OCG. The sensitivity for the detection of stones is quite high in both examinations and slightly higher for ultrasound. Both have certain advantages and some limitations. The OCG requires some patient preparation and the use of ionizing radiation. On the other hand, it demonstrates not only gallbladder morphology but function. Ultrasound does not demonstrate function but is highly sensitive in the detection of stones and can give additional information regarding the surrounding organs. Little or no patient preparation is necessary for ultrasound examination.

On OCG examination with opacification of the gallbladder, noncalcified stones show as filling defects of varying number and size (Fig. 6-30). A single stone may be present, or the gallbladder may be distended with numerous stones. Stones may be sandlike, rounded, or faceted. On ultrasound examination, the presence of acoustic shadowing in the dependent portion of the gallbladder is typical of gallstones. The com-

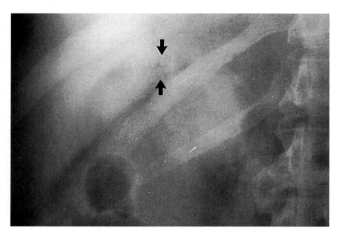

Fig. 6-28   A coned-down view of the right upper quadrant demonstrates a subtle stellate lucency *(arrows)* representing gas within a large, fissured gallstone, the Mercedes-Benz sign.

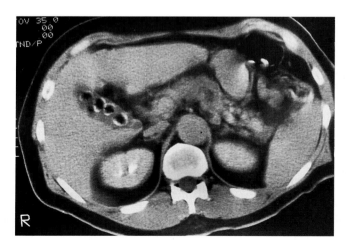

Fig. 6-29   CT through the liver demonstrates numerous gallstones, calcified in their rim with internal fissures and gas collections resulting in the Mercedes-Benz sign seen on plain film.

position of the gallstone does not appear to be a factor in the degree of acoustic shadowing present. On occasion, gallstones will float, particularly pure cholesterol gallstones. The layering out process can be observed in both ultrasound and OCG studies. A striking finding on OCG occurs when multiple small stones layer out and form a radiolucent band across the gallbladder lumen (Fig. 6-31).

New approaches to gallstone therapy have led to a mild resurgence in use of the OCG. Methods for chemical stone dissolution and biliary lithotripsy have been major topics for discussion, both in the medical literature and the lay media in the last decade. Initially, oral bile salts were used in an attempt to dissolve gallstones. Success was quite limited, not always reproducible, and recurrence common. Newer, direct dissolving agents have been developed, the most noteworthy of which is methyl-tert-butyl ether (MTBE). Dissolution of gallstones utilizing MTBE does require the direct application of the chemical to the gallstones, which in turn requires a percutaneous transhepatic route or endoscopic cannulation of the cystic duct. Infusion and aspiration of MTBE follows, resulting in complete dissolution of the stones in 30% to 60% of patients. Stone recurrence is a problem following MTBE treatment, more so in patients with multiple stones.

Length of hospital stay is often greater for MTBE treatment than for laparoscopic cholecystectomy, particularly if the transhepatic percutaneous route is undertaken. A small number of patients (5% to 10%) will experience complications related to transhepatic puncture or cystic duct perforation.

The first extracorporeal shock-wave lithotripsy (ESWL) treatments were undertaken in the mid-1980s following success in renal stone therapy. The goal of ESWL is to shock and fragment gallstones into tiny fragments that can pass through the biliary system into the gut or be dissolved more easily by MTBE. Focused shock waves, generated either by electromagnetic or piezo-ceramic techniques, are utilized to produce a high pressure shock effect over an area of several centimeters. The tissue damage to the gallbladder and adjacent organs is minimal and, with the exception of the occasional case of mild pancreatitis, appears to be of little consequence. The amount of fragmentation appears to depend upon the number, size, and composition of the stones. Best results are obtained in patients with a limited number of small, noncalcified stones. The recurrence rate of gallstones after complete clearance is significant, ranging between 10% and 15%. Combining ESWL with powerful dissolving agents like MTBE appears to give a slightly higher rate of success. The unresolved question is the relative cost of different therapies with the advent of laparoscopic surgery. In general, the enthusiasm for ESWL seen during the 1980s has waned significantly. Clearly, in symptomatic patients for whom surgery is contraindicated, it does represent a very encouraging alternative.

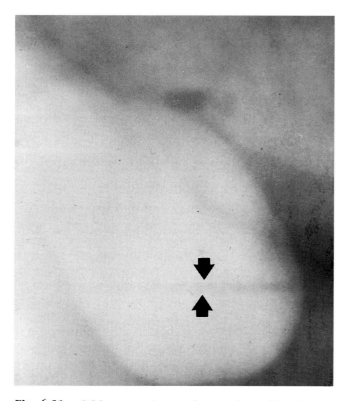

Fig. 6-31 OCG on a patient in the upright position demonstrates numerous tiny cholesterol stones layering out, forming a linear radiolucent band *(arrows)* across the lumen of the gallbladder.

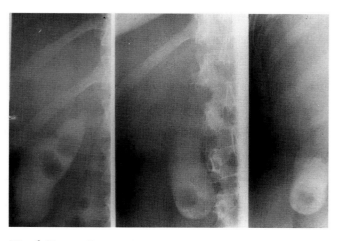

Fig. 6-30 Gallstones: OCG demonstrates good opacification of the gallbladder that has at least two rounded mobile lucencies within it.

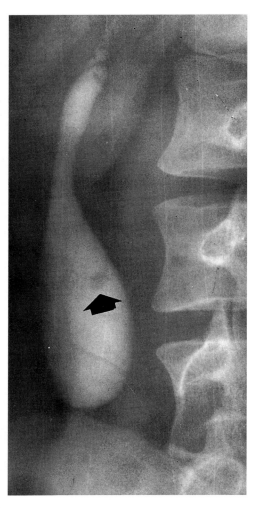

Fig. 6-32   OCG on a patient with a single, nonmobile filling defect within the gallbladder *(arrow)* found to represent a solitary cholesterol polyp.

Nonadenomatous Polyps

The most common cause of polypoid (nonmobile) filling defects within the gallbladder is cholesterol polyps (Fig. 6-32). These polyps arise from a condition of the gallbladder known as cholesterolosis in which deposits of cholesterol and cholesterol precursors are found within the gallbladder wall. The typical OCG and ultrasound findings are similar to those of a gallstone, with the exceptions that the lesion is fixed on the gallbladder wall and there is no acoustic shadowing on ultrasound. The morphological changes can be either a focal buildup forming a discrete cholesterol polyp or diffuse surface deposition over the gallbladder mucosa, giving rise to an unusual surface texture and pattern sometimes referred to as strawberry gallbladder.

Cholesterolosis and its manifestations are part of a larger group of conditions often referred to as the hy-perplastic cholecystoses, first described by Jutras in 1960. Under the same heading, he also included adenomyomatosis as well as several rare and unusual conditions. The validity and significance of the latter conditions have been questioned and, for the most part, cholesterolosis and adenomyomatosis are considered to be the only two important conditions under the hyperplastic cholecystoses classification. Jutras used the term hyperplastic cholecystoses to describe a group of gallbladder disorders that had common functional abnormalities such as hyperconcentration, hyperexcretion, and hypercontractibility. Adenomyomatosis will be discussed in more detail in upcoming sections.

Other nonadenomatous polypoid lesions of the gallbladder are rare. These include such lesions as lipomas, leiomyomas, fibromas, hemangiomas, and neurofibromas. Carcinoid tumors of the gallbladder have been reported. On rare occasion, granular cell myoblastomas (also a rare finding in the esophagus) have also been described in the gallbladder.

In addition to the above, an unusual but troublesome filling defect in the gallbladder is, on rare occasion, seen as a result of a gallstone adherent to the gallbladder mucosa.

Adenomatous Polyps

True epithelial adenomas are uncommon. When present, they can occur as either sessile or pedunculated filling defects. They can occur in any portion of the gallbladder, and multiplicity is a frequent finding. The possibility that gallbladder adenomas represent a definite precursor to carcinoma, such as in the colon, still lacks convincing scientific support. However, the presence of carcinoma-in-situ in some reported cases of gallbladder adenomas does make it a real possibility.

Carcinoma of the Gallbladder

It is estimated that approximately 6000 people will die in the United States in 1992 as a result of gallbladder carcinoma. The incidence is higher in females and among native American Indians and Hispanics.

This continues to be one of the more dismal malignant neoplasms, with a 5-year survival rate between 2% and 4%. If the patient is symptomatic, prognosis is always grave. On the other hand, patients who are asymptomatic and whose lesions are discovered fortuitously have a higher 5-year survival rate. The etiology of gallbladder cancer is poorly understood. It must include the possibility of malignant degeneration of gall bladder adenomas. The development of gallbladder cancer in patients with calcified gallbladder walls (porcelain gallbladders) is thought to be extremely high, ranging between 20% and 30%.

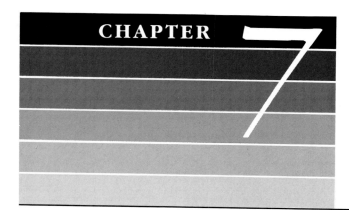

CHAPTER 7

The colon and rectum are two of the more common sites for disease in the gut, with a wide spectrum of disease processes encountered on a daily basis in medical practice. However, the steady increase in the incidence and mortality resulting from colorectal cancer has focused both the medical and lay community's attention on early detection and potentially effective screening strategies for this disease. Despite the refinement of air-contrast barium enemas (ACBE) and the advent of colonoscopy, there has been no discernible change in the overall survival or mortality rates in the last 40 years nor have any of these screening strategies, put forth at various times by various groups, proved to be very efficient or cost effective.

As a result, the question of an efficient and cost-effective method of screening may be considered unanswered at this time. It appears possible that the barium enema, whose demise was announced by our gastroenterology colleagues in the late 1970s and early 1980s, is still quite useful. Indeed, the barium enema could be a better and more cost-effective method of examining the colon than previously realized and may potentially play a role in future screening strategies. However, before we see that, many questions regarding screening for colorectal cancer remain to be answered, including; among the choices or combination of choices for screening, what is the most cost-effective method? Or even more fundamental, does any form of widespread screening for colorectal cancer actually reduce mortality in the population, such as has been shown with mammography for breast cancer or the Pap test for cervical cancer?

Much remains to be done; many questions are yet unanswered. Hopefully, a coordinated, well-planned, multi-sited national study of the efficacy and instru-ments of colorectal screening will be forthcoming in the coming decade and will shed light on these controversial areas.

EXAMINATION TECHNIQUES

Double-Contrast Barium Enema

Although the number of barium enemas has declined over the last decade, the double-contrast barium enema (DCBE) study remains one of the mainstays in the diagnostic evaluation of the colon. The three types of contrast enemas utilized today are the DCBE, the single-contrast barium enema (SCBE), and the water-soluble contrast enema. It is beyond the scope of this book to instruct in the technique and mechanics of how to do these examinations. However, it is important to discuss certain general principles regarding how a radiologist will decide which type of examination is to be used in a given clinical situation.

The DCBE is, for all practical purposes, considered the standard radiological examination of the colon (Fig. 7-1). However, there are still very good indications for both the SCBE and the water-soluble contrast enema. The issue, of course, rests upon pre-examination diagnostic goals. In patients with bleeding, mild to moderate degrees of diarrhea, nonspecific abdominal pain, or who might be at risk for polyp or cancer development, the DCBE study will be utilized. These patients require an efficient bowel preparation for which a variety of commercially prepared products are available. The PEG (polyethylene glycol) electrolyte solution for colonic lavage is becoming the most popular.

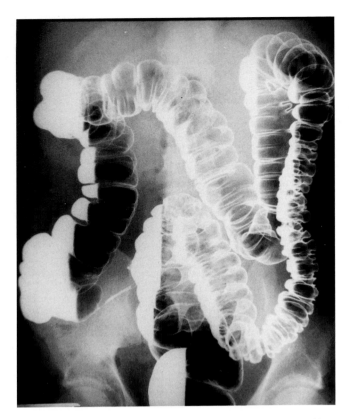

Fig. 7-1   A right decubitus film from a DCBE. Decubitus films with compensation filtration are the most important overhead views in this examination.

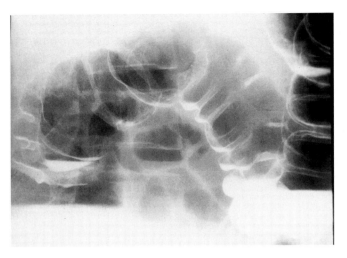

Fig. 7-2   Air-contrast examination in which residual fluid makes coating of the ascending and transverse colon ineffectual. Lesions can easily be missed under these circumstances. Rotating the patient and washing the area with barium can result in additional coating.

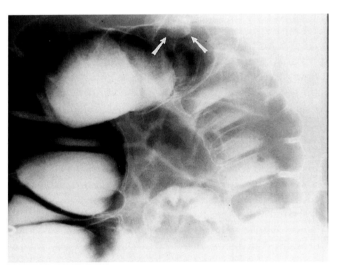

Fig. 7-3   Same patient as shown in Fig. 7-2. Because of the wetness and poor coating of the right colon, the patient was rotated and additional barium was allowed to wash over the area, demonstrating a rounded polyp on the superior margin of the hepatic flexure *(arrows)*.

It is the same preparation commonly used for colonoscopy. The tendency of this type of bowel preparation to leave the colon clean but wet can be dealt with by the administration of bisacodyl suppositories at appropriate intervals before the examination (Figs. 7-2 and 7-3). The use of all bowel preparations should be made with some knowledge of the patient's current clinical status and the diagnostic questions to be addressed. In some instances, particularly in inflammatory bowel disease or bowel obstruction, colonic bowel preparation may require modification, or in some cases, be totally omitted.

Double-contrast technique consists of administering a high-density, low-viscosity barium into the colon followed by air insufflation and the demonstration of the entire mucosal surface of the rectum and colon. In the well-prepared patient, this is a sensitive examination detecting cancer approximately in 94% of cases. It is also able to detect early mucosal inflammatory changes. The guiding principle in the performance of this, like all radiological procedures, is to achieve a high-quality examination that results in maximum information about the state of the patient's colon. Having

said this, it should also be a high priority of the examining radiologist to attempt to achieve this goal with certain well-founded patient concerns in mind.

The technologist who prepares the patient for the examination will, no doubt, explain the examination in detail and do much to allay most of the patient's concerns. Nevertheless, it is inadvisable for a radiologist to first meet the patient while that patient is on the fluoroscopic table with a rectal tube in place. Despite the acknowledgment that it is an efficient examination for the detection of disease, the barium enema, over the decades, has achieved a notorious reputation among lay people as a well-devised form of medical torture. With this in mind, it is the wise radiologist who will endeavor to utilize every psychological and physical advantage in attempting, to some extent, to debunk this reputation, while at the same time not sacrificing the efficiency of the examination.

The psychological state of the patient is often crucial to the successful completion of the study, and this is particularly the case in the more difficult examinations. Thus, it is not unreasonable to greet the patient before the examination, elicit a brief history, explain the examination, and address whatever concerns the patient may have regarding the study. It is also important that the radiologist not lose sight of patient anxiety, discomfort, and embarrassment that are commonly associated with this procedure. All of these issues can be addressed during the course of the examination. The number of films, fluoroscopic time, and overall radiation exposure should be kept to the minimum necessary to achieve an efficient examination. The radiologist should strive to ensure that the amount of time the patient spends on the fluoroscopic table is as short as possible. Concerns with patient dignity and embarrassment should be dealt with by making sure the patient is properly draped at all times. Many radiologists have perfected the procedure to the point where they are able, in many instances, to remove the rectal tip relatively early in the examination. This results in a significant decrease in patient discomfort and an increased patient tolerance for the remainder of the study.

For similar reasons, some radiologists prefer the tableside fluoroscopic examination over remote control facilities. In some cases, the patient will need to be talked through the difficult parts of the examination, and being beside the patient with a hands-on directive approach can make the difference between success and failure. A spectral voice emanating from a loudspeaker somewhere in the room while the table moves and the overhead tower arcs above the patient will do little to allay the anxieties of many patients. Of course, there is controversy and disagreement on this issue. Nevertheless, it is clear that the patient is the center of the radiological practice, and it is reasonable therefore to expect that radiologists should practice patient-centered rather than machine-centered radiology. Moreover, there is perhaps no other area in radiology where this can be practiced with such gratifying results as fluoroscopy.

Single-Contrast Barium Enema

In most large medical centers, approximately 85% of barium enema studies are double-contrast examinations. However, 15% of the patients will have well-defined reasons for using the single-contrast barium enema. Before the study, the radiologist should carefully review the goals of the study to establish the technique to be undertaken. In patients in whom colonic obstruction must be excluded, a single-contrast examination will suffice to address the question. In many cases, these patients have undergone incomplete bowel preparation or none at all.

In questionable cases of diverticulitis, some radiologists will prefer the single-contrast examination, feeling that the radiological findings of diverticulitis are better demonstrated with a single-contrast study. This is based on the supposition that dilute barium will flow more readily into intramural or paraluminal tracts or abscesses than will the more viscous double-contrast barium.

In instances where patients are impaired and cannot move or roll to the extent required for a successful DCBE study, a single-contrast study should be seriously considered. This is particularly the case in older, debilitated, severely mentally retarded, or extremely ill patients. Although a double-contrast examination has been shown to be more sensitive for the detection of both inflammatory and polypoid processes, a bad double-contrast examination is worse than a bad single-contrast examination. This is a good rule of thumb to remember, and given a choice in a situation where a very limited or poor DCBE is possible, one should opt for the single-contrast study.

Water-Soluble Contrast

There is a limited role for the water-soluble contrast enema. This is almost entirely for the evaluation of a patient with suspected perforation. Quite frequently these patients have experienced recent trauma, instrumentation or surgery. The water-soluble contrast enema may also be utilized in the evaluation of a colon in which the potential for perforation may be high. This would include patients with colonic dilatation and particularly a cecum that may be acutely dilated to a preperforation state.

Computed Tomography and Magnetic Resonance Imaging

The role of computed tomography (CT) is becoming more important in colonic diagnosis. The ability of CT imaging to detect bowel wall thickening makes it slightly more sensitive in the detection of diverticulitis than is the barium enema. In addition, paraluminal abscesses are readily identified with CT. The ability to evaluate adjacent structures is an added dimension of the examination. Although the occasional dramatic demonstration of a colonic malignancy with CT is encountered, there is no role, at the moment, for CT in the primary evaluation of colonic polyps and masses. Although CT is able to demonstrate bowel wall thickening to advantage, the evaluation of inflammatory disease within the colon or adjacent small bowel will require additional examinations, either colonoscopy or barium studies.

The role of magnetic resonance imaging (MRI) in colorectal imaging is extremely limited at this time. However, there is increasing interest and activity in the use of MRI in evaluating rectal tumors for staging purposes. Although there is some evidence to suggest that MRI may be slightly superior to CT in evaluating the extent of tumor invasion of pelvic structures, it apparently is less reliable in the detection of abnormal nodes.

Ultrasound

Except for abscess detection, there is a relatively little role for conventional ultrasound in the evaluation of colonic abnormalities. Although some early success has been reported using conventional ultrasound to examine water-filled colons, its potential as a routine method of colon evaluation is questionable. However, the use of endoscopic sonography in the evaluation of rectal disease has increased in some medical centers with early results suggesting that it is as accurate, if not more accurate than CT, in the detection of disease, evaluation of the extent of disease, and in determining the absence or presence of regional lymph nodes. This is a safe examination with no significant complications reported to date.

SOLITARY FILLING DEFECT

Adenoma
Carcinoma
Lipoma
Leiomyoma
Carcinoid Tumor
Lymphoma
Colonic Duplication
Inverted Appendiceal Stump
Unusual Diverticulum
Foreign Bodies

The radiological problems of the colon and rectum will be discussed as they relate to standard intraluminal contrast examinations of the colon. Other imaging techniques will be included as part of the relevant discussion of the radiological problem under consideration.

Filling defect is a term historically rooted in the development of the SCBE and suggests displacement of barium by a space-occupying entity. Hence, for a focal area, a thinner barium column is presented for the x-ray beam to penetrate, resulting in less attenuation and producing a focal lucency. The term is used frequently when describing polypoid lesions on double-contrast studies, although technically these are usually not filling defects in the strict definition.

The radiological problem of an intraluminal filling defect presents a wide variety of diagnostic possibilities and can be divided into benign neoplastic, malignant neoplastic, and a wide assortment of miscellaneous causes. Inflammatory causes of a solitary filling defect are rare.

Adenoma

Most adenomatous polyps are solitary. However, in the presence of carcinoma, the incidence of multiple

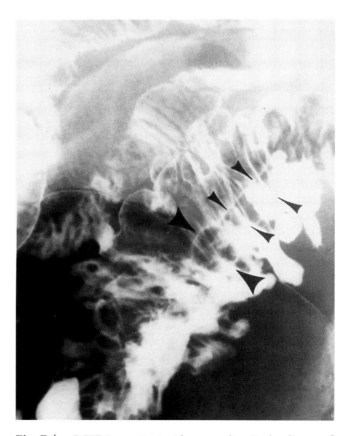

Fig. 7-4   DCBE in a patient with severe diverticular disease of the sigmoid colon. A polyp on a long stalk is present *(arrowheads)* but obscured by the multiple diverticula.

adenomatous polyps increases. Approximately 25% of patients with colorectal cancer will have one or more adenomatous polyps elsewhere in the large bowel. There is also a suggestion that the presence of multiple hyperplastic polyps may be associated with an increase in the number of adenomas. Moreover, the chance for multiplicity clearly increases with age.

Adenomatous polyps histologically fall within the classification of tubular, tubulovillous, and villous adenoma. The villous adenoma tends to have the greatest malignant potential, while the tubular adenoma has the least. Most adenomatous polyps are tubular adenomas and frequently are smooth-surfaced or lobulated. They may be sessile or pedunculated, having a stalk of varying lengths (Figs. 7-4 and 7-5). The stalk is usually composed of normal mucosal tissue and is often associated with larger polyps. Progressive peristaltic activity results in stretching of the base of the polyp and, over a prolonged period of time, elongation into a well-defined stalk. The villous adenoma has the typical frond-like papillary surface, often described by pathologists as being "velvety" in nature. They are almost always sessile and the amount of lobulation may be considerably more than seen with the tubular adenoma. These surface characteristics, so familiar to radiologists, hold true for polyps greater than 1 cm but are less reliable for smaller lesions.

The frequency of adenomatous polyps in the general population has been found to vary markedly from study to study. Autopsy studies may provide the most consistent data, placing the incidence between 10% and 30% of the population. The incidence increases significantly with age.

Various studies have indicated that most adenomatous polyps are found in the rectosigmoid region. It has been estimated that as many as 50% of adenomas occur in this area, although in recent years some research has suggested a so-called "proximal migration" of colonic polyps. This may represent a combination of an increasingly aging population and improvements such as colonoscopy and DCBE in examining the colon.

It is now widely accepted that the great majority of colorectal cancers result from malignant transformation of benign adenomatous polyps, the adenoma-carcinoma sequence. Estimations of the risk of malignant degeneration are imprecise; however, the well-differentiated tubular adenomas have a smaller risk than the more volatile villous adenomas. The incidence of cancer is 0.01% in polyps less than 5 mm and about 1.0% in polyps 1 cm or smaller. In polyps greater than 2 cm, the incidence increases to 30% to 40%. The time progression of adenoma to carcinoma evolution is estimated at between 10 and 15 years, although startling exceptions are encountered from time to time (Figs. 7-6 and 7-7).

Clinically, most adenomas are asymptomatic. By far the most common presentation will be rectal bleeding, either occult or overt. Additionally, polyps can act as

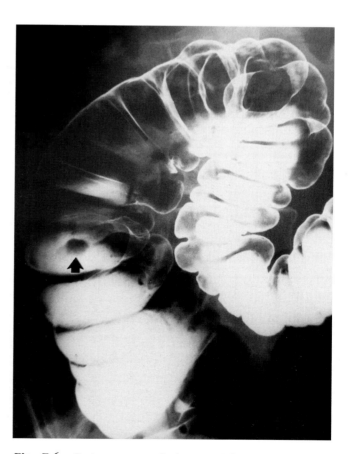

Fig. 7-6 Barium enema discloses a 1.5 cm pedunculated polyp in the ascending colon *(arrow).*

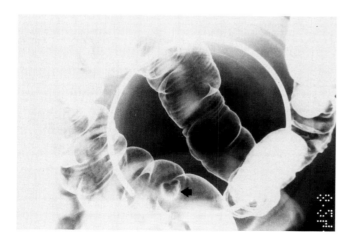

Fig. 7-5 A sessile sigmoid polyp *(arrow)* is demonstrated on a DCBE *(arrow).*

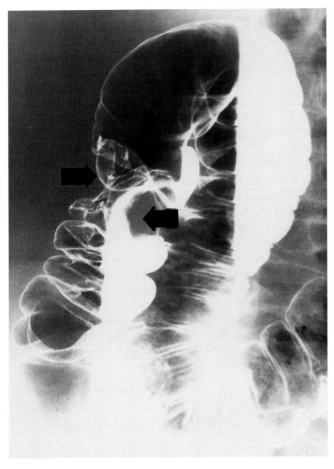

Fig. 7-7   In the same patient as Fig. 7-6, a DCBE obtained less than 2 years later reveals an annular carcinoma at the site of the polyp on the earlier examination.

the lead point for intussusception although this is unusual in the colon. The classical association of large villous adenomas with loss of fluid and electrolytes (especially potassium) is infrequently encountered.

The detection rate of polyps is higher with double-contrast technique than with single-contrast technique. However, a high kilovoltage (kV), full-column technique, utilizing fluoroscopic manipulation and compression, may have an equally high yield for polyps greater than 1 to 2 cm. Polyps less than 1 cm are detected with less frequency in both types of studies, although the ability to detect smaller polyps appears to be significantly higher in double-contrast studies than in single contrast studies.

The radiographic appearance of polyps on full-column, single-contrast studies is often that of the traditional filling defect. The demonstration on double-contrast studies is somewhat more complex, as this technique provides the ability to literally see through the colon, observing both mucosal surfaces at the same time. As a result, the polyp can be seen profiled, en face, or tangentially, resulting in different well-known appearances, such as the Mexican hat sign or the bowler hat sign (Fig. 7-8). Evaluation of the polyp should include size, the presence or absence of a stalk or pedicle, description of the surface features, and the presence or absence of ulceration. With respect to size, it should be remembered that at least a 25% magnification distortion, on average, should be figured into the final estimation of the polyp size.

Interestingly, the polyp that often provides the most difficulty in radiological diagnosis during DCBE is the polyp on a long stalk (Fig. 7-9). Because it shifts posi-

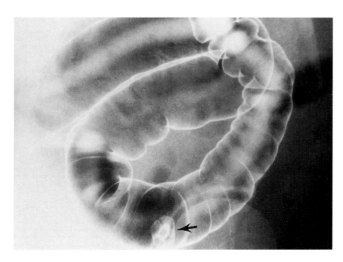

Fig. 7-8   Sigmoid spot film demonstrates a polyp (*arrow*) with a central "ring shadow" representing barium coating of the short stalk of the polyp. This configuration is sometimes known as the Mexican hat sign.

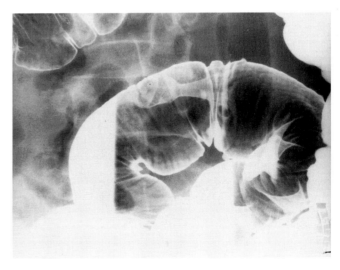

Fig. 7-9   Decubitus view demonstrates a polyp on a stalk. Because of the length of the stalk, the polyp shifts with changes in the patient's position.

tion with the various views, it may be misinterpreted as residual stool. Occasionally, these polyps can be quite large, reminding us that the interpretation of double-contrast studies must, by necessity, include a meticulous evaluation of the various lines and contours of the colon. There is a dictum in GI radiology, that double-contrast radiology of the colon is an excellent examination, with the only difficulties being lesions that are extremely tiny or those that are extremely large. This can, on occasion, become an embarrassing reality.

Carcinoma

It is estimated that approximately 155,000 to 160,000 new cases of colorectal carcinoma will be diagnosed in 1992. Approximately two thirds of these will be in men. The incidence of colon cancer is approximately 2½ times that of rectal cancer. Only breast and lung cancer exceed colorectal cancer in terms of cancer deaths. In 1992, approximately 60,000 deaths will be attributable to colorectal cancer. The overall mortality associated with this disease has not significantly changed since the 1930s, and the mean 5-year survival rate is about 40% to 50%. However, for any given patient, survival will depend on how early the lesion is diagnosed. The Duke's classification, on which the staging of colorectal carcinoma is based, reflects both the extent of tumor involvement and the prognosis. Duke's stage A represents lesions confined to the bowel wall and has an 85% 5-year survival rate. Duke's stage B represents lesions that have extended through the bowel wall, and these are associated with a 70% 5-year survival rate. With Duke's stage C representing metastatic lesions to regional lymph nodes, the survival rate falls to 33%. Distant metastatic disease, Duke's stage D, has a 5% 5-year survival rate. It has been estimated that as many as 40% to 50% of patients will have hepatic metastatic disease at the time of diagnosis.

The disease continues to be mainly one of Western industrialized nations. It is a disease of older people, with the median patient's age at diagnosis in the 60s.

The etiological and epidemiological data associated with this disease are ponderous and cannot be addressed in detail. It is clear that the issues and controversies surrounding the possible etiologies are becoming more openly discussed in the lay media as the nation becomes more conscious of nutrition and health. The controversy surrounding suspected etiologies and associated risk factors includes dietary intake with particular emphasis on increasing the ingestion of dietary fiber and decreasing the ingestion of animal fats. Recent observations have been put forth suggesting that intake of vitamin C or aspirin on a regular basis may

confer some degree of protection. These are interesting possibilities but require considerable further investigation.

There are, however, some things about which we are more certain and one is that most colorectal cancers progress through the adenoma-to-cancer route. A few may arise de novo from dysplastic changes within the mucosal surface, although this is felt to be uncommon in patients without inflammatory bowel disease (IBD). We know that IBD, in particular, ulcerative colitis carries a higher risk for the development of colorectal cancer. We know that certain familial polyposis syndromes carry an extremely high if not absolute certain risk of cancer. We also know that colorectal cancer can run in certain families, and that in approximately 25% of new cases there will be a family history of colorectal cancer. Furthermore, it has been estimated that individuals who are first-generation relatives of patients with colorectal cancer have a 10% to 15% increased risk above that of the general population.

The clinical presentation of colorectal carcinoma is, to a large extent, dependent upon the site of the lesion. During early stages of growth, the patient may be asymptomatic, or there may be undetected occult bleeding. The most insidious lesions usually arise from the right side of the colon. This occurs because the wider luminal diameter, greater distensibility of the right colon, and the more liquid nature of the colonic content on the right side delay the onset of obstructive symptoms and allow the lesion to become larger and invasive before the diagnosis is finally made. (Fig. 7-10). Patients with right-sided lesions often present with bleeding. They may experience crampy, nonspecific right-sided abdominal pain. However, by far, the most common presenting problem is usually iron deficiency anemia as a result of chronic blood loss. Tumors on the left side, in the descending and sigmoid colon, tend to present earlier. This is a result of the smaller luminal diameter of the colon in this region and the firmer colonic content. Changes in the luminal diameter, secondary to tumor growth, will most commonly result in obstruction. Lesions in the rectum commonly present with bright red bleeding and changes in bowel habits. Generally, lesions in the distal colon are detected earlier and survival is somewhat better. Approximately 50% of lesions are found distal to the mid-descending colon. On rare occasions, colonic adenocarcinoma can perforate, and the patient may present with a pericolic abscess.

Given the impact of this disease in terms of the morbidity and mortality, a complete examination of the colon is required. Although flexible sigmoidoscopy can examine up to 50 cm, this will still result in approximately half of the lesions being undetected. Colonoscopy permits direct examination of the mucosal sur-

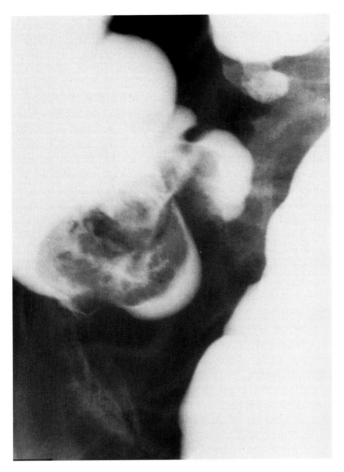

Fig. 7-10 Single-contrast examination of the colon reveals a large, lobulated cecal mass representing an adenocarcinoma. The mass is ulcerated on its surface and is nonobstructing.

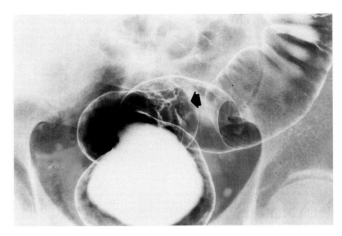

Fig. 7-11 Spot film from a DCBE reveals a focal area of raised, irregular mucosa with radiation towards a small, central mound *(arrow)*. Biopsy revealed villous adenoma with malignant degeneration.

face of the entire length of the colon. However, the examination is incomplete in 10% to 30% of attempts. Colonoscopy is a relatively expensive undertaking, although it can be of considerable value because it permits removal of polyps and the retrieval of tissue specimens for pathological diagnosis.

The DCBE is a relatively low cost examination with a high rate of detection for colorectal cancers (approximately 94%) and an extremely low rate of incomplete exams. Moreover, this examination is considerably safer than instrumentation, having one tenth the incidence of bowel perforation associated with colonoscopy.

Problems associated with DCBE relate to bowel preparation and coexistent diverticular disease. Both of these factors can render the examination less sensitive. The presence of extensive diverticular disease in the sigmoid region results in such significant bowel distortion that it may be virtually impossible to identify a polypoid lesion. It is possible that single-contrast compression views of this area would be much more useful in detecting polypoid lesions in this situation. Additionally, residual stool can be troublesome. Double-contrast examinations ought to include decubitus views which can often sort out these problems. Other areas of difficulty include the ileocecal region and the medial wall of the ascending colon where subtle or occult lesions can hide. The majority of missed colorectal carcinomas on double-contrast examination have been shown to be errors of perception. The importance of meticulous and careful analysis of double-contrast views of the colon cannot be overestimated. It goes without saying that interpretation of these studies is an exercise in self-discipline and concentration.

The radiological findings of colorectal cancer can include a number of configurations, from round polypoid filling defects to encircling, constricting lesions. They can also be seen as raised, ulcerated masses or as irregular, villous-appearing lesions (Fig. 7-11). The more subtle lesions may be manifested as distortions in the normal haustral pattern or bowel wall contours.

Frequently CT evaluation of the abdomen may reveal a soft-tissue mass adjacent to or within the colonic lumen (Fig. 7-12). One should take care to not misinterpret a prolapsed ileocecal valve or stool as a cecal mass (Figs. 7-13 and 7-14). There may be evidence of extension of the tumor beyond the wall, or involvement of adjacent organs, such as lymph nodes or the liver. Ultrasonography may demonstrate a large hypoechoic mass with some central echoes representing thickened bowel wall and the central lumen respec-

The polyps tend to be most numerous in the small bowel, although colonic polyps are not uncommon. Patients are often middle-aged and present with diarrhea relating to an associated protein-losing enteropathy. Although the initial reports considered the polyps to be adenomas, subsequent studies have consistently demonstrated a lesion resembling a juvenile polyp with hamartomatous and inflammatory elements. Occasional reports of colon cancer in patients with this condition have raised the question of whether there may be a slightly increased risk.

From a clinical perspective, the chronic diarrhea appears to present more of a threat to the patient's health than the presence of GI polyps.

Cowden's syndrome Cowden's syndrome is uncommon and is characterized by multiple harmartomatous polyps of the esophogus, stomach, small bowel, and colon. The polyps themselves are not known to be associated with any clinical symptomatology. The significant aspect of the syndrome is the extra-gastrointestinal manifestations, which include skin changes, perioral papillomas, faciotrichilemmomas, thyroid abnormalities including goiter and cancer as well as an increased risk of breast cancer.

Neurofibromatosis Neurofibromatosis (von Recklinghausen's disease) is a condition in which the most well-known manifestations are multiple subcutaneous neurofibromas. Involvement of the gut with disseminated neurofibromatosis is unusual but does occur. Although involvement of the gut is usually associated with the cutaneous manifestations, the disease may also be confined to the GI tract. Most of the reports of colonic involvement occur in children. They usually present with intussusuception or rectal bleeding. There is some slight increased risk of malignant degeneration.

Pseudopolyps

Pseudopolyps are polypoid protrusions into the lumen of a colon exhibiting the changes of severe inflammatory bowel disease (IBD) and are truly named, in that they are not polyps in the typical sense. The pseudopolyp is actually residual edematous mucosa sitting, like an island, on a sea of surrounding ulceration. The denuding of the adjacent mucosa and the swelling of the remaining island of mucosa result in the classical polypoid appearance of the pseudopolyp.

Pseudopolyps may be seen in virtually any IBD involving the colon, although by far the most common is ulcerative colitis. Pseudopolyps are a particularly prominent feature of toxic megacolon.

Postinflammatory Polyps

The appearance of colonic postinflammatory polyps is a direct effect of IBD and in particular ulcerative co-

litis. It may be seen less commonly in Crohn's disease and other inflammatory conditions of the colon.

These polyps are, in fact, composed of normal mucosa. They are often filiform or comma-shaped in configuration and tend to be mostly found in the distal colon. These projections of normal mucosa into the lumen occur as a result of mucosal healing following severe IBD. They represent what were, during the height of the inflammatory process, pseudopolyps. Once the healing process begins, reepithelialization of the surrounding ulcerated areas occurs. This reepithelialization process extends into the undermined base of the pseudopolyp. As a result, when healing is complete, a projection of normal mucosa, usually in a filiform shape and often readily identifiable, is seen (Fig. 7-25). This may be seen on a background of normal colonic mucosa or recurrent disease.

Unusual presentations of postinflammatory polyposis include mucosal bridges, which are occasionally seen, and represent reepithelialization of a thin strip of via-

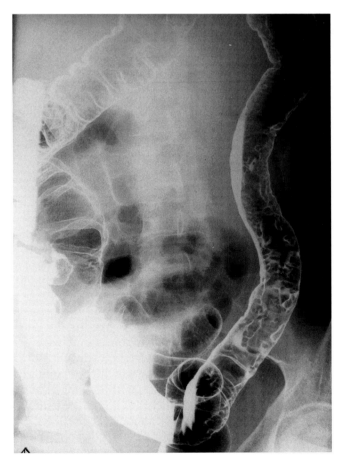

Fig. 7-25 DCBE on a patient with a previous history of ulcerative colitis reveals tubular-appearing left colon with numerous filiform filling defects representing postinflammatory polyposis.

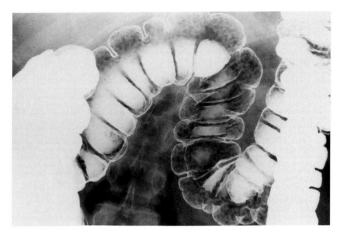

Fig. 7-26   Numerous, tiny filling defects are seen throughout the colon in this adult patient, representing a prominent lymphoid follicular pattern.

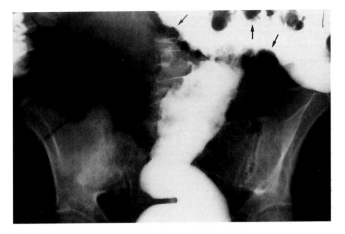

Fig. 7-27   Barium enema reveals numerous marginal nodular filling defects, some of which have the appearance of thumbprinting *(arrows)*. However, the filling defects are air-filled and represent pneumatosis coli.

ble mucosa that has been totally undermined by ulceration. Additionally, large masses of postinflammatory polyps have been reported, having, in some instances, the appearance of a large villous tumor. These have been called giant postinflammatory polyps.

Lymphoid Hyperplasia/Lymphoid Follicular Prominence

The diagnosis of nodular lymphoid hyperplasia (NLH) presents something of a dilemma. This diagnostic title suggests a disease, whereas the presence of prominent lymphoid follicles throughout the colon is usually a normal finding in children and seen with much more frequency than previously thought in adults.

In most instances, these small lymphoid nodules of the colon are considered a normal variant. They usually measure 1 to 3 mm and are rounded elevations of the mucosa with poor definition of the borders (Fig. 7-26). They tend to occur in areas where lymphoid follicles are most numerous, such as the ileocecal area and rectum. However, they can also be seen distributed throughout the entire colon. When these nodules are larger than 3 mm, the condition is commonly referred to as lymphoid hyperplasia and characterized radiologically by a tiny central barium-filled dimple seen on ACBE. This is not a disease but, more likely, the reaction of the lymphoid follicles to an adjacent inflammatory or infectious process, although the process may not always be apparent. The presence of nodular lymphoid hyperplasia in the small bowel and possibly the colon of patients with hypogammaglobulinemia and associated giardiasis has also been noted. There has been

suggestion over the years that lymphoid hyperplasia may represent the earliest changes of IBD or lymphatic disease, although this is quite speculative and has never been proven.

Pneumatosis Cystoides Coli

Pneumatosis coli is manifested by two distinctive patterns. The condition is characterized by air in the bowel wall. The most common form is subserosal cystic blebs (Fig. 7-27). The actual cause is unknown. Speculation has largely centered on coexistent chronic obstructive pulmonary disease in which microruptures of the alveoli occur and air dissects through the vascular-bronchial interstitial pathways to the mediastinum, down the mediastinum into the retroperitoneum, and into the root of the mesentery. Further dissection of air occurs along the leaves of the mesentery until it reaches the peritoneal surface of the bowel. Most of the subserosal cystic air collections are seen in the distal colon, with abrupt termination at the peritoneal reflection off the rectum. The oxygen is largely absorbed, and the remaining gas is primarily nitrogen. Another condition that has been associated with this is scleroderma. These patients are almost always asymptomatic and the findings usually incidental. On rare occasion, if a subserosal cyst is sufficiently large, there can be stretching of the overlying mucosa and potential ulceration and bleeding. Additionally, the subserosal blebs on occasion can rupture, and the patient can have a benign pneumoperitoneum. Such a finding can often cause confusion in the emergency department.

Another, more ominous form of pneumatosis coli is the presence of linear intramural collections of air.

These are not subserosal in location, but usually submucosal. This finding is most frequently associated with underlying acute vascular insults to the bowel, ischemia and infarction. Air that has percolated into the submucosa, as result of a loss of mucosal integrity, will, like food nutrients, be taken up in the portal venous system and transported through the mesenteric veins to the portal vein. From there, it can be carried into the intrahepatic portal venous system. This can be identified on plain radiographs as tiny, branching, tubular collections of air in the periphery of the liver. In most instances, at the time of radiological evaluation, these patients are sufficiently toxic to confidently make the diagnosis. However, the findings of air in the bowel wall may precede by several hours the onset of catastrophic decline in the patient's physical status. There may be little more than complaints of abdominal pain in some patients undergoing major bowel infarction who will not survive 24 hours. This may be especially true in older individuals.

A major pitfall for the radiologist is the discovery of extensive linear submucosal air collections or air within the portal venous system in a relatively asymptomatic patient. Some conditions that may manifest a benign form of this pneumatosis coli, unrelated to bowel wall ischemia or necrosis, include GI surgery, pyloric obstruction, peptic ulceration, instrumentation, and mucosal trauma. In these situations, the cause of this condition is related to mechanical and surgical factors rather than bowel necrosis. However, linear pneumatosis on plain film or abdominal CT should always lead to an immediate consultation with the referring clinician.

Metastatic Disease

Metastatic spread of tumor to the colon and rectum can produce a variety of radiological findings and clinical symptomatology. The spread to the colon may occur as a result of seeding through the intraperitoneal pathways, local contiguous spread, or hematogenous dissemination. Tumors that can spread in such a manner and produce multiple and, on rare occasion, solitary filling defects include breast cancer, malignant melanoma, and bronchogenic carcinoma. Radiographic appearances are quite variable and may include well-defined intramural polypoid masses or large, bulky, irregular masses with superficial ulceration. Lesions originating in the ovary and stomach most commonly spread through the intraperitoneal pathways and result in narrowing and stricture. Involvement of the rectum by cervical cancer or prostatic cancer usually results from contiguous invasion.

Colitis Cystica Profunda

Colitis cystica profunda (CCP) is an unusual nonneoplastic condition characterized by the presence of mucus-filled cysts in the submucosa and is usually confined to the rectum or distal sigmoid. The radiographic appearance can be variable, with a classical description of numerous, smooth polypoid lesions that may be indistinguishable from adenomatous polyps. Occasionally, the polyps can be clustered and irregular, even assuming a masslike configuration that requires differentiation from malignant neoplasm. Clinically, these patients present with rectal bleeding and passage of excessive mucus per rectum.

The etiological basis of the condition is quite confusing. It is felt by some to originate as a primary focal glandular abnormality of the distal large bowel and rectum. Conversely, there is also a fairly convincing argument that this is a variant of the solitary rectal ulcer syndrome. Solitary rectal ulcer syndrome is probably a result of chronic internal rectal prolapse. This causes superficial ulceration, interval episodes of inflammation, and healing, with invagination of the glandular structures that become cystic over a period of time.

Kaposi's Sarcoma

For decades, Kaposi's sarcoma has been known as an indolent cutaneous neoplastic disease of older men and was considered uncommon. However, with the advent of AIDS, it has come to the forefront of diagnostic considerations. Of patients with AIDS 30% to 40% of patients with AIDS have Kaposi's sarcoma somewhere in the GI tract. Virtually all cases of Kaposi's sarcoma of the gut are associated with AIDS. The lesions can affect the esophagus, stomach, small bowel, or colon. They may predate the cutaneous lesions. Barium enema will commonly demonstrate multiple nodular lesions, usually in the distal colon. Infiltrative or irregular masses can also be seen.

These patients may present with GI bleeding as a result of ulceration of the larger nodules. In some instances, this may be the presenting complaint before the diagnosis of AIDS is known. The presence of Kaposi's sarcoma within the bowel is indicative of poor prognosis, and few of these patients will survive beyond 12 to 18 months following diagnosis.

Colonic Lymphoma

In most instances, lymphoma will be indistinguishable from primary adenocarcinoma. However, on occasion, this lesion may present as multiple nodular polypoid lesions within the colon, usually on the right side (Fig. 7-28).

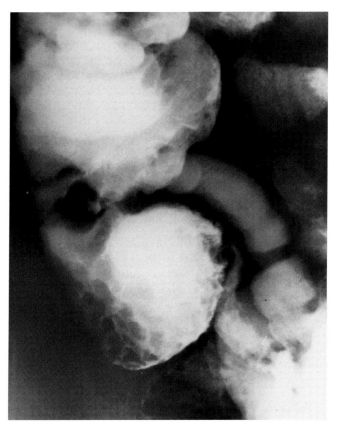

Fig. 7-28 Spot film of the cecum demonstrates multiple mucosal nodules in the cecal tip, giving a somewhat mosaic pattern and representing lymphoma. Other conditions that can give a similar appearance include ischemic changes, Crohn's disease, and *Yersinia* colitis.

EXTRINSIC DEFECTS

Liver
Gallbladder
Spleen
Abdominal/pelvic masses

Extrinsic defects affecting the colon may fall within the normal or abnormal category. In the normal category, one can expect to see impressions from the right lobe of the liver, particularly a Riedel's lobe, where the inferior aspect of the right lobe is somewhat elongated and impresses the ascending colon. A patulous or prominent gallbladder may be seen impressing the superior margin of the proximal transverse colon. Splenic impressions are common, but their presence does not necessarily indicate splenomegaly. Occasionally, individuals with a very prominent sacral promontory will demonstrate some posterior impression at the rectosigmoid junction.

Virtually, any intraabdominal mass can result in colonic displacement or compression. This ranges from abscesses, the most common of which are due to diverticular, periappendiceal and pelvic inflammatory disease, to cystic lesions, most commonly of the ovary. Significant cystic disease of the kidney can also impress the colon. Intraabdominal tumor masses can compress, displace, or invade the colon.

ULCERATION

Ulcerative Colitis
Crohn's Disease
Viral Colitis
Bacterial Colitis
Ischemic Colitis
Amebiasis
Radiation Colitis
Tuberculosis
Solitary Rectal Ulcer Syndrome
Trauma
Behçet's Disease
Diversion Colitis
Gonorrheal Proctitis

Ulcerative Colitis

Of the group of diseases generally known as IBD, ulcerative colitis and Crohn's disease represent the two most important conditions (Table 7-2). Ulcerative colitis is a mucosal disease that involves the colon distally and may progressively advance to affect the proximal colon. The disease, if limited to the rectum at the time of diagnosis, is referred to as ulcerative proctitis.

The cardinal clinical features are diarrhea and rectal bleeding. The severity of the clinical presentation will often be dependent upon the amount of large bowel involved. Approximately one third of patients will have pancolonic involvement at initial presentation. The disease can present as an acute process, a recurrent process, or a chronic ongoing condition. It is mostly a disease of young people, although it can be seen in any age group. The pathological characteristic of the disease is continuous and concentric superficial involvement of the bowel wall with inflammatory changes, mostly limited to the mucosa. In severe fulminating disease, the extent and depth of disease can significantly increase and become transmural as in the case of toxic megacolon.

When early active disease is present, the mucosal surface will become hyperemic, granular, and edematous. Tiny punctate ulcers may also be seen in the acute phase. The haustral pattern is usually diminished

widespread amebiasis can occur. The protozoan is ingested as a cyst in food or water and eventually passes into the small bowel and colon where the cyst dissolves and the uninuclear trophozoite form is released. These motile organisms invade the colonic mucosa causing hyperemia and edema. Progression of the infectious process results in mucosal ulcers. The cecum and ascending colon are the areas most commonly affected within the colon. Involvement of the adjacent distal ileum is unusual.

In addition to widespread mucosal inflammation and ulceration, a more localized, masslike form of the process, an ameboma, is occasionally identified. An ameboma is a marked, localized reaction involving extensive granulomatous type of inflammation, thickening of the bowel wall, and narrowing of the lumen. The configuration of an ameboma may look like carcinoma on endoscopic or radiological examination. Fortunately, amebomas are uncommon and seen in less than 0.5% of cases.

The barium enema often shows severely inflamed spastic bowel with widespread ulceration. In the early stages, superficial discrete ulcers may be identified on ACBE. The disease tends to be more prevalent in the proximal portions of the colon. In severe disease, there can be marked edema of the bowel wall, thumbprinting, and even toxic dilatation (Fig. 7-39). The radiological findings are not specific, and any stage of the examination can resemble Crohn's disease or ulcerative colitis. Distinction between amebiasis and inflammatory

bowel disease is crucial, as patients with amebiasis who are inadvertently treated with steroids may decline rapidly. The definitive diagnosis is made by detecting the organisms in the stool or endoscopic aspirate.

A helpful but not specific radiological finding is the conical-shaped cecum resulting from diffuse inflammation and spasm of the cecal tip. However, other conditions such as Crohn's disease, tuberculosis, actinomycosis, and even adjacent appendiceal disease can also result in a conical cecum.

Radiation Colitis

Inflammatory changes secondary to radiation are most commonly seen in the rectum and sigmoid colon, usually as a result of radiation therapy for pelvic neoplastic disease. This appears to be most commonly associated with treatment of carcinoma of the cervix. Acute changes are nonspecific and mostly consist of edema and erythema. In more severe radiation damage or chronic radiation damage, the colon tends to lose its haustral pattern and become somewhat tubular (Fig. 7-40). Rectal folds may completely disappear. Fre-

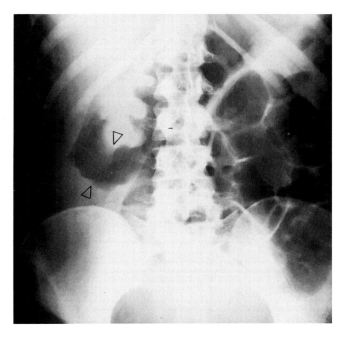

Fig. 7-39   Plain film of the abdomen on a patient with fulminant amebic colitis. Note the narrowing of the proximal transverse colon and the prominent nodularity (thumbprinting) in this region (*arrowheads*).

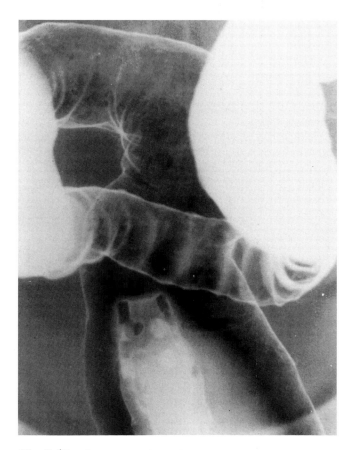

Fig. 7-40   Rectosigmoid spot film from a patient with chronic radiation proctitis and sigmoiditis. There is a general loss of the haustral pattern with a somewhat tubular appearance of the bowel.

quently, there is widening of the presacral space. Ulceration may be present to varying degrees in both the acute and chronic phases.

Tuberculosis

Tuberculosis involving the GI tract can be either primary or secondary. The primary involvement, usually associated with the ingestion of nonpasteurized milk, is rarely seen in Western countries today. But *Mycobacterium tuberculosis* primarily involving the lungs can secondary infect the GI tract as a result of swallowed organisms in the sputum. The disease tends to occur around the ileocecal region, possibly because of the abundant lymphoid tissue in that area. Clinical presentation tends to be nonspecific with the most common presenting complaints being abdominal pain, weight loss, fever, and diarrhea. The radiological evaluation may be helpful in identifying an inflammatory mucosal process but is not diagnostic. The radiological appearance can mimic Crohn's disease, including mucosal ulceration, fold thickening, and occasionally stricture. The terminal ileum is commonly involved. In patients with known primary pulmonary tuberculosis, these findings would raise the diagnostic possibility of GI tuberculosis. However, the definitive diagnosis is made by identification of the organism.

The incidence of GI tuberculosis has increased with an increasingly large AIDS population in the community. In addition to *Mycobacterium tuberculosis*, another form of tuberculosis that has been seen with increasing frequency in these patients is *Mycobacterium avium-intracellulare* (MAI). This organism is generally nonpathological. However, in immunoimpaired patients, such as patients with AIDS, MAI infections primarily involving the respiratory tract are seen with increasing frequency. In such patients, this organism may occasionally found to be the basis of GI infection as well.

Solitary Rectal Ulcer Syndrome

Solitary rectal ulcer syndrome, an unusual and somewhat confusing disorder, was first described in the early 1800s. It is most commonly seen in young or middle-aged adults, and the presenting findings are rectal bleeding and mucous discharge. Many patients will also report difficulty passing stool. Ulcers frequently can be identified, although commonly there is more than a solitary ulcer present.

Multiple etiological theories have been suggested. Perhaps the most important is the association of internal rectal prolapse and difficult rectal evacuation. The disease may be associated with or identical to the condition known as colitis cystica profunda.

Radiologically, inflammatory changes including ulceration can be identified along the anterior rectal wall. The rectal valves will often appear thickened, and a polypoid inflammatory mass may also be identified and may mimic neoplastic disease.

Trauma

Although colorectal trauma may result from a variety of causes, such as gunshot wounds, stabbing, or blunt trauma, the majority of cases are probably iatrogenic. These can occur as a result of the traumatic effect of a barium enema tip on the rectal mucosa or intracolonic instrumentation, such as results from sigmoidoscopy or colonoscopy. Frequently, these instruments may cause mucosal lacerations but infrequently result in serious complications, such as perforation.

Behçet's Disease

Behçet's disease is a condition of unknown etiology characterized by four main clinical findings. These include apthous ulcers of the mouth, eyes, skin, and genitalia. It tends to be more common in men between the ages of 40 and 50 years. GI involvement occurs in less than half the patients and tends to be a minor manifestation of the condition. However, in a small number of patients, colonic involvement can be severe, and significant ulceration may be seen.

The radiological evaluation may be confusing, as the condition can simulate either Crohn's disease or, in some cases, ulcerative colitis. Additionally, because both of these idiopathic IBDs are known to have extracolonic manifestations that involve the eyes and skin, patients with Behçet's disease may carry the diagnosis of IBD for some time.

Diversion Colitis

In patients who have had their fecal stream diverted as the result of a proximal colostomy or ileostomy, a nonspecific inflammation involving the diverted portion of the colon may be seen, representing what has been called diversion colitis.

The radiological evaluation of the excluded colonic segment will show acute inflammatory changes very similar to mild acute ulcerative colitis. This curious condition usually spontaneously regresses when the ostomy has been taken down and the fecal stream reestablished.

Gonorrheal Proctitis

Gonorrhea is a relatively common sexually transmitted infectious disease that involves the mucous membranes of the urethra, vagina, and cervix. Rectal involvement can occur in women either as a result of infected vaginal discharge and secondary rectal infection or primarily as a result of anal intercourse. In men, it always results from direct sexual contact and is seen in the homosexual population. The radiological findings are those of superficial inflammatory changes involving the mucosa of the rectum with fold thickening and areas of punctate ulceration (Fig. 7-41). The appearance may be identical to ulcerative proctitis seen early in the development of ulcerative colitis. In addition, other infectious processes such as *Campylobacter* and viral proctitis can give a similar picture.

COLONIC NARROWING

Adenocarcinoma
Diverticulitis
Postinflammatory Strictures
Ischemic Colitis
Adjacent Inflammatory Neoplastic Disease
Endometriosis
Lymphoma
Lymphogranuloma Venereum
Actinomycosis
Extrinsic Compression
Carcinoid

Adenocarcinoma

Although the physical manifestations of colonic adenocarcinoma are numerous, one of the more common is focal irregular narrowing, classically described as the "apple core" configuration or the English equivalent, the "napkin ring" (Fig. 7-42). This lesion will involve a short segment of colon, frequently with some degree of proximal dilatation or obstruction, especially in the sigmoid colon.

Annular lesions tend to be relatively uncommon in the rectum, where large bulky polypoid lesions are considerably more frequent (Fig. 7-43). Rectal lesions also occur in a slightly older age group and are associated with a more aggressive course and slightly decreased survival time.

Diverticulitis

Diverticulitis represents one of the two common complications of diverticulosis of the colon (the other being bleeding), and as such, the underlying condition of diverticulosis requires some understanding before this complication can be fully understood.

Diverticular disease of the colon is a condition of

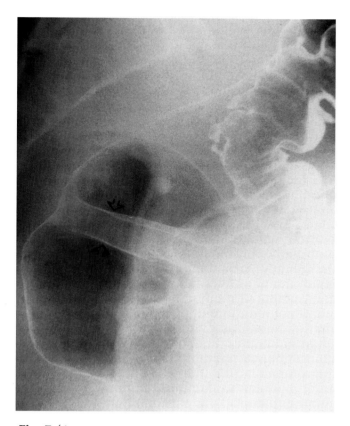

Fig. 7-41   Spot film of the rectum of a patient with known gonorrheal proctitis. Note the thickening of the rectal folds (*arrows*) and the granular appearance of the mucosa.

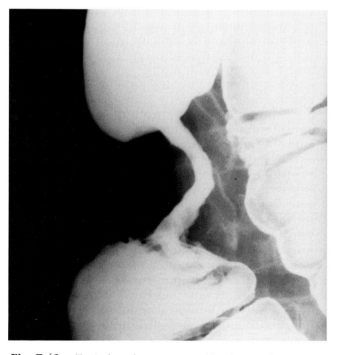

Fig. 7-42   Typical apple core or napkin ring configuration of an annular carcinoma of the colon.

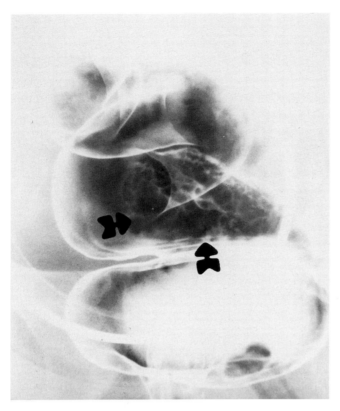

Fig. 7-43 An air-contrast view of rectal carcinoma *(arrows)* demonstrates a large, bulky polypoid lesion with a villous appearance.

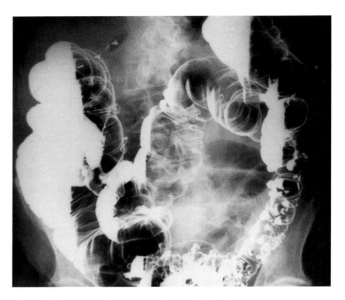

Fig. 7-44 Decubitus view from DCBE demonstrates marked diverticular changes concentrated in the sigmoid region, resulting in considerable distortion of the bowel and difficulty in evaluating the area.

twentieth-century industrialized nations and was a relatively uncommon before this century. Diverticula can occur anywhere in the colon but most commonly in the sigmoid region (Fig. 7-44). These diverticula develop at the site of penetrating blood vessels entering the bowel wall. The mucosa and submucosa of the bowel wall tend to protrude through these natural areas of wall weakness. This anatomical relationship of diverticula to penetrating blood vessels accounts for the high incidence of hemorrhage associated with diverticula formation.

The etiological origins of diverticula formation appear to be related to abnormally high intraluminal colonic pressures and abnormally prolonged colonic transit times. Chronic disease results in muscular thickening, and when severe diverticulosis is present, there can be diffuse narrowing even without the presence of diverticulitis.

The incidence is thought to be slightly more common in women than in men and most definitely increases with age. At age 60, 60% to 70% of patients examined by barium enema will have some degree of diverticula formation. There is also some suggestion that

the disease may be occurring in increasingly younger individuals.

As previously mentioned, this condition appears to be most commonly seen in Western industrialized nations and is almost unheard of in Africa and the Far East. This is thought to relate to differences in the fiber content of the diet and to significant differences in colonic transit times. It has also been observed that long-time vegetarians appear to have a decreased incidence of diverticular disease.

It is probably safe to suggest that most patients with uncomplicated diverticulosis are asymptomatic. On the other hand, there is a poorly defined group of patients who experience lower abdominal pain, exacerbated by dietary intake and known under the diagnostic label of irritable bowel syndrome. Whether the so-called irritable bowel syndrome is a manifestation of colonic intraluminal pressure abnormalities leading to diverticula formation or whether it is a coexisting condition is not absolutely clear, and there is, in fact, difficulty in defining the irritable bowel syndrome. There have been assertions that a correlation exists between the two conditions, although this remains controversial.

Patients who develop complications associated with diverticulosis most frequently develop rectal bleeding. Indeed the most common cause of massive lower GI bleeding is diverticulosis.

Much the same way that appendicitis develops, diverticulitis can occur when a diverticulum becomes occluded by stool, and peridiverticular inflammatory changes associated with microperforations can occur.

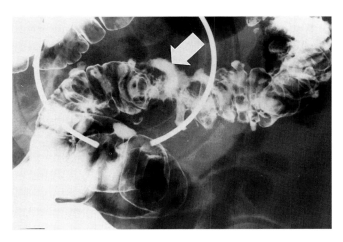

Fig. 7-45   Spot film from DCBE reveals multiple diverticula in the sigmoid region with narrowing and irregularity. A lenticular collection of barium *(arrow)* represents a pericolic abscess secondary to diverticulitis.

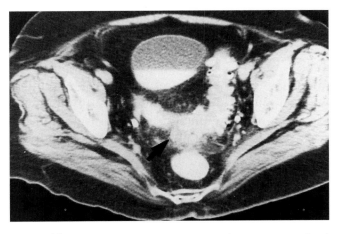

Fig. 7-46   CT scan through the pelvis demonstrates a focal area of sigmoid colon where the bowel margin becomes quite blurred *(arrow)*. There is also increased density in the pericolic area and in the surrounding mesenteric fat. These are typical findings of diverticulitis.

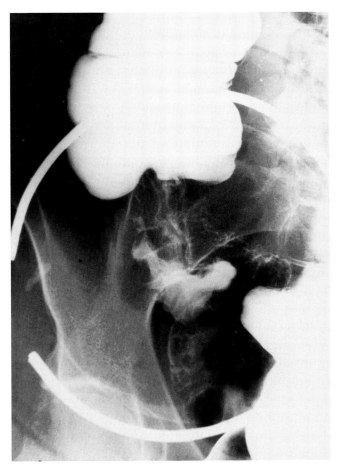

Fig. 7-47   Patient with persistent colonic stricture located just above the ileocecal valve. The mucosa appears to be intact, and this stricture was found to be inflammatory in nature, representing CMV colitis.

These can go on to frank pericolic abscess formation (Fig. 7-45). Areas of narrowing may occur as a result of spasm associated with the inflammation, even in the early changes of diverticulitis without abscess formation. With the presence of abscess formation, the narrowing results from a combination of spasm and mass effect. CT is very useful in the evaluation of diverticulitis, demonstrating thickened edematous bowel wall and pericolic abscesses. The barium enema findings are narrowing and spasm, mass effect, and barium in intramural tracts or pericolic abscess. (Fig. 7-46).

Postinflammatory Strictures

A number of inflammatory conditions can cause focal stricturing and narrowing of the colon. They may occur during the acute phase (Figs. 7-47 and 7-48), but commonly are seen as a sequela to chronic disease.

Colonic strictures can be seen in less than 10% of patients with chronic ulcerative colitis (Fig. 7-49). They rarely result in obstructive changes. Additionally, in patients with severe chronic ulcerative colitis, the

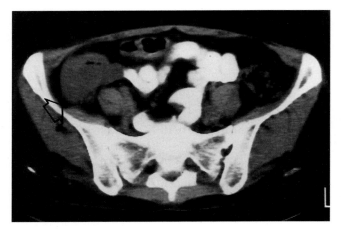

Fig. 7-48 CT scan through the upper pelvis in the same patient as shown in Fig. 7-47. Note the marked thickening of the colonic wall (*arrow*) just above the ileocecal valve.

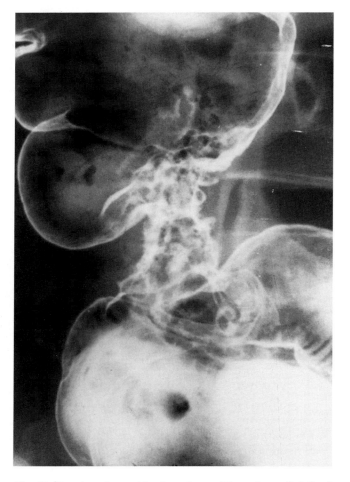

Fig. 7-49 A patient with ulcerative colitis and a well-defined stricture located just above the ileocecal valve, secondary to focal inflammatory changes.

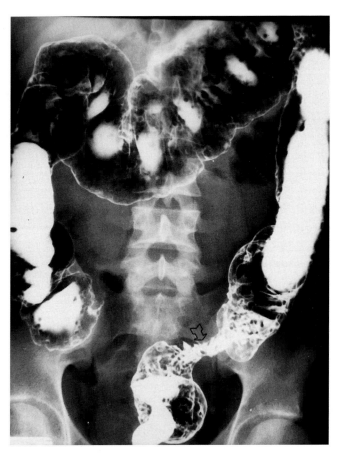

Fig. 7-50 DCBE in a patient with chronic ulcerative colitis. Widespread postinflammatory polyposis is seen along with a strictured segment *(arrow)* in the sigmoid colon.

narrowing may be more diffuse, involving a long segment of the colon (Fig. 7-50).

Because of the transmural inflammatory changes associated with Crohn's disease, areas of focal stricture are slightly more common (Fig. 7-51). The strictures may be asymmetric, reflecting the asymmetric involvement of the bowel at that level.

One of the more common causes of narrowing in the rectum and sigmoid area is radiation colitis. Radiation therapy is usually performed for neoplastic disease of the pelvis. The involved bowel in the radiation port undergoes degrees of vascular injury. Diffuse or focal areas of narrowing are encountered.

Other unusual causes of colonic stricture include amebic, bacterial, and viral colitides.

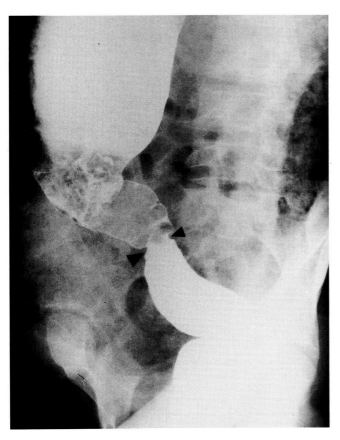

Fig. 7-65 Barium enema (same patient as Fig. 7-64) demonstrates an area of transition in the distal sigmoid, representing the zone of transition *(arrowheads)* from normal to aganglionic colon in a patient with Hirschsprung's disease.

muscular disorder of the GI tract involving all parts of the gut. Some of these patients will have colonic distention without acute clinical findings. However, many of these patients will have chronic abdominal complaints, including distention, chronic abdominal pain, and constipation. A plain film of the abdomen will often show marked colonic distention, and without a clinical history, the radiologist may be obligated to consider differential considerations that include colonic volvulus or obstruction secondary to inflammatory or neoplastic disease.

DIMINISHED HAUSTRAL PATTERN

Chronic ulcerative colitis
Crohn's disease
Scleroderma
Cathartic colon
Radiation

A number of conditions, many of which have been previously discussed, can result in a diminished haustral pattern and a tubular appearance of the colon. These include idiopathic inflammatory processes, such as ulcerative colitis and Crohn's disease as well as bacterial and viral colitides.

In addition, the fold pattern may appear diminished in scleroderma, in which the haustral pattern may assume an asymmetric saccular pattern. Similar changes can be seen in the small bowel. Chronic laxative abuse and resultant cathartic colon will also demonstrate a diminished haustral pattern.

Any chronic or healed inflammatory process involving the colon, such as chronic or healed ulcerative colitis, or the chronic stages of radiation colitis can result in diminished or absent haustral pattern.

THICKENED HAUSTRAL FOLDS

Ischemic colitis
Intramural bleeding
Inflammation
Toxic megacolon
Pseudomembranous colitis
Typhlitis
Pneumatosis coli

A number of conditions can result in varying degrees of thickening of the haustral folds. These can be mild thickening to marked fingerlike indentations of the bowel margin known as thumbprinting. In general, the causes of fold thickening and thumb printing are a result of thickening, hemorrhage or malignancy. Hemorrhage is seen most commonly as a cause of thumbprinting resulting from ischemic colitis. However, thumbprinting resulting from intramural hemorrhage may be entirely indistinguishable from severe inflammation and marked edematous changes such as might be seen in fulminating IBD or toxic megacolon. The clinical history is extremely helpful in sorting out these problems.

Ischemic colitis is a condition seen in the elderly population, with most of the patients being over 70 years of age. The condition relates to an acute reduction of the splanchnic blood flow and is commonly seen, or distal to, in the watershed areas between the inferior mesenteric artery and the superior mesenteric artery circulations. However, more extensive colitis involving longer segments is common.

The exact causes for this diminished blood flow may be multiple. Conditions such as acute hypotensive episodes, underlying vasculitides, or mechanical causes such as herniation or volvulus have been implicated.

There is an increased incidence in patients ischemic colitis undergoing hemodialysis. The rectum is rarely involved because of the abundant collateral circulation.

The finding of thumbprinting on either a plain film or during a barium enema examination, is most often seen in the transverse or descending portions of the colon and represents intramural hemorrhage. This finding is present in about 20% to 25% of patients. The patients frequently present with painless rectal bleeding. Over half of the cases are transient and reversible. Slightly less than half of the cases will develop complications, usually focal stricture, or more seriously, bowel necrosis, which will require surgical intervention. Interestingly, the site of complications is most commonly in the sigmoid colon.

Toxic megacolon (TMC) is an acute complication of fulminating inflammatory disease of the colon that involves the entire thickness of the bowel wall (Fig. 7-66). Tissue cohesion is severely impaired, and perforation is a common result. TMC is most frequently seen as a complication of ulcerative colitis although it occurs with less frequency in Crohn's disease and in bacterial colitis. It has also been reported in pseudomembranous colitis as well as ischemic colitis.

The condition is characterized by a dilated transverse colon with marked thickening and nodularity of the haustral pattern. Multiple nodular filling defects can also be seen profiled and en face, representing pseudopolyps. The reason these changes are mostly seen in the transverse colon is because the transverse colon represents the most anterior portion of the colon in the supine patient. As a result, air gathers in the transverse colon and the findings are most apparent in this region. In fact, toxic megacolon may involve the entire colon and even portions of the distal small bowel. Additionally, it should be remembered that a few cases of toxic megacolon have been reported in which the transverse colon is not significantly dilated. Although radiographically these cases may appear similar to ischemic colitis, the clinical presentation makes differentiation relatively easy. Patients presenting with toxic megacolon are systemically toxic and usually have a history of IBD.

Although the barium enema has been implicated in the development of TMC in patients with IBD, this probably is more of a temporal relationship than cause and effect. However, when presented with plain films of a severely ill patient with findings suggesting TMC, contrast examination of the colon is contraindicated due to the high risk of perforation.

Pseudomembranous colitis may also present with plain films demonstrating a thickened nodular fold pattern within the colon. This finding occurs as a result of the marked edema and the presence of adherent pseudomembranes along the mucosal surface. This condition, although uncommon, can result in a

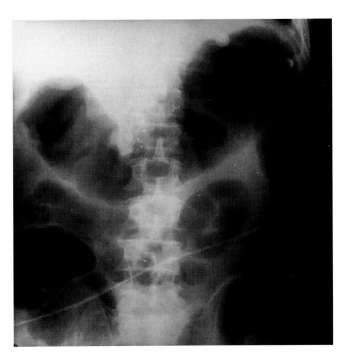

Fig. 7-66 Plain film of the abdomen of a patient with severe inflammatory bowel disease demonstrates dilatation of the colon, particularly in the transverse region, with thickening and nodularity of the folds typical of toxic megacolon.

potentially deadly illness. It has been referred to as antibiotic colitis and is thought to represent a complication of chronic antibiotic therapy. Clinically, the patient often experiences diarrhea with occasional bleeding and abdominal pain. The onset of symptoms is usually within 2 to 3 days following the commencement of antibiotic therapy. Although the condition was initially associated with lincomycin and tetracycline, it is now known that virtually any antibiotic can trigger the disease.

The underlying cause is thought to represent an acute change of the bacterial colonic flora and an overgrowth of the bacterium, *Clostridium difficile,* which is known to produce toxins absorbed across the colonic mucosa. The finding of marked bowel wall and haustral thickening with nodularity and possible thumbprinting in a patient with suspected pseudomembranous colitis should give sufficient warning to the radiologist to avoid doing a barium enema examination. These patients also run an increased risk of perforation.

Other conditions that may mimic thumbprinting include lymphoma, carcinoma, metastatic extension from the serosal surface, amyloid infiltration of the bowel, and in the cecal region, typhlitis.

Typhlitis, sometimes known as neutropenic entero-

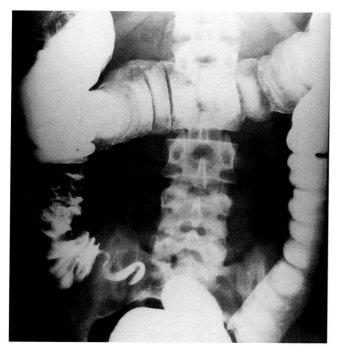

Fig. 7-67   A young patient with leukemia presents with right lower quadrant abdominal pain. Barium enema demonstrates inflammatory and spastic changes involving the cecum and a portion of the ascending colon, representing typhlitis.

colitis, is a condition occasionally encountered in patients undergoing treatment for hematological malignancies, particularly leukemia and lymphoma (Fig. 7-67). The patients are often neutropenic, and changes are most commonly seen in the terminal ileum, cecum, and proximal ascending colon. Marked focal changes of inflammation that can progress to bowel wall necrosis are the manifestations of this condition, and the clinical findings may simulate acute appendicitis.

An interesting condition that, to the inattentive observer, can simulate the appearance of haustral fold thickening and possible thumbprinting is pneumatosis coli. The haustral folds may appear thickened and nodular, but careful attention to the films will disclose that this is the result of cystic collections of air in the bowel wall (see Fig. 7-27).

ABNORMALITIES OF POSITION

Malrotation

Degrees of colonic malrotation can occur and are usually of little clinical significance (Fig 7-68). These result from the counterclockwise rotation that occurs as the midgut returns from the umbilical sac into the abdomi-

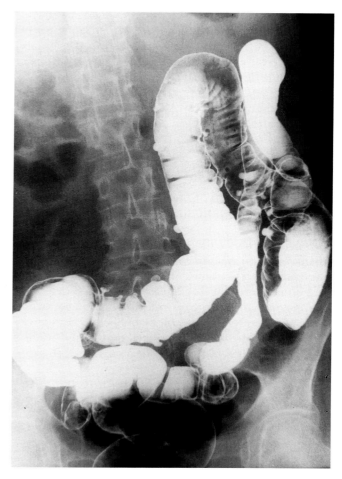

Fig. 7-68   Barium enema in a patient with malrotation demonstrates both flexures on the left side of the abdomen. The cecum is in its expected location.

nal cavity between 6 and 12 weeks of embryonic life. The amount of rotation may be incomplete, and fixation of the ascending portion of the colon either absent or limited. This can cause considerable mobility of the cecum and ascending colon. This condition may potentially predispose to internal torsion abnormalities, such as cecal or transverse colon volvulus. Complete failure of rotation, or nonrotation, is not common. When it does occur, the entire colon will be seen on the left side of the abdomen and the small bowel on the right side.

Hernias

Hernias, both of the inguinal and femoral canals, can include segments of colon, most commonly sigmoid. However, the cecum and appendix can also be involved. Internal hernias can involve the colon. These include mesenteric hernias, diaphragmatic hernias, or even herniation through the foramen of Winslow into the lesser sac. Hernias through the diaphragm can occur as a result of traumatic defects in the diaphragm or as a result of congenital defects, such as Morgagni's hernia anteriorly or Bochdalek's hernia of the posterior diaphragm. These herniations may exist for long periods of time with no symptoms. However, strangulation or obstruction of the bowel can occur and result in a surgical emergency.

Herniation of portions of both small bowel and colon through the anterior abdominal wall is relatively common. This includes umbilical hernias and postoperative incisional hernias. Spigelian hernia is an unusual form of ventral hernia in which a defect occurs along the linea semilunaris located in the abdominal wall lateral to the rectus abdominis muscle. The herniated portions of bowel pass through the transverse and internal oblique muscle layers but remain beneath the overlying intact external oblique muscle. As a result, the hernia is difficult to clinically detect and quite fretent abdominal pain is reported in some patients. Radiographically, bowel seen on plain film, CT, or barium enema lying laterally to the rectus muscle outside the expected confines of the peritoneal cavity suggests the diagnosis.

MISCELLANEOUS

Presacral Widening

The presacral, retrorectal space normally measures up to 1.5 cm. However, a number of conditions can result in abnormal widening of the presacral space. Most of these conditions involve the rectum itself, and ab-normal rectal findings are usually present on the barium enema examination.

The most common cause of presacral widening is inflammatory disease involving the rectum and colon. This is a common finding in ulcerative colitis but can also be seen in Crohn's disease when it involves the rectum (Fig. 7-69). Formation of perirectal fistulous tracts or abscesses in Crohn's disease can result in further widening of the presacral space. Other inflammatory conditions of the rectum including lymphogranuloma venereum, radiation proctitis, viral (i.e., CMV) proctitis (Fig. 7-70), and rarely ischemic disease can result in increased presacral space size.

Neoplastic disease arising from the colon, such as carcinoma of the rectum, will also be an important cause of an enlarged retrorectal space. The most common malignant lesion is adenocarcinoma, which usually results in a large, bulky lesion. However, the mass of the lesion plus the perirectal extension can combine to cause significant widening of the presacal space. Other rare malignancies of the rectum include lymphoma and cloacogenic carcinoma, both of which might produce similar appearances.

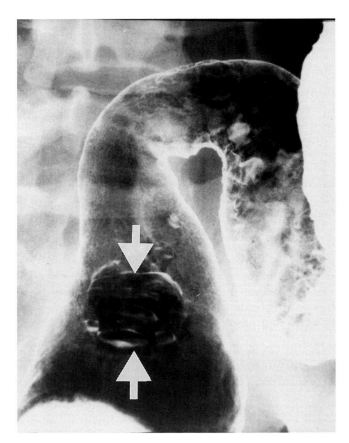

Fig. 7-70 Rectal spot views in a patient with CMV proctitis demonstrate numerous ulcerations, including a huge, superficial ulcer in the rectum (arrows).

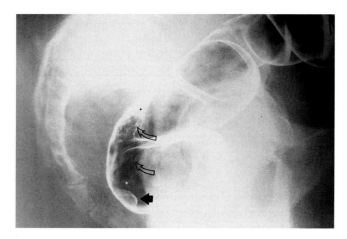

Fig. 7-69 Spot film of the rectum demonstrates inflammatory changes of the rectum (curved arrows) associated with widened presacral space. Also note a small adenomatous polyp (arrow).

Cystic lesions that contribute to presacral widening are dermoid cysts (sacral teratoma), and less commonly, rectal duplications (enteric cysts) (Fig. 7-71).

Lesions arising from the sacrum itself can also contribute to a widened presacral space. These include infectious processes, such as osteomyelitis of the sacrum, metastatic disease, primary bone tumors, and neurogenic tumors arising from the sacrum. Chordomas are seen in the cervical and sacrococcygeal regions of the spine. These are slow-growing lesions, usually resulting in destructive changes in the sacrum, and mass effect with anterior extension and displacement of the rectum, and widening of the presacral space.

Malignant neoplastic lesions arising from structures around the rectum can, by contiguous extension, encircle and deform the rectum and widen the presacral space. This is not common, but is occasionally seen in prostatic carcinoma in men and cervical carcinoma in women (Fig. 7-72).

Pelvic abscesses with extension into the pouch of Douglas can result in widening of the presacral space on barium enema examination. Although the abscess itself may not extend beyond the confines of the peritoneal recess into the actual presacral space, the effect of adjacent inflammation presumably results in sufficient edema in the region to separate the rectum and sacral margin. A common example of this would be periappendiceal abscess with pus collections in the lower pelvic recesses. Both pelvic inflammatory disease and diverticulitis may have similar effects.

Fistulous Connections and Sinus Tract Formation

Fistulous connections and sinus tract formation are the hallmarks of Crohn's disease. Full-thickness involvement of bowel wall by the disease and extension beyond the wall to the adjacent mesentery and mesenteric fat often result in matting and bonding together of several loops of bowel. Mucosal ulcerations progress, deepen, penetrate, and eventually communicate with the adjacent adherent loops of bowel. This is frequently seen in the right lower quadrant, with fistulous tracts between ileal loops and adjacent ileum, cecum, and ascending colon. These fistulous communications can also extend to the skin, particularly in the postoperative patient. Enteric-colonic fistulous formation does not necessarily present a problem in itself and, in some instances, may actually relieve the potential for obstruction. However, the development of abscess cavi-

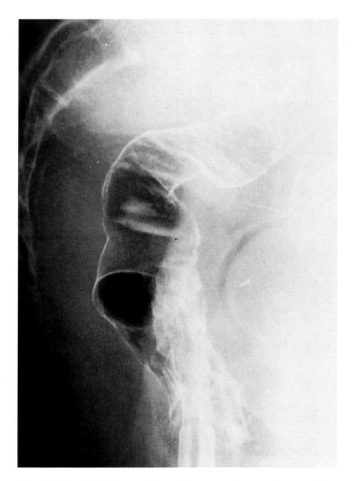

Fig. 7-72 DCBE in a patient with aggressive carcinoma of the cervix. The lesion has invaded the perirectal region with widening of the presacral space.

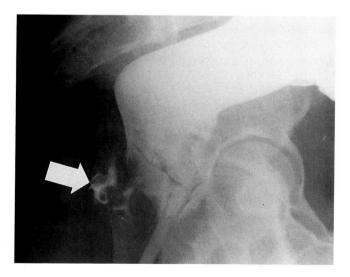

Fig. 7-71 Presacral space is widened secondary to a rectal duplication. There is some communication between the enteric cyst and the bowel lumen, with contrast seen within the duplication *(arrow)*.

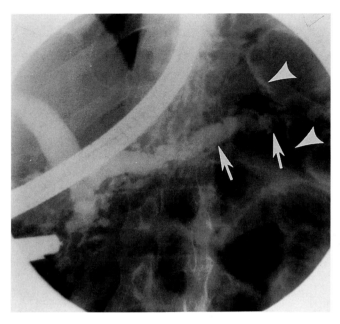

Fig. 7-73   ERCP in a patient with chronic pancreatitis. The pancreatic duct is ectatic and dilated *(arrows)*. There is communication with the splenic flexure of the adjacent colon, and contrast is seen on the colonic mucosa *(arrowheads)*, confirming a pancreaticocolonic fistula.

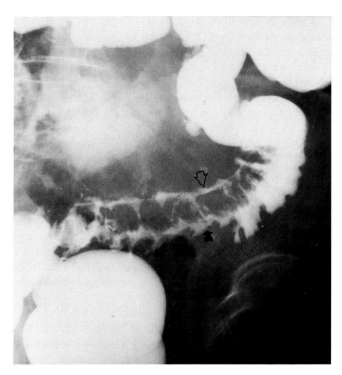

Fig. 7-75   Well-defined example of double-tracking on a barium enema. The narrowed, irregular lumen is seen *(closed arrow)*. Parallel to this is the intramural tract of barium *(open arrow)*.

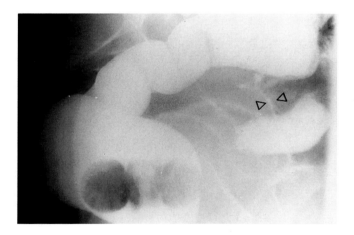

Fig. 7-74   SCBE in a patient with radiation colitis and a narrow fistulous communication *(arrowheads)* to the bladder.

ties along the tract, the diverting and bypassing of a significant amount of bowel resulting in malnutrition, or extension of the fistula to the skin or adjacent organs can represent serious complications.

Fistulous communications between the stomach and the colon result from either inflammatory or malignant disease arising in the stomach or colon. The large, penetrating benign gastric ulcer seen in patients on steroids or high doses of aspirin that communicates with the colon is rarely encountered today. Malignant lesions arising from the greater curvature of the body and fundus of the stomach or the splenic flexure of the colon can form a gastrocolic fistula.

Patients with chronic pancreatitis, on rare occasion, develop a fistulous communication from the pancreatic duct to the colon (Fig. 7-73).

Sinus tracts and fistulous communications are not uncommon in patients with diverticulitis. The fistulous communications often are from colon to bowel loop, particularly adjacent small bowel. However, fistulous tracts may also develop between the colon and the vagina or the bladder.

On occasion, radiation colitis can result in a fistulous communication between adjacent bowel or other structures, such as the bladder or vagina (Fig. 7-74).

An interesting variation of sinus tract formation is the intramural sinus tract, sometimes referred to as "double-tracking", which is most commonly seen in diverticulitis (Fig. 7-75). However, this can also be seen to a lesser extent in patients with Crohn's disease. Patients with carcinoma of the colon may also have short, irregular intramural sinus tracts (Fig. 7-76).

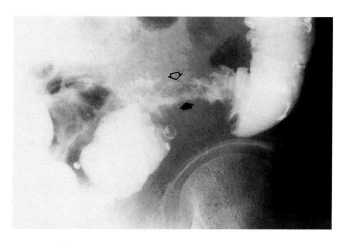

Fig. 7-76 A patient with adenocarcinoma of the sigmoid colon and an apple core type of constricting lesion. Note the narrowed lumen *(closed arrow)* and the adjacent, thin, poorly defined periluminal tract *(open arrow).*

Actinomycosis with colonic involvement frequently results in sinus or fistulous tracts and communication with adjacent organs or the skin. This organism's blatant disregard for fascial planes is a hallmark of its natural history, and fistulous communications are a common manifestation (Fig. 7-77). Fistula and sinus formation is also a common finding with lymphogranuloma venereum (Fig. 7-78).

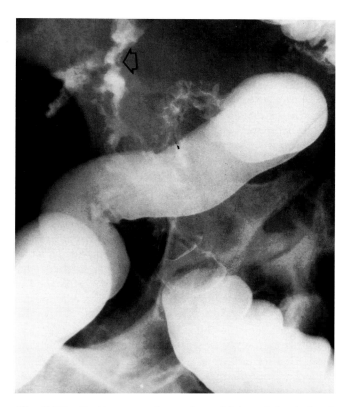

Fig. 7-77 Barium enema in a patient with intraabdominal actinomycosis involving the sigmoid colon, with resultant spasm, narrowing, and development of a branching sinus tract *(arrow)* extending from the affected sigmoid colon.

Appendix

The normal appendix originates between the cecal tip and the ileocecal valve. It is a structure of variable length, measuring anywhere from 4 to 12 cm. In a significant number of cases (approximately 25%), the appendix may be retrocecal in position, and the tip of the appendix, on occasion, may be located in the right upper quadrant of the abdomen below or at the margin of the liver. Filling of the appendix during a barium enema study occurs in approximately 60% of cases. If a postevacuation film is obtained, one can expect to see additional filling in another 20% to 25% of patients.

The most common condition of the appendix is appendicitis, resulting from occlusion of the appendiceal lumen by a fecalith and development of inflammatory changes within the obstructed appendix. The appendiceal wall becomes thickened, hyperemic, and edematous. Clinical presentation is usually suggestive of the diagnosis. Progression of the inflammatory process can result in perforation with periappendiceal abscess formation or free perforation and generalized peritonitis. On barium enema, spasm at the cecal tip or mass effect

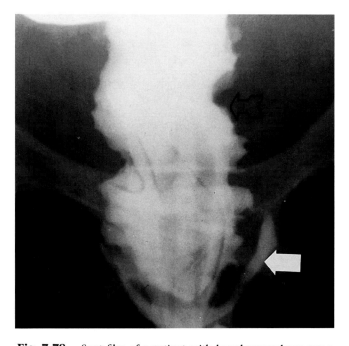

Fig. 7-78 Spot film of a patient with lymphogranuloma venereum demonstrates marked irregularity and ulceration of the rectal margin *(open arrows)* as well as prominent bilateral perirectal sinus tracts *(closed arrow).*

from the adjacent abscess may be the expected findings. Incomplete filling of the appendix during barium enema does not exclude appendicitis. However, complete filling and demonstration of the bulbous tip of the appendix does rule out the diagnosis.

Crohn's disease of the terminal ileum or cecum may also, by extension, involve the appendix (Fig. 7-79). Isolated appendiceal involvement is extremely rare.

The most common cause of a filling defect at the tip of the cecum is previous appendectomy with an inverted appendiceal stump. Frequently, this inverted stump is smooth and in its expected location. On occasion, the stump can appear lobular and require colonoscopy to differentiate it from a neoplasm. Occasionally, a true neoplasm may be found arising from the appendiceal stump. There is no reason to suspect that this is any more than coincidental nor is there evidence to suggest any increased risk of malignancy at the site of the inverted stump. On occasion, a filling defect at the base of cecum, sometimes with concentric circles arising from the center of the filling defect, can be seen and is the result of appendiceal intussusception. This frequently is asymptomatic and transient, although occasionally it can be associated with acute appendicitis. A similar "coil-spring" appearance can also be seen after appendectomy.

A mucocele of the appendix is another cause of a filling defect at the appendiceal origin. The most widely held etiology for this condition is aseptic obstruction of the appendiceal lumen with mucus accumulation and cyst formation. Most of these lesions are asymptomatic. Occasionally, the mucocele can calcify

in its wall. Rupture of an appendiceal mucocele can lead to the condition known as pseudomyxoma peritonei, in which spillage of the mucocele content results in massive accumulations of thick gelatinous adhesive type of ascites.

An interesting and rare type of appendiceal mucocele is myxoglobulosis, in which numerous, tiny cohesive translucent globules are mixed with the liquid mucous content of the mucocele. These globules can calcify and, on positional views of the abdomen, may be seen to move within the mucocele.

The most common of appendiceal neoplasms is the carcinoid. The appendix, in fact, represents the most common site of carcinoid development within the GI tract. Over 90% of GI carcinoids arise from either the appendix or the distal ileum. These lesions are almost always benign and rarely cause the carcinoid syndrome. The discovery is usually incidental during surgery or autopsy.

Primary malignant neoplasm of the appendix is unusual and is invariably adenocarcinoma. Frequently, this results in gradual luminal obstruction and may

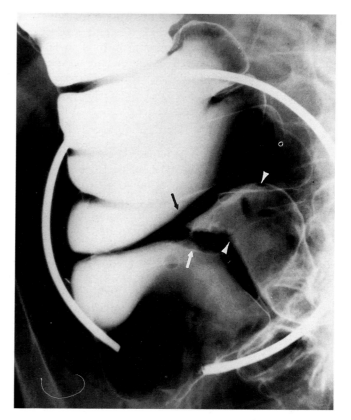

Fig. 7-80 Spot film from a barium enema demonstrates the normal and most common configuration of the ileocecal valve. Note the smooth V-shaped configuration of the valve *(arrows)* and the normal bird's-head configuration of the terminal ileum *(arrowheads)* as it enters the valve.

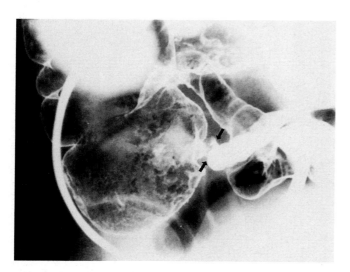

Fig. 7-79 Spot film of the cecum on a patient with Crohn's disease. Inflammatory involvement of the cecum, more severe on its medial aspect around the origin of the appendix, is seen. There is also involvement of the first several centimeters *(arrows)* of the appendix.

present as acute appendicitis. The diagnosis is frequently intraoperative or postoperative.

Ileocecal Valve Enlargement

The appearance of the ileocecal valve can be quite variable, from a small polypoid filling defect on the first transverse fold within the colon to the more typical lip-like valvular configuration (Fig. 7-80). The normal valve may also have a rosette configuration. It is commonly located on the medial side of the cecum, although there can be variation. The valve can be seen on the lateral margin of the cecum in some patients. The size of the normal valve can also be quite variable. The upper limits of normal for the vertical diameter of the valve is probably 3 to 4 cm. Generally speaking, the valve should be measured during full cecal distention. It is not uncommon to see prominence of the valve on a postevacuation film as compared with the distended cecal views. This is because there are degrees of ileal prolapse through the valve when the cecum is collapsed, accentuating the size of the valve.

Reflux of barium across the ileocecal valve into the terminal ileum is a common phenomenon on SCBE, probably occurring in more than 75% of the cases. Fortunately, this is not the case with double-contrast technique, and reflux into the terminal ileum with obscuration of the sigmoid colon occurs with considerably less frequency. The exact reason for this is unclear. It may relate to the smaller amounts and the more viscous nature of the barium used in double-contrast work.

The most common benign neoplastic lesion of the ileocecal valve is the lipoma, which is seen as a rounded, well-circumscribed, smooth mass arising from one of the valvular lips. This should be differentiated from lipomatous valvular infiltration, which is not a neoplastic process (Fig. 7-81). In the latter condition, the valve may appear large and lobulated along both lips. There is also a change of valvular configuration with compression. Both benign adenomas and adenocarcinomas can arise from the ileocecal valve. Like most cecal or right-sided lesions, a valvular malignancy can grow to sizeable proportions before becoming symptomatic, as a result of the fluid nature of the bowel content at this level (Figs. 7-82 and 7-83).

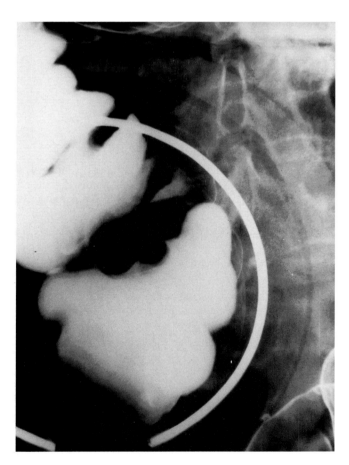

Fig. 7-81 A patient with lipomatous infiltration of the ileocecal valve. The valve is enlarged and nodular. Compression may cause the valve to change shape.

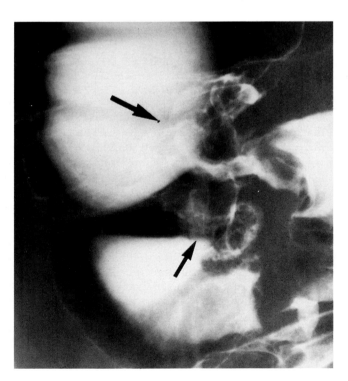

Fig. 7-82 A large polypoid carcinoma arising from the ileocecal valve *(arrows)*. Note the narrowing of the lumen of the valve and the adjacent terminal ileum into which the tumor has extended. This patient is not obstructed.

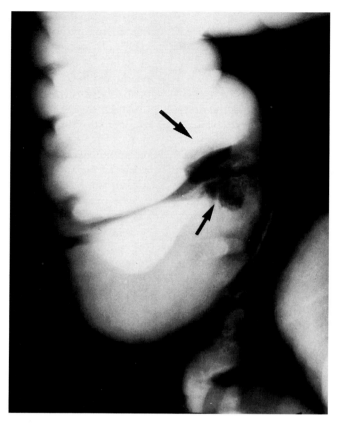

Fig. 7-83   An anemic patient examined with barium enema was found to have a lobulated lesion arising from the ileocecal valve *(arrows)* that proved to be a villous adenoma.

Inflammatory changes involving the terminal ileum and the cecum can also involve the valve. This is particularly the case in Crohn's disease, where involvement of the ileocecal valve frequently indicates involvement of the terminal ileum. *Yersinia,* which involves the distal ileum, may also result in inflammatory changes of the valve.

In ulcerative pancolitis, inflammation in the cecal region can result in incompetence of the valve and unimpeded reflux into the terminal ileum. The ileum tends to appear large and distended but is usually not involved in the primary inflammatory process.

Inflammatory conditions that involve the ileocecal region, including tuberculosis, amebiasis, and typhoid fever, can also involve the ileocecal valve.

SELECTED READING
Colon

Balthazar EJ, Megibow AJ, Hulnick D, et al: Carcinoma of the colon: detection and preoperative staging by CT, *AJR* 150:301-306, 1988.

Balthazar EJ, Megibow A, Schinella RA, et al: Limitations in the CT diagnosis of acute diverticulitis: comparison of CT, contrast enema, and pathologic findings in 16 patients, *AJR* 154:281-285, 1990.

Balikian JP, Uthman SM, Khouri NF: Intestinal amoebiasis, *AJR* 122:245-256, 1974.

Bartram CI: Radiology in the current assessment of ulcerative colitis, *Gastrointest Radiol* 1:383-392, 1977.

Bernstein MA, Feczko PJ, Halpert RD, et al: Distribution of colonic polyps: increased incidence of proximal lesions in older patients, *Radiology* 155:35-38, 1985.

Campbell WL, Wolff M: Retrorectal cysts of developmental origin, *AJR* 117:307-313, 1973.

Cho CK, Morehouse HT, Alterman DD, et al: Sigmoid diverticulitis: diagnostic role of CT—comparison with barium enema studies, *Radiology* 176:111-115, 1990.

Chrispin AR, Fry IK: The presacral space shown by barium enema, *Br J Radiol* 36:319-322, 1963.

Claymon CB. Mass screening for colorectal cancer: are we ready? *JAMA* 261:609, 1989.

deLange EE, Fechner RE, Edge SB, et al: Preoperative staging of rectal carcinoma with MR imaging: surgical and histopathologic correlation, *Radiology* 176:623-628, 1990.

Dworkin B, Winawer SJ, Lighdale CJ: Typhlitis: report of a case with long-term survival and a review of the recent literature, *Dig Dis Sci* 26:1032-1037, 1981.

Feczko PJ, Halpert RD: Reassessing the role of radiology in hemocult screening, *AJR* 146:697-701, 1986.

Fishman EK, Kavuru M, Jones B, et al: Pseudomembranous colitis: CT evaluation of 26 cases, *Radiology* 180:57-60, 1991.

Fleischer DE, Goldberg SB, Browning TH, et al: Detection and surveillance of colorectal cancer, *JAMA* 261:580-585, 1989.

Frager DH, Goldman M, Beneventano TC: Computed tomography in Crohn disease, *J Comput Assist Tomogr* 7:819-824, 1983.

Gelfand DW, Wu WC, Ott DJ: The extent of successful colonoscopy: its implication for the radiologists, *Gastrointest Radiol* 4:75-78, 1979.

Glotzer DJ, Glick ME, Goldman H: Proctitis and colitis following diversion of the fecal stream, *Gastroenterol* 80:438-441, 1981.

Golstein SJ, MacKenzie Crooks DJ: Colitis in Behçet's syndrome, *Radiology* 128:321-323, 1978.

Greenall MJ, Levine AW, Nolan DJ: Complications of diverticular disease: a review of the barium enema findings, *Gastrointest Radiol* 8:353-358, 1983.

Greenstein AJ, Janowitz HD, Sachar DB: The extra-intestinal complications of Crohn's disease and ulcerative colitis: a study of 700 patients, *Medicine* 55:401-412, 1976.

Halpert RD: Toxic dilatation of the colon, *Rad Clin North Am* 25:147-155, 1987.

Jackman RJ, Mayo CW: The adenoma-carcinoma sequence in cancer of the colon, *Surg Gynecol Obstet* 93:327-330, 1951.

Jones IT, Fazio VW: Colonic volvulus: etiology and management, *Dig Dis* 7:203-209, 1989.

Keller CE, Halpert RD, Feczko PJ, et al: Radiologic recognition of colonic diverticula simulating polyps, *AJR* 143:93-97, 1984.

Kelvin FM, Gardiner R, Vas W, et al: Colorectal carcinoma missed on double contrast barium study: a problem in perception, *AJR* 137:307-313, 1981.

Kelvin FM, Max RJ, Norton GA, et al: Lymphoid follicular pattern of the colon in adults, *AJR* 133:821-825, 1979.

Kelvin FM, Oddson TA, Rice RP, et al: Double contrast barium enema in Crohn's disease and ulcerative colitis, *AJR* 131:207-213, 1978.

Laufer I, Costopoulos L: Early lesions of Crohn's disease, *AJR* 130:307-311, 1978.

Laufer I, Mullens JE, Hamilton J: Correlation of endoscopy and double-contrast radiography in the early stages of ulcerative and granulomatous colitis, *Radiology* 118:1-5, 1976.

Lennard-Jones JE, Morson BC, Ritchie JK, et al: Cancer in colitis: assessment of the individual risk by clinical and histological criteria, *Gastroenterology* 73:1280-1289, 1977.

Maglinte DT, Keller KJ, Miller RE, et al: Colon and rectal carcinoma: spatial distribution and detection, *Radiology* 147:669-672, 1983.

Megibow AJ, Balthazar EJ, Kyunghee CC, et al: Bowel obstruction: evaluation with CT, *Radiology* 180:313-318, 1991.

Moss AA: Computed tomography in the staging of gastrointestinal carcinoma, *Radiol Clin North Am* 20:761-780, 1982.

Munyer TP, Montgomery CK, Thoeni RF, et al: Post inflammatory polyposis (PIP) of the colon: the radiologic-pathologic spectrum, *Radiology* 145:607-614, 1982.

Muto T, Bussey HJR, Morson BC: The evolution of cancer of the colon and rectum, *Cancer* 36:2251-2270, 1975.

Ott DJ, Gelfand DW, Wu WC, et al: Sensitivity of double-contrast barium enema: emphasis on polyp detection, *AJR* 135:327-330, 1980.

Peskin GW, Orloff MJ: A clinical study of 25 patients with carcinoid tumors of the rectum, *Surg Gynecol Obstet* 109:673-682, 1959.

Rifkin MD, Ehrlich SM, Marks G: Staging of rectal carcinoma: prospective comparison of endorectal US and CT, *Radiology* 170:319-322, 1989.

Rose CP, Stevenson GW, Somers S, et al: Inaccuracy of radiographic measurements of colon polyps, *J Can Assoc Radiol* 32:21-23, 1981.

Rubesin SE, Levine MS, Bezzi M, et al: Rectal involvement by prostatic carcinoma: barium enema findings, *AJR* 152:53-57, 1989.

Sauerbrei E, Castelli M: Hypogammaglobulinemia and nodular lymphoid hyperplasia of the gut, *J Can Assoc Radiol* 30:62-63, 1979.

Schuffler MD, Rohrmann CA, Templeton FE: The radiologic manifestation of idiopathic intestinal pseudo obstruction, *AJR* 127:729-736, 1976.

Stanley RJ, Melson GL, Tedesco FJ: The spectrum of radiographic findings in antibiotic-related pseudomembranous colitis, *Radiology* 111:519-524, 1974.

Thoeni RF, Petras A: Detection of rectal and rectosigmoid lesions by double-contrast barium enema examination and sigmoidoscopy, *Radiology* 142:59-62, 1982.

Van Fleet RH, Shabot MJ, Halpert RD: Adenocarcinoma of the appendiceal stump, *South Med J* 83:1351-1353, 1990.

Index

A

Pneumatosis coli, 233
Pneumatosis cystoides coli, 210-211
Pneumatosis cystoides intestinalis, 100
Pneumatosis intestinalis, 106-107
Pneumobilia, 175
Pneumocolon, peroral, 83-84
Polyp
    colonic
        adenomatous, 196-199
        hyperplastic, 205
    esophageal, 5
    gallbladder and, 184
    gastric, 53
        adenoma and, 54
        fibroid, 54-55
        hyperplastic, 55
    Peutz-Jeghers syndrome and, 99-100
    of small bowel, 100
        fibroid, 98
Polypoid carcinoma, gastric, 57-58
Polypoid lesion
    bile duct, 165
    duodenal adenoma as, 75
    ectopic pancreas as, 53
Polyposis
    familial, 206
    juvenile, 206, 208
Porcelain gallbladder, 189
Portal hypertension, 73
Portal vein, 151
Portal venous air, 150-151
Portography, computed tomography arterial, 129,
        138-139
    regenerating nodules and, 147
Positioning, for gastric examination, 33-35
Postcholecystectomy syndrome, 191
Postcricoid defect, 9
Postinflammatory condition
    colonic polyps as, 209-210
    colonic strictures as, 223-224
Postoperative condition
    biliary, 166
    cholecystectomy and, 174-175, 191
    esophageal surgery and, 30-31
    gastric, 66-68
    of pancreas, 126
    of small bowel, 107-108
Pouch of Douglas, abscess into, 235
Pregnancy, fatty liver and, 131
Presacral widening, 234-235
Proctitis, gonorrhea, 220-221
Progressive systemic sclerosis, 88
Proliferative disorder, spleen and, 153
Protozoan infection, spleen and, 153
Pseudocalculus, biliary, 164
Pseudocyst
    pancreatic, 119-120, 122
    of spleen, 154-155
Pseudodiverticulum, esophageal, 24
Pseudohypertrophy, lipomatous, of pancreas, 114

Pseudolymphoma, gastric, 49, 60
Pseudomass, gastric, 66
Pseudomembranous colitis, 232
Pseudoobstruction, intestinal, 41, 230-231
Pseudopolyps, colonic, 209
Pyloric stenosis, 38

R
Radiation injury
    colonic
        colitis as, 219-220, 224
        fistula and, 236
    esophageal fistula caused by, 13-14
    gastric, 45
    of small bowel, 92
    spleen and, 153
Radionuclide scan
    biliary system and, 162
    of gallbladder, 178
    of liver
        hemangioma and, 137
        thoratrast and, 150
Rectum
    cloacogenic carcinoma of, 201
    colorectal carcinoma and, 199
    presacral widening and, 234
    solitary ulcer of, 220
Reflux
    gastroesophageal
        fluoroscopy of, 2
        gastric examination and, 34
        postoperative, 67-68
    ileocecal valve and, 239
Reflux esophagitis, 5
    thoracic esophagus and, 15
    ulceration caused by, 13
Regenerating nodule, hepatic, 147
Regional enteritis; *see* Crohn's disease
Remnant gastritis, 66-67
Resection of small bowel, 107
Rest, pancreatic, 125
    duodenal filling defect and, 74
Retention cyst
    esophageal, 8
    pancreatic, 120
Retrograde cholangiopancreatography, endoscopic, 112,
        161
    common bile duct stone and, 162, 163
    pancreas divisum and, 125
    pancreatic carcinoma and, 116
    pancreaticolonic fistula and, 236
    pancreatitis and, 113
    sclerosing cholangitis and, 167
Retroperitoneal tumor, gastric compression from, 43
Reverse figure 3 configuration of duodenal fold, 72
Ring, esophageal, 27
Rokitansky-Aschoff sinuses, 186
Roundworm infestation of small bowel, 89, 90,
        197
Rupture of hepatic abscess, 145